Working in community-based settings? Here are some "must have" references!

Psychosocial Nursing for General Patient Care, 2nd Edition
By Linda M. Gorman, Marcia L. Raines and Donna F. Sultan.

Diseases and Disorders: A Nursing Therapeutics Manual, 2nd Edition
By Marilyn Sawyer Sommers and Susan A. Johnson.

Community-based Nursing Practice: Learning Through Students' Stories
By Jeanne M. Sorrell and Georgine M. Redmond.

Community-based Nursing Curriculum: A Faculty Guide
By Georgine M. Redmond and Jeanne M. Sorrell.

Coping with Chronic Illness: Overcoming Powerlessness, 3rd Edition
By Judith Fitzgerald Miller.

Family Health Care Nursing: Theory, Practice, and Research, 2nd Edition
By Shirley May Harmon Hanson.

Nurses and Families: A Guide to Family Assessment and Intervention, 3rd Edition
By Lorraine M. Wright and Maureen Leahey.

Transcultural Health Care: A Culturally Competent Approach
By Larry D. Purnell and Betty J. Paulanka.

Buy Today!

Available from your local health science bookstore or from F. A. Davis.

To order online, go to **www.fadavis.com** or call our Customer Service Department at 800-323-3555. In Canada call 800-655-1148.

For more information about these books and others, visit our online store at www.fadavis.com.

F. A. DAVIS COMPANY

0802-0A

LINDA M. GORMAN, RN, MN, CS, OCN, CHPN

Palliative Care/Hospice Clinical Nurse Specialist
Cedars-Sinai Medical Center
Los Angeles, California

Assistant Professor
University of California, Los Angeles
Los Angeles, California

Certified Clinical Nurse Specialist
Adult Psychiatric/Mental Health Nursing

MARCIA L. RAINES, PhD, RN, MN, CS

Chair and Professor
California State University, San Bernardino
San Bernardino, California

Certified Clinical Nurse Specialist
Adult Psychiatric/Mental Health Nursing

DONNA F. SULTAN, RN, MS

Mental Health Counselor, RN
West Valley Mental Health Center
Los Angeles County Department of Mental Health
Los Angeles, California

Psychosocial
Nursing
for General Patient Care

SECOND EDITION

 F. A. DAVIS COMPANY • Philadelphia

F.A. Davis Company
1915 Arch Street
Philadelphia, PA 19103
www.fadavis.com

Printed in the United States of America

Last digit indicates print number: 10 9 8 7 6 5 4 3 2

Acquisitions Editor: Joanne DaCunha
Developmental Editor: Diane Blodgett
Cover Designer: Louis Forgione

As new scientific information becomes available through basic and clinical research, recommended treatments and drug therapies undergo changes. The author(s) and publisher have done everything possible to make this book accurate, up to date, and in accord with accepted standards at the time of publication. The authors, editors, and publisher are not responsible for errors or omissions or for consequences from application of the book, and make no warranty, expressed or implied, in regard to the contents of the book. Any practice described in this book should be applied by the reader in accordance with professional standards of care used in regard to the unique circumstances that may apply in each situation. The reader is advised always to check product information (package inserts) for changes and new information regarding dose and contraindications before administering any drug. Caution is especially urged when using new or infrequently ordered drugs.

Library of Congress Cataloging in Publication Data

Gorman, Linda M.
    Psychosocial nursing for general patient care / Linda M. Gorman, Marcia L. Raines, Donna F. Sultan.—2nd ed.
        p. cm.
    Previous ed. published with title: Davis's manual of psychosocial nursing for general patient care.
    Includes bibliographical references and index.
    ISBN 0-8036-0802-0 (pbk. : alk. paper)
        1. Psychiatric nursing—Handbooks, manuals, etc. 2. Nursing—Social aspects—Handbooks, manuals, etc. I. Luna-Raines, Marcia. II. Sultan, Donna. III. Gorman, Linda M. Davis's manual of psychosocial nursing for general patient care.

RC440 .G659 2002
610.73'68—dc21

                                                                                    2001047637

PREFACE

Having worked in a variety of specialty areas over the years as staff nurses, clinical nurse specialists, educators, and managers, we realize that nurses aspire to become highly proficient in their area of practice but that psychosocial skills are often more difficult to perfect. Very often nurses feel inadequately prepared to deal with complex behaviors and psychiatric problems. Even nurses who practice in the psychiatric setting find themselves dealing with unique situations that challenge their level of expertise. And yet, a large percentage of nurses' time is spent dealing with these issues.

Psychosocial Nursing for General Patient Care bridges the gap between the information contained in large, comprehensive psychiatric nursing texts and the information needed to function effectively in a variety of healthcare settings. The clinician can refer to this book to find the information to effectively handle specific patient problems. The nursing student can use this book as a review of basic psychosocial information that will be useful throughout nursing school curriculum.

The concise, quick reference format allows the nurse to easily find information on a specific psychosocial problem commonly seen in practice. In addition to common psychosocial problems, psychiatric disorders are explained and discussed. Information on etiology, assessment, age specific implications, nursing diagnosis and interventions, patient/family education, pharmacologic approaches, and community-based care is provided.

Today's fast-paced healthcare environment demands quick assessment and treatment plans that are realistic, cost-effective, and outcome driven. The information contained in this book is readily applicable to all patient care settings.

Each psychosocial problem includes a section on common nurses' reactions to the patient behaviors that may result from the problem. Nurses often think they should have only acceptable and "proper" emotional reactions to their patients. The nurses may deny certain feelings and have unrealistic expectations of themselves. These factors impact how the nurse then responds to the patient's problems. The more aware the nurse becomes of how one reacts to a patient's behaviors the easier it will be to accept one's own feelings and understand how these feelings affect the patient and influence interventions.

This second edition provided us with the opportunity to add chapters on two important areas: culture and end-of-life care. In addition, chapters now include information on alternative and complementary approaches where appropriate. Nurses need to be familiar with the herbal products and nonpharmacologic approaches that patients use and how these choices can impact other treatment modalities. The increased emphasis on care outside of the acute hospital has been expanded in this edition as well. Many of the chapters now have specific interventions identified for patients receiving home healthcare, outpatient care, and care in long-term care settings. Pharmacologic approaches that have changed so much in the last few years have been revised and expanded throughout this new edition.

This is now our third collaboration as authors. The writing of our books has seen us through many of life's changes and challenges, including marriage, birth, death of parents, and personal illness. We all have had to face these while trying to maintain a healthy balance and get the books done on time. We want to recognize the roles our families, friends, and colleagues have had in encouraging us through the revision of this manuscript. We want to thank our three contributors—Yoshi Arai and Margaret Mitchell for their excellent chapters and Susan McGee for her work in revising some chapters. We also want to thank Joanne DaCunha of F.A. Davis and our editor, Diane Blodgett, for keeping us on track. We particularly want to recognize the nurses we have worked with over the years. They have taught us so much about the demands and rewards of our profession. That is the foundation of this book.

Linda M. Gorman

Marcia L. Raines

Donna F. Sultan

CONTRIBUTORS

YOSHINAO ARAI, RN, MN, CS
Mental Health Counselor, RN
Harbor-UCLA Medical Center
Los Angeles County Department of Mental Health
Los Angeles, California

Clinical Nurse Specialist
Pharmacology Research Center
Harbor-UCLA Research and Education Institute
Los Angeles, California

SUSAN J. McGEE, RN, MSN
Assistant Professor of Nursing
California State University, San Bernardino
San Bernardino, California

MARGARET L. MITCHELL, RN, MN, MDIV, MA, CNS
Senior Mental Health Counselor, RN
Treatment Authorization Request Unit
Los Angeles County Department of Mental Health
Los Angeles, California

CONSULTANTS

MARCIA G. BOWER, RN, CS, MSN, CRNP
Nurse Practitioner
Chandler Hall
Newtown, Pennsylvania

PATRICIA R. DEAN, RN, MSN, CARN
Associate Professor
Florida State University
Tallahassee, Florida

LORETTA GILLIS, RN MSCN
Professor
St. Francis Xavier University
Antigonish, Nova Scotia, Canada

KIM HAYES, RN, MPA, MS
Assistant Professor, Nursing
Central Ohio Technical College
Newark, Ohio

ALICE H. SINCLAIR, RN, MSN
Supervisor, Adult Education, Health Occupations
Burlington County Institute of Technology
Medford, New Jersey

ANN G. ROSS, RN, MN
Retired, Professor
Shoreline Community College
Seattle, Washington

CONTENTS

Introduction to Psychosocial Nursing for General Patient Care

LEARNING OBJECTIVES

➤ Define psychosocial nursing care.
➤ Describe the impact of patient behavior problems in a managed-care setting.
➤ Describe how patient education is part of psychosocial care.
➤ Describe resources the nurse can use when planning for patients across care settings.

Every day nurses are confronted with psychosocial patient problems and crises and must find a way to deal with them. Nurses often must care for patients with:

• Intense emotional responses to illness
• Personality styles that make care difficult
• Psychiatric disorders
• Stresses and family problems that affect patients' reactions to illness or hospitalization

Nurses who are proficient in managing patients' physical health problems may be less prepared to manage emotional problems. The ability to recognize behaviors that suggest psychosocial problems and to develop skills to manage them effectively can not only improve the patients' chances of healing but reduce frustration for nurses.

Psychosocial care emphasizes interventions to assist individuals who are having difficulty coping with the emotional aspects of illness, life crises that affect health and health care, or psychiatric disorders. For example, problems with depression, anger, substance abuse, or grief can influence response to illness or to the healthcare system. Psychosocial care focuses on the effects of stress in psychologic and physiologic illness and on the intrapsychic and social functioning of individuals responding to stress.

The nurse has a responsibility to facilitate each patient's adaptations to his or her unique stresses by helping and supporting the person in his or her environment, level of wellness, and adjustment to the illness or condition. Identifying the patient's coping responses, maximizing strengths, and maintaining integrity will help the nurse meet this responsibility.

NURSES' POSSIBLE REACTIONS

A factor whose importance cannot be overlooked in psychosocial care is becoming aware of one's own reactions to patient behaviors. These reactions will influence the nurse-patient relationship, assessment findings, and selection of potential interventions. They can help or hinder the relationship. Recognizing the influence of these reactions can help the nurse to:

- Increase awareness of his or her own reactions that influence objectivity
- Identify reactions frequently experienced by other nurses to ease feelings of guilt and resentment
- Increase understanding of colleagues' reactions to enhance the work environment
- Facilitate self-support by reducing self-criticism and reinforcing skills
- Select better assessment tools to identify patients' dilemmas and responses
- Recognize how personal reactions to patients can influence assessment, planning, and effective interventions

THE ROLE OF PSYCHOSOCIAL NURSING IN MANAGED-CARE SETTINGS

Some patients require many more resources because of psychosocial and psychiatric problems. A patient's emotional reactions can increase length of stay, contribute to noncompliance, and drain physical and emotional resources. Once these patient problems are identified, the nurse needs to use skills to meet the patient's needs while making judicious use of available resources.

Managed care is a system whereby controls are exerted over access, use, quality, and effectiveness of health services. Managed care has led to shortened hospital stays and limitations in available resources. Outpatient programs and home health care are being used more to address problems in place of inpatient care. To work within this system, the nurse must quickly identify the patient's needs, establish a realistic plan of care, implement interventions, and evaluate outcomes all within a predetermined length of time. Psychosocial and psychiatric patient problems complicate the demands made on the nurse in an already stretched healthcare environment and can negatively affect patient outcomes. When the nurse has skills readily at hand to identify problems and intervene effectively, patient outcomes can be improved and nurse satisfaction will be enhanced.

Managed care has also increased the focus on outcome-focused interventions to address key problems in a shorter time frame. Clinical pathways, also called care maps, are often used to drive this process. These pathways are abbreviated plans of care to achieve goals within a designated length of stay. Psychosocial and psychiatric problems often have to be addressed to keep on target with the pathway.

LIFE SPAN ISSUES

Although each individual is unique, we all share certain patterns and common links throughout the life cycle. Psychosocial development proceeds through a series of stages and developmental crises. Each phase of the life span presents new challenges, experiences, and problems. Many psychosocial problems have their origins in developmental crises that remain unresolved or that are resolved with negative outcomes. Problems such as depression and grief affect individuals differently in each stage of life. Childhood, adolescence, and old age are times of particular vulnerability.

Interventions in this book are geared to adults, but many of them can be adapted to children. To adapt an intervention to a pediatric population, the nurse must consider children's developmental and cognitive levels and incorporate them in the care plan and consult specialists in pediatrics if necessary.

COLLABORATIVE INTERVENTIONS

Our complex healthcare system relies on a variety of healthcare professionals to meet patients' needs. Obviously, the nurse does not work in a vacuum, but must participate in the interdisciplinary team and be aware of other disciplines as resources for psychosocial intervention. The nurse also needs to know when work needs to be shared or delegated through referrals. For example, social workers may be helpful because they are often familiar with psychotherapists and community support groups for emotional problems. The nurse should be aware of agency policies regarding referrals to psychotherapists. Some may require a doctor's order. Other resources include physicians, pharmacists, clergy, dietitians, and others, depending on the specialty and setting. Knowing when and how to access them and work effectively with them will improve patient outcomes and enhance the working environment.

PATIENT EDUCATION

Patient education is an important component of psychosocial care. Nurses are required to incorporate appropriate patient education in their practice. To provide adequate education, the nurse needs to be aware of how psychosocial issues influence learning. For example, assessing the patient's anxiety level or disturbed thoughts will influence timing of teaching as well as the type of information. Patient education can enhance independence and control, patient and family involvement in the treatment plan, preparation for possible emotional changes, coping skills, and responses to medications. It can be important in reducing length of stay and helping patients to take more responsibility for their own care.

Many factors can impact effective patient education including patients' cultural beliefs and language as well as knowledge of and access to computer technology.

WHEN TO CALL FOR HELP

Many difficult, challenging situations require a number of complex skills. While continuing to gain knowledge in identifying and intervening in psychosocial care, nurses also need to recognize their limitations and be able to recognize patient behaviors that may precede or currently signal a dangerous or emergency situation. Knowing when to call for help and how to use resources is essential in providing quality, cost-effective care.

CHARTING TIPS

Changes in patients' emotional responses and behaviors and their response to interventions and education are significant and must be noted in the medical record. Increased computerized documentation presents new challenges to identify behavioral problems succinctly.

COMMUNITY-BASED CARE

Many patients require care across various settings. In most cases, acute hospital care is now a small part of the treatment plan and eventually ends. To ensure continuity of care, planning for the next level of care should begin as early as possible. While the patient is in the acute setting, this planning needs to begin on admission. Long-term care, outpatient rehabilitation, other outpatient programs, and home health care are now used for many patients. Nurses in all these settings must also consider planning for the next level of care.

Many home health agencies now have psychiatric nurses on staff. Box 1–1 lists possible interventions by psychiatric home care nurses. These nurses can be helpful in evaluating response to psychotropic medications, confusion, psychotic behavior, and suicide risk. Patients may need referrals to other levels of care, such as psychiatric hospitalization or convalescent care, and assistance with financial support. Other professionals such as social workers, case managers, and counselors can help ensure safe and effective home care. Other resources including support groups, hotlines, and even telemedicine increase access to care.

BOX 1–1. Interventions by Psychiatric Home Care Nurses

- Crisis intervention
- Suicide risk assessment
- Management of psychiatric medications and blood level monitoring
- Administration of long-acting injectable psychiatric medications
- Counseling and education
- Assessment of patient and family coping
- Safety assessment

DSM-IV

The American Psychiatric Association (APA) has developed a classification system for mental disorders. It is the most widely accepted system in the United States today and is published and revised periodically as the Diagnostic and Statistical Manual. The current (fourth) edition was published in 1994 and is referred to as DSM-IV. This reference provides clinicians with guidelines, specific criteria, and accepted terminology. Throughout this book, you will see references to the criteria published in DSM-IV. These criteria are used to prevent negatively labeling or incorrectly categorizing patient behaviors as psychiatric disorders. In 2000, the American Psychiatric Association published a revised version called DSM-IV-TR, meaning text revision that is also referenced in this book.

OVERVIEW OF THE BOOK

Chapters 2 through 6 cover basic skills and emphasize the need for psychosocial assessment and culturally sensitive care. Chapters 7 through 19 address specific problems commonly encountered by nurses. Nursing interventions are provided for major nursing diagnoses. Chapter 20 reviews the medications that the nurse may be using to manage behavioral symptoms.

Psychosocial Response to Illness

LEARNING OBJECTIVES

➤ Describe the role of self-esteem, body image, powerlessness, and guilt in the patient's emotional response to illness.
➤ Describe the role of Maslow's Hierarchy of Needs in explaining a patient's response to illness.
➤ Define defense mechanisms and describe examples of each.
➤ Describe commonly used coping mechanisms.

Any illness has some psychological impact. Illness threatens the individual and evokes a wide array of emotions, such as fear, sadness, anger, depression, despair, and loss of control. Each individual who faces an illness responds differently according to personality, previous life experiences, and coping style. Denial, noncompliance, aggression, and threats of suicide may be some of the more maladaptive responses that the nurse may face in caring for ill individuals. Most often these responses are temporary and subside with time. However, they can also be chronic maladaptive behavioral responses that the patient uses whenever he or she experiences a stressful situation. There is often no way of knowing on first meeting a patient whether his or her response is temporary or habitual.

All behavior is an attempt to communicate needs. To determine underlying motivation, identifying the need can be a first step to understanding. Maslow's Hierarchy of Needs (1954) provides a framework within which to begin examining the motivation (Fig. 2–1). Maslow identified five levels of needs. Each type of need, starting at the most basic physiologic level, must be met before one can move on to the next level.

Professional nursing uses a holistic framework by which it views the individual and his or her environment in its entirety. The influence of the mind as well as the body is recognized in the development of and response to illness. It is known that the response to stress involves the immune and neuroendocrine systems. Emotional response to stress suppresses the immune system, stimulates the cardiovascular system, and alters secretions of hormones that influence the body's response to the illness.

Stress cannot be avoided. It is a normal part of living. It does not matter if a stressor is pleasant, such as an upcoming holiday, or unpleasant, such as illness, disability, or hospitalization. What is critical is the individual's perception of the intensity of the stressor requiring readjustment and his or her capacity to adjust to it.

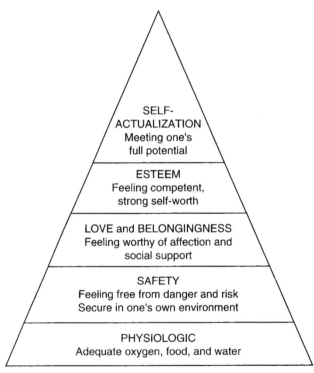

FIGURE 2–1. Maslow's Hierarchy of Needs

KEY ISSUES IN RESPONSE TO ILLNESS

ALTERED SELF-ESTEEM

Self-esteem is the individual's personal judgment of his or her own worth. The roots of self-esteem are in early parental and social relationships as well as in the person's perception of goal attainment and his or her own ideal. Maslow places self-esteem at a very high level, indicating that this need can be accomplished only when the more basic needs are fulfilled. Self-esteem increases as the individual achieves personal goals. High self-esteem indicates that the individual has accepted his or her good and bad points and knows that he or she is loved and respected by others. High self-esteem also implies a sense of control over personal destiny. Feeling good about one's self influences many aspects of life, including dealing with others, managing conflict, standing up for one's own beliefs, taking risks, and believing in one's ability to handle adversity.

Throughout life, both internal and external factors influence self-esteem. For instance, falling in love or graduating from school promotes positive self-esteem, whereas illness can represent a threat to self-esteem. Illness and disability often require a person to alter or even abandon personal goals and may strongly influence the person's view of himself or herself. Some people are able to adjust readily and create new, more realistic goals with little impact on self-esteem. Others may struggle with the changes and be unable to regain the previous level of self-esteem. Serious illnesses such as prostate or breast cancer, heart disease, or stroke not only require adaptation of personal goals but often distort the deeper sense of self. This is a major contributor to depression. But the desire to maintain a strong sense of self is a powerful drive, and over time many people adapt to changes in health.

ALTERED BODY IMAGE

Body image is the mental picture a person has of his or her own body. It significantly influences the way a person thinks and feels about his or her body as a whole, its functions, and the internal and external sensations associated with it. It also includes perceptions of the way others see the person's body and is central to self-concept and self-esteem. Often a person's belief about his or her body mirrors self-concept. This is evident when an individual seeks out cosmetic surgery to alter his or her appearance. However, when the self-concept is poor, even cosmetic surgery may not change the person's body image. This person may continue to struggle with low self-esteem even though the physical "imperfections" are changed.

A person's body image changes constantly. Illness, surgery, and weight loss or gain can have a major influence on the view of self. Amputation, colostomy, and dependence on equipment such as dialysis are examples of obvious external changes that influence body image. Some conditions such as a myocardial infarction may not cause obvious external body changes, but the individual may now view his or her body as weak. Altered body image may contribute to lowered self-esteem and, possibly, depression.

POWERLESSNESS

Powerlessness is a perceived lack of personal control over certain events and over one's self. Individuals need to maintain a sense of power and control over their destiny and environment. Loss of this sense of control can negatively affect an individual's view of his or her effectiveness. Illness consistently forces the individual to face his or her powerlessness over a situation.

Entry into the healthcare system adds to this sense of powerlessness. Now, in addition to facing the feeling of helplessness over the illness, the person is being subjected to following the orders of strangers, complying with others' schedules, and losing privacy. As soon as the hospitalized patient gives up his or her clothes and puts on a hospital gown, he or she is reminded of the sense of powerlessness within the new role. Resisting a doctor's orders and even refusing pain medication suggest that the patient is attempting to maintain some sense of control and fight off feelings of powerlessness. Helping these patients to maintain some sense of power and control is an important nursing intervention. Individuals who chronically view themselves as helpless may be more prone to depression and vulnerable to victimization by others who try to control them.

LOSS

Actual or potential loss is any situation in which something a person values is rendered or threatened to be rendered inaccessible. Loss occurs throughout life as we experience changes in relationships, inability to reach an expected goal, and disappointment in others. Any time we have an emotional investment in someone or something, we are vulnerable to losing it. This includes loss of a body part or body function. All losses in life can contribute to loss of hopes, dreams, and goals and require some period of grieving as the individual adapts to the new situation. The degree of response to the loss depends on the amount of value the individual places on whatever is lost. Eventually the individual will go on to develop new attachments and goals. Maladaptive responses to loss can include anger, guilt, depression, and, possibly, suicidal thoughts.

HOPELESSNESS

Hope is fundamental to life. No matter how bad the situation may be, the ability to hope for improvement will help an individual get through it. Hopelessness is the sustained subjective state in which an individual sees no alternatives or personal choices available to solve problems or to achieve desired goals. Lack of hope can develop from an overwhelming loss of control and is related to a sense of despair, helplessness, apathy, and depression.

The person without hope is unable to mobilize enough energy to even establish personal goals and may be unable to recognize or accept help or new ideas. Serious illness alone usually does not cause hopelessness. Usually deep personal feelings of loss, depleted emotional reserves, and an overwhelming sense of powerlessness also contribute. To regain a sense of hope, the individual needs to view the situation differently, alter negative goals and expectations, and, possibly, create new ones. For example, a terminally ill patient, rather than hoping to cure the illness, may need to refocus on achieving a pain-free state or making contact with family members. For some individuals, hopelessness can lead to discovery of alternatives that will add meaning and purpose to life. Spiritual crises may be related to hopelessness as well.

GUILT

Guilt is self-blame and regret for some real or perceived action. It is a painful emotion that can negatively influence feelings, behaviors, and relationships with others. Conflicts within relationships can occur when an individual feels guilty about resentment that his or her needs are not being met.

Nurses frequently observe behavior in patients or their families that seems to be motivated by guilt. Examples include family members who suddenly hover over an ill patient or make numerous demands on the staff and unjustly accuse them of providing inadequate care, or the patient who refuses to ask for help. Self-blame is another frequent behavior motivated by guilt. For example, a wife may blame herself for not taking her husband to the doctor sooner or a patient may blame himself for the stress his illness is causing his wife. Survivor guilt is often seen in people who survive traumatic events in which others are killed or injured.

ANXIETY

Anxiety is a universal, primitive, unpleasant feeling of tension and apprehension. It may be an early warning signal of possible danger. Anxiety is an important motivator of behavior that makes people act or change to reduce the uncomfortable feelings of tension. Low to moderate levels of anxiety can enhance learning and action. More severe anxiety may be reduced by using defense or coping mechanisms as the unconscious self tries to protect us from this discomfort.

DEFENSE MECHANISMS

Defense mechanisms protect the individual from threats, feelings of inadequacy, and unacceptable feelings or thoughts. They are unconscious mental processes used to reduce anxiety and conflict by modifying, distorting, and rejecting reality (Table 2–1). Because they are unconscious, the individual is not aware of how these mechanisms affect thoughts, feelings, and behavior. In some ways, they are used to alter reality to make the situation more acceptable. Without these mechanisms, the threatening feelings might overwhelm and paralyze the individual and interfere with daily living. Essential, adaptive defense mechanisms help to lower anxiety so that goals can be achieved. We could not survive without them. However, they are used too extensively, they can contribute to highly distorted perceptions and interfere with normal functioning and interpersonal relationships. Excessively distorted defense mechanisms can be characterized as psychiatric disorders.

An individual's repertoire of defense mechanisms is learned through child-

TABLE 2–1. COMMON DEFENSE MECHANISMS

Defense Mechanism	Definition	Example
Denial	Attempt to remove an experience or a feeling from consciousness	After a diagnosis of terminal condition, the patient does not exhibit any expected emotional reaction and states that diagnosis is not true.
Displacement	The belief that one would be in great danger if true feelings about someone were known to that person, which causes the individual to discharge or displace feelings onto a third person or object	A family member is angry at the patient for not taking better care of himself and feels too guilty to express this to the ill person. Instead, he expresses anger at the nursing staff for giving inadequate care.
Identification	Accepting the other person's circumstances as though they were one's own	A man's wife died a very painful death from cancer. When he is diagnosed with cancer, he experiences extreme anxiety because he has accepted his wife's experiences as if he had lived them.
Intellectualization	Separating emotion from an idea or thought because emotionally it is too painful	A patient discusses the physiology of his leukemia at length without any emotional reaction.
Isolation	Blocking out feelings associated with an unpleasant or threatening situation or thought	A nurse caring for critically ill patient who is the same age provides care without experiencing the emotions related to tragedy of the patient's situation.
Projection	Transferring or blaming others for one's own unacceptable ideas, impulses, wishes, or feelings	After a myocardial infarction, a patient relates that his wife is coping poorly with his condition. This patient's anxiety may be too great and threatening to face, so he places his own fears onto his wife.
Rationalization	Substituting acceptable reasons for the true reasons for personal behavior because admitting true reasons is too threatening	Smoker continues to smoke despite physician's warning because he knows many people who smoke and have no ill effects.
Reaction formation	Actions that are opposite of the true, unacceptable feelings that the person is experiencing	A woman has negative feelings about her pregnancy but then lavishes constant attention on her newborn.
Regression	Reverting to earlier patterns of development as a way to reduce anxiety and demands on one's self	During serious illness, a patient exhibits behavior more appropriate for a younger developmental age, such as excessive dependency.

Defense Mechanism	Definition	Example
Repression	Forcibly dismissing unacceptable thoughts, feelings, impulses, or memories from consciousness	A person is unable to recall feelings of hostility toward a sibling or specific memories from childhood.
Sublimation	Expressing repressed urges or desires in socially acceptable ways	An angry person writes a poem about his reactions to his feelings.

hood experiences. Each time a defense mechanism reduces uncomfortable anxiety feelings, it provides positive reinforcement.

COPING MECHANISMS

Coping mechanisms are usually conscious methods that the individual uses to overcome a problem or stressor. They are learned adaptive or maladaptive responses to anxiety based on problem solving, and they may lead to changed behavior. They involve higher levels of emotional and ego development than defense mechanisms. However, overuse of coping mechanisms such as overeating or smoking can create problems. In addition, unconscious mechanisms can also play a role in using or selecting a specific coping mechanism. Inappropriate coping mechanisms can be readily changed because the patient is usually aware of using them.

Some common coping mechanisms include:

- Talking problems out with others and gaining new insights by looking at or coping with the problem
- Expressing intense emotion by crying, yelling, or laughing
- Seeking comfort from friends, favorite foods, cigarettes, treasured objects, or mind-altering substances
- Using humor to discharge tension in a way that avoids fully acknowledging a difficult situation
- Exercising or performing manual labor
- Problem solving using a series of strategies and step-by-step approaches to the resolution of a problem
- Sleeping
- Avoiding upsetting situations, for example by feigning illness, to avoid a confrontation

Psychosocial Skills

Providing psychosocial care requires a combination of astute psychosocial assessment skills, experience in performing mental status examinations, and using therapeutic communication.

PSYCHOSOCIAL NURSING ASSESSMENT

Psychosocial information must be part of every patient assessment to develop a nursing diagnosis, goals, and interventions. Psychosocial problems influence the selection of a diagnosis and treatment of the illness. With a thorough assessment, the nurse can determine the patient's needs, problems, and potential problems and identify patients who are at a higher risk for developing more serious problems. A psychosocial assessment includes information on the patient's sociocultural background, emotional and biologic aspects of current problems, history, spiritual and philosophical beliefs, and family issues.

To perform a thorough psychosocial assessment, the nurse uses many skills. The first is the ability to establish a rapport with the patient. Showing an interest in what the patient is saying, asking appropriate questions, and making observations help to put the patient at ease and enable him or her to divulge personal information. Box 3–1 offers suggestions for creating an appropriate interview environment.

The psychosocial assessment focuses on the effect of the illness on the patient and family rather than on physical symptoms. This assessment begins the process of identifying key nursing diagnoses. In addition, it provides important information for the patient's treatment plan. The assessment should include:

Lifestyle information: Determine with whom the patient lives, significant relationships, available support people, marital status, occupation, religion, and other important components of the patient's lifestyle.

Normal coping patterns: Identify which coping mechanisms the patient uses when under stress and in past illnesses or hospitalizations. What happened the last time the patient was under severe stress? How is the patient currently coping?

Understanding of current illness: Ask the patient about his or her understanding of the diagnosis or reason for seeking medical attention. Determine how the patient views the illness affecting his or her life.

Personality style: After interacting with the patient, identify any important personality traits that may affect his or her care or compliance, such as a tendency to be dependent, hostile, dramatic, or critical.

BOX 3–1. Creating an Appropriate Interview Environment

- Create a quiet, private environment.
- Minimize interruptions if possible.
- Maintain appropriate eye contact.
- Sit at eye level with the patient.
- Ask open-ended questions to encourage the patient to talk.
- Avoid writing a lot of notes during the interview.
- Demonstrate an interest in the patient's concerns.
- Ask the patient's permission to be interviewed.
- Indicate acceptance of the patient by avoiding criticism, frowning, or demonstrating shock.
- Avoid asking more personal questions than are actually needed.
- Determine whether the family can provide information if the patient is unable to communicate.
- Maintain confidentiality.
- Be aware of your own biases and discomforts that could influence the assessment.

History of psychiatric disorder: If the patient is currently taking medications for psychiatric problems, be sure to ask why he or she is taking them. Consider asking if the patient has experienced any psychiatric symptoms, such as depression. If his or her behavior indicates a psychiatric disorder, explore this further.

Recent life changes or stressors: Determine if there have been any major changes or traumatic events recently (especially in the last year). Keep in mind that these changes may be both positive and negative, such as moving to a new house or area, a death in the family, a job or role change, or recent birth of a child.

Major issues raised by current illness: Determine how this illness has affected the patient's lifestyle or sense of self, including areas such as self-esteem, body image, loss of intimacy, role changes, and change in family dynamics.

Mental status examination: Perform the mental status examination to help identify dysfunction in emotional, cognitive, or behavioral spheres.

THE MENTAL STATUS EXAMINATION

The mental status examination is used to determine whether or not there are abnormalities in the patient's thinking and reasoning ability, feelings, or behavior. Nurses often perform quick mental status examinations every time they see their patients without realizing they are doing it. Changes in a patient's appearance, memory, emotions, or thinking can be observed while the nurse is making quick rounds or having a social conversation with the patient. A more formal mental status examination can be part of a psychosocial assessment in a new patient, or it may be done when changes in the patient's condition are seen.

The mental status examination includes observations and questions in the following categories: appearance, behavior, and speech; thoughts; mood and affect; ability to perform abstract reasoning; memory; intelligence; concentration; orientation; judgment; and insight (Table 3–1 and Fig. 3–1).

To gather a comprehensive evaluation, review all the categories of the examination. Congruence or discrepancies between sections may reveal important information. Note inappropriate responses as well as the absence of the usual anticipated responses. For example, a patient may relate that the physician says her cancer has metastasized too much to consider surgery (thought). This clear and coherent thought, expressed in a droning, monotonous voice (speech) without any apparent intensity, distress, or expression of emotion (mood) may suggest that the patient is denying her illness. A patient who may be experiencing an extreme stress response to his or her illness may be unable to verbalize any expected concerns (thoughts), but may become increasingly anxious or depressed (mood and/or emotions) with increasing restlessness (behavior). Choosing an appropriate nursing diagnosis will depend on integrating all these observations along with knowledge of the patient's usual responses to stress.

Changes in mental status are often caused by alterations in the psychological or physical state. For example, behavioral changes such as confusion, de-

TABLE 3–1. MENTAL STATUS EXAMINATION AND RELATED DEFINITIONS

Category	Description	Related Definitions
Appearance	Describe what patient looks like including dress, posture, grooming.	
Behavior	Describe behavior, motor activity, mannerisms.	*Catatonic:* Remaining totally immobile *Posturing:* Assuming inappropriate or bizarre positions *Compulsions:* Insistent, repetitive unwanted actions
Speech	Describe how patient speaks; list barriers to communication.	*Perseveration:* Mechanical repetition of words, thoughts *Pressured:* Highly accelerated rapid speech *Loose associations:* Absence of logical connections between thoughts *Flight of ideas:* Rapidly jumping from one thought to another with minimal links *Tangential:* Talking around main point *Word salad:* Unconnected words and phrases without meaning or logic *Thought blocking:* Stopping suddenly in the middle of verbalizing a thought and staring into space *Neologism:* Making up new words only speaker understands
Mood/affect	Describe the emotions that are apparent from facial expressions, motor behavior, words used.	*Labile:* Emotions that change quickly and unpredictably *Flat affect:* No demonstration of any feeling *Blunted affect:* Constricted display of emotions *Anhedonia:* Absence of any pleasure *Inappropriate affect:* Emotions displayed not fitting with topic discussed *Ambivalence:* Contradictory feelings experienced simultaneously
Thoughts	What are themes in conversation? Does patient make sense? Is patient preoccupied with certain thoughts?	*Hallucinations:* Sensory perceptions (auditory, visual, gustatory, olfactory, tactile) without external stimuli, e.g., hearing nonexistent voices. *Illusions:* Misinterpretations of real external sensory stimuli, e.g., seeing a ghost in a shadow

Category	Description	Related Definitions
		Delusions: False, fixed beliefs not alterable by logical explanations
		Obsessions: Unwanted, distressing recurring thoughts
		Phobia: Irrational fear of a specific situation, accompanied by avoidance of the phenomenon feared
		Depersonalization: Sense of not being real; sense of being detached from one's body or self
		Magical thinking: Believing that thinking about something happening is the same as doing it
		Grandiosity: Exaggerated beliefs in own worth and/or abilities
		Paranoia: Unwarranted belief that others have harmful intentions to person
Ability to abstract	Describe the patient's ability to define similarities between objects or explain a proverb.	*Concrete description:* Sees objects in very definite simple ways, e.g., sees an apple and an orange as "round" rather than the overall category "fruit"
		Abstract ability: Can generalize the meaning of a concept and find meaning in symbols, e.g., "still water runs deep" means that quiet people have depth rather than lakes are deep bodies of water
Memory	Describe patient's ability to repeat the names of 3 objects immediately after being told and again in 5 minutes.	
Intelligence	Describe patient's level of knowledge, language, understanding of instructions.	
Concentration	Describe patient's ability to focus on a single thought without becoming distracted.	*Serial 7s:* Test to determine the patient's ability to concentrate by having him or her continually subtract from 100 by 7 (93, 86, etc.)
Orientation	Describe patient's awareness of person and surroundings. A person is fully oriented when he or she is aware of person, place, time and situation.	*Orientation to person:* Knows his or her name
		Orientation to place: Knows where he or she is (Ask for specific location.)

(Continued)

**TABLE 3–1. MENTAL STATUS EXAMINATION
AND RELATED DEFINITIONS (*Continued*)**

Category	Description	Related Definitions
		Orientation to time: Knows the date, day of week, year; most serious impairment is if the patient cannot identify year
		Orientation to situation: Knows what is wrong with him or her, why he or she is receiving care, the circumstances of current situation
Judgment	Describe patient's ability to use common sense to make reasonable decisions.	
Insight	Determine patient's understanding of factors contributing to his or her condition.	

pression, delirium, or even psychosis may be signs of drug toxicity, electrolyte imbalance, or intracranial bleeding (Table 3–2).

THERAPEUTIC COMMUNICATION

Therapeutic communication, the essence of the helping relationship, occurs when the nurse communicates with the patient in a manner that facilitates acquiring information and understanding the patient's concerns and problems. It is the art of reaching a person by means of verbal and nonverbal messages. Acceptance, respect, honesty, trust, concern, protection, and support must all be present for communication to be therapeutic. Therapeutic communication allows the patient to share feelings, feel accepted, and look at problems from a new perspective. It should not be confused with counseling, which focuses on interpretation and the process of communication rather than the content. The patient should also expect confidentiality to be maintained (Tables 3–3 and 3–4).

Because nonverbal language is such a major part of any communication, the nurse needs to be aware of how his or her body language may enhance or inhibit therapeutic communication. Studies consistently support the concept that the way in which we communicate is much more powerful than the content of our words. Nonverbal communication includes eye contact, body movements, facial expressions, gestures, and posture. Facial expressions are probably one of the most important sources of communication. Posture can communicate interest, tension, or boredom. A person's walk can convey anxiety or confidence. Eye contact can be comforting and supportive or invasive and threatening. Gestures such as placing a hand on the patient's arm during intense emotions can be very supportive, especially in contrast to standing away from the patient with your arms crossed in a judgmental way.

Mental Status Examination Answer Sheet

Circle the correct words or fill in the blanks.

Appearance

Neat   clean   disheveled   poor grooming   erect posture   good eye contact

inappropriate makeup, _____

Behavior

Calm   appropriate   restless   agitated   compulsions   unusual actions

_____

Speech

Appropriate   pressured   loose association   loud   soft   mute

_____

Mood

Appropriate   labile   flat   depressed   worried   anxious   angry

hopeless_____

Thoughts

Appropriate   low self-esteem   suicidal ideations   hallucinations   delusions,

phobias _____

FIGURE 3–1. Mental Status Examination Answer Sheet (*Continued on Next Page*)

OTHER PSYCHOSOCIAL SKILLS

In addition to therapeutic communication, nurses use several other skills to help patients find new ways of coping with illness and the problems it causes. Many of these are used without the nurse's even being aware of using them. Perfecting the following techniques can greatly enhance your ability to meet the psychosocial needs of your patients.

Ability to abstract

Impaired   Yes   No

Memory

Impaired recent memory   Yes   No

Impaired past memory   Yes   No

Number of objects able to remember after 5 minutes_____

Estimated Intelligence

Below average   average   above average

Concentration

Able to focus,   easily distractible _____

Able to subtract backwards by 7's from 100 correctly until number_____

Orientation

Person_____Time_____

Place_____ Situation_____

Judgment

Realistic decision making   Yes   No

Insight

Good   fair   poor

Summary of Impressions:

FIGURE 3–1. (*Continued*)

Acceptance: Demonstrating an interest in a patient's behavior and feelings communicates to the patient that he or she is valued. You can
demonstrate acceptance of the patient by listening to him or her even
if you disagree with the ideas being communicated. It is important not
to criticize or judge the patient. Acceptance reinforces self-esteem.

Reassurance: Providing support by giving your attention to matters that
are important to the patient reinforces emotional security and helps
reduce the patient's anxiety. With less anxiety to deal with, he or she

TABLE 3–2. MENTAL STATUS CHANGES CAUSED BY ELECTROLYTE IMBALANCE

Electrolyte Imbalance	Possible Cause	Mental Status Changes
Calcium (Blood Level: 8.5–10.5 mg/dL)		
Hypercalcemia	Hyperparathyroidism	Loss of energy
	Lung, breast cancer	Depression
		Confusion
		Irritability
Hypocalcemia	Hypoparathyroidism due to calcium deficiency, lack of dietary vitamin D, or iatrogenic causes	Reduced concentration and intellectual function
		Emotional lability
		Depression
		Psychosis (if surgical excision of a parathyroid gland)
Sodium (Blood Level: 135–145 mEq/L)		
Hypernatremia	Dehydration caused by excessive water loss (diarrhea, vomiting, diuresis)	Irritability
		Hyperactive intellectual function
	Restricted fluid intake	Stupor
	Diabetes insipidus	
Hyponatremia	Severe dietary sodium restriction	Depression
	Addison's disease	Lethargy
	Excessive water intake	Withdrawal
		Anorexia
Phosphorus (Blood Level: 2.6–4.5 mg/dL)		
Hypophosphatemia	Gram-negative septicemia	Apprehension
	Alcohol withdrawal	Irritability
	Intravenous hyperalimentation	Numbness
	Low dietary intake	Stupor
Potassium (Blood Level: 3.5–5 mEq/L)		
Hyperkalemia	Renal disease	Weakness
	Potassium-sparing diuretics	Dysphagia
	Increased IV intake	
Hypokalemia	Renal disease	Mood and personality change
	Cushing's syndrome	Tearfulness
	Potassium-wasting diuretics	Hopeless
	Vomiting	Helplessness
	Diarrhea	
Base Bicarbonate (Blood Level: 24 mEq/L, pH 7.38)		
Alkalosis	Prolonged vomiting	Decreased intellectual function
	Large intake of sodium bicarbonate	Apathy
		Delirium
	Hyperventilation	Stupor
Acidosis	Severe emphysema	Decreased intellectual function
	Status asthmaticus	Drowsiness
	Renal failure	Confusion
	Diabetes mellitus with ketosis	Delirium

Source: Reprinted with permission from Barry, P: Psychosocial Nursing Assessment and Intervention (3rd ed). Philadelphia, JB Lippincott, 1989.

TABLE 3–3. THERAPEUTIC COMMUNICATION TECHNIQUES

Technique	Definition	Example
Empathy	The helper becomes keenly attuned to the patient's feelings to understand them fully while maintaining a sense of one's own separateness	In response to a patient's recounting the recent loss of a baby, the nurse says, "You must have felt very disappointed."
Open-ended questions	Questions structured to encourage the patient to share information and feelings	"How did you feel when the doctor told you of your diagnosis?"
Closed-ended questions	Information-gathering questions that require only a one-word or very brief answer	"Where does it hurt?"
Active listening	Accepting what the speaker has said, analyzing it, and reflecting back your understanding of what was heard	"From what I understand, you are planning to stop coming to counseling."
Clarification	Increasing the understanding of what the patient is trying to communicate	"I'm not sure I understand what happened next. Could you go over it again?"
Silence	Allowing time for the patient to gather thoughts and ponder a topic without interruption (This can communicate acceptance and concern.)	
Reflection	Verbally giving back the feeling part of the patient's communication to help focus on the feeling tone	"You sound very worried about the test results."
Nonverbal communication	Overt behavior that indicates listening and attention	Maintaining eye contact, learning forward, keeping facial expressions appropriate for the emotions being expressed, keeping a comfortable distance.
Congruent communication	Body language, facial expression, and verbal content all expressing the same thing	Nurse's physical appearance, voice, and emotional reaction all communicate that she or he is listening, accepting, concerned, and understanding.

can spend more time on effective problem solving and healing. However, avoid false reassurance because it can reinforce a sense of distrust in the nurse if unexpected events occur.

   Enhancing self-esteem: Increased self-esteem gives the patient a sense of control and hope. This will help reduce anxiety and give the patient more time for problem solving and healing. Techniques to reinforce

TABLE 3–4. BARRIERS TO THERAPEUTIC COMMUNICATION

Technique	Possible Result	Example
Giving advice	Inhibits communication and sharing feelings. Patient may think you are not listening.	"You should go back to school."
False reassurances	May communicate that you do not fully understand the patient's feelings.	"I'm sure you'll do just fine."
Judgment	Patient will sense your disapproval.	"How can you still smoke when your husband has lung cancer?"
Leading statements	Inhibits communication by possibly imposing feelings on the patient that he or she may not have.	"I'm sure you must have felt depressed after the divorce."
Multiple questions	Patient may not know what to answer first.	"Whom do you live with? Is that the way you want to live?"
Why question	May inhibit communication by threatening the patient. Often we may not know why we do the things we do or feel the way we do.	"Why do you feel that way?"
Parroting	Continually repeating what the patient says may appear to be too mechanical and frustrate the patient.	*Patient:* "I'm worried about the test results." *Nurse:* "You're worried about the test results?"

positive self-esteem include focusing on patient's positive traits and accomplishments, providing opportunities for the patient to demonstrate skills and abilities successfully, and emotional support and reassurance.

Expression of feelings: Providing an environment in which a patient can feel safe and comfortable to express emotions, including sorrow or anger, and to verbalize disagreement, fear, and disappointment is essential for both enhancing a therapeutic relationship and allowing the patient to solve problems.

Role modeling: The nurse can exhibit more socially acceptable ways of performing a certain role or demonstrating a certain behavior. When the patient sees how effective these behaviors are, he or she can more easily understand how to use them and emulate the behaviors. For example, the nurse can communicate assertively with a family member who may be intimidating the patient. When the patient sees how that family member responds to assertive behavior, he or she may adopt that method of interaction. The nurse also provides a role model for adopting a healthy lifestyle by eating healthy foods, not smoking, and exercising,

Role playing: Role playing is acting out other methods of response to a situation. It can be done to increase one's own or another's understanding of the other's point of view or to practice appropriate responses, such as assertiveness. This is done with a supportive person playing the part of someone you want to communicate with in a new way.

Stress management: Accepting stress as a fact of life and managing it using specific, tested techniques can reduce feelings of anxiety. The techniques are meant to promote a feeling of calm and a sense of control over the situation. Common stress management techniques include physical interventions such as taking deep breaths, exercising, and avoiding caffeine; and psychological interventions such as counting to 10, avoiding additional stressors, maintaining a positive attitude, and seeking out emotional support.

Assertiveness: Assertiveness is the use of behavioral techniques that allow the individual to stand up for his or her rights without infringing on the rights of others. To gain expertise in using assertive behavior, role playing and practicing with others is useful. You may try role-playing assertive responses to common situations in a supportive environment, such as asking for a refund or telling a colleague that you are not satisfied with the quality of work performed.

Limit setting: Limit setting is a form of behavior modification rather than a punishment and is used for times when acceptance of the patient's behavior is no longer appropriate. To set limits on behavior, you need to clearly define the desired behaviors and the consequences of not conforming to them. Then you must be prepared to follow through with the stated consequences. If appropriate limits are not set to control the patient's inappropriate behavior, it can escalate and possibly lead to injury and resentment from those who feel manipulated by the patient.

Deescalation: These techniques are also used to reduce anxiety and slow down the emotional response to it, such as aggressive behavior. Useful techniques include removing the patient from volatile situations and using appropriate medication and physical restraints.

Confrontation: At times it is necessary to make direct statements that challenge the patient's behavior or beliefs. Confrontation is a verbal message designed to help the other person recognize inconsistencies or inappropriate behavior. It can assist the patient in gaining insight. However, it can also be so threatening that it could precipitate a crisis situation, so be sure to consult with specialists before using this method.

Empathy: Communicating an understanding of how the client feels indicates that the nurse shares the feelings. Empathy differs from sympathy in that empathy does not indicate sharing of personal feelings.

Silence: Sometimes saying nothing for a few moments can communicate more than words. This can convey support, acceptance, and concern and give the patient time to compose himself or herself.

Relaxation techniques: The nurse can use a variety of techniques, including deep breathing, imagery, and muscle relationship. See Appendix A for more details.

ASSESSING USE OF COMPLEMENTARY AND ALTERNATIVE THERAPIES

Americans are using complementary and alternative therapies in increasing numbers. The Journal of the American Medical Association reported in 1998 that 42 percent of consumers use some of these therapies, which include dietary supplements, folk remedies, and herbal products. Complementary approaches are defined as those used in addition to conventional treatment. Alternative ones are used in place of conventional therapies. See Appendix B for a listing of commonly used approaches. Many of these are used to treat emotional problems such as anxiety and depression.

Healthcare professionals need to incorporate assessment of these approaches in their care. Eisenberg (1998) found that fewer than 40 percent of patients tell their healthcare provider about products they are using. Patients often do not tell their provider that they are using herbs or megavitamins because they believe the products are harmless or think their healthcare provider will discourage the use of such products.

The Food and Drug Administration now tracks the adverse drug reactions of herbal products, and the public needs to be aware of possible drug interactions or negative effects. Impurities, lack of regulation in dosing, and lack of knowledge about interactions with other prescribed medications can create complications. For example, St. John's wort, which is often used for depression, interacts with some HIV protease inhibitors, making them less effective.

The increased use of these herbal products reflects the public's wish for more control, incorporation of cultural values, and hope in their care. Nurses, as patient advocates, need to be sensitive to these approaches and incorporate them in the plan of care where possible. Routine questions about use of herbs and supplements should be part of the routine nursing assessment.

Nurses' Responses to Difficult Patient Behaviors

LEARNING OBJECTIVES

➢ List qualities expected in a "good" patient.
➢ Describe how the concept of a "difficult patient" reflects both the patient's behavior and the nurse's interpretation of that behavior.
➢ Identify the process of evaluating what patients may be communicating by difficult behavior.
➢ List types of nurses' responses that may impair awareness of the dynamics of problematic patient behavior.
➢ List resources available in most healthcare agencies for psychosocial support.

Nurses often see patients behaving at their worst because they are stressed and overwhelmed by their illness or hospitalization. These nurse-patient relationships may change as the patient's healthcare needs change, requiring different types of involvement. Optimally, each nurse should respond positively to each patient, but human nature makes that all but impossible. The next best strategy, then, is to learn the most effective ways to deal with patients who are "difficult," usually defined by the amount of trouble and distress that the staff has in managing them. They often exhibit problem behaviors such as anger, regression, and out-of-control or manipulative behaviors (Fincannon, 1995). Nursing interventions may make the problem worse if staff members are unable to differentiate their responses to the behavior from their response to the person. If you think of these patients as having "difficult-to-care-for behaviors" rather than as "difficult patients," you may find that the staff's frustration decreases and more effective care strategies are identified. Sometimes the patient uses these objectionable behaviors, with or without being aware of it, to regain personal equilibrium and to reduce anxiety and fears and maintain control. Thus, although these behaviors may cause stress for the staff, they work "just fine" for the patient. In addition, some patients are totally unaware that they are affecting the staff negatively. Nurses who learn effective skills to deal with these problem behaviors may experience a sense of enhanced competence, and improved patient outcomes will follow.

NURSE-PATIENT INTERACTIONS

The nurse-patient interaction is based on the continuous flow of communication between the nurse and patient with input from both. The nurse's therapeutic use of self is the basic tool that enhances the interaction. Communication skills, an awareness of how personal responses can influence the patient, and a good knowledge base combine to enhance a positive nurse-patient interaction.

Difficult patient behaviors can negatively influence the nurse-patient interaction and, possibly, the quality of nursing care. Whenever a relationship is disrupted, the nurse needs to identify the source of the problem. Does it originate in the patient, in the nurse, or in both? For example, a demanding patient who constantly rings the call bell may be communicating the fear that she will not recover and is seeking reassurance that someone will respond if she needs it. If the nurse interprets this behavior to mean that the patient feels that the nurse is doing his or her job poorly, he or she may become frustrated and angry. The nurse needs to assess the situation objectively to determine if the patient is truly looking for reassurance or if the nurse is just not as tolerant as usual because of the workload. Responding without assessing the situation could inhibit favorable nurse-patient interactions and negatively affect the patient's outcome. To be effective, the nurse must treat the behaviors as symptoms and assess their cause. The nurse needs to explore his or her own attitudes and reactions, which may be unwittingly initiating or perpetuating the undesired behavior. Better understanding can lead to a greater acceptance of both the patient's and the nurse's feelings to create a more positive cycle of nurse-patient interactions. Table 4–1 compares the ways in which assessment and appropriate interventions can significantly alter patient outcomes.

Sometimes the only effective way to change a patient's behavior is for the nurse to change his or her response. If there is still no resolution of the situation, the nurse should seek the advice or interventions of other available resources to help understand the patient's behavior and the nurse's response to it and then select more effective interventions. If the patient continues to manifest difficult behaviors despite all efforts, the nurse should focus on self-awareness to remain objective.

TABLE 4–1. THE NURSING PROCESS WITH DIFFICULT PATIENT BEHAVIORS

Assessment Step	Positive Cycle	Negative Cycle
Assessment	Nurse assesses patient's and his or her own understanding of what is happening. Nurse evaluates if he or she is stereotyping or reacting personally. Nurse gets assistance and support.	Patient does not explore issues. Patient responds only to surface level of communication. Patient reacts personally. Nurse complains to staff about patient.
Intervention	Nurse responds accurately and with empathy to patient.	Nurse avoids or rejects patient. Nurse is unable to control patient's behavior.
Patient outcome	Patient feels heard, accepted, and understood, resulting in less anxiety. Difficult behavior decreases. Patient can participate more fully in health care.	Patient feels alienated with escalation of undesirable behaviors. Potential exists for negative health outcome.

ROLE EXPECTATIONS

Clarifying the nurse's intertwining role expectations of the patient in the sick role and himself or herself as the helper can provide a useful perspective. Keep in mind that nurses have chosen their roles as helpers but most patients have not deliberately chosen to become patients. A nurse may have chosen this profession for the personal satisfaction and self-esteem resulting from attaining a high level of expertise. The patient, on the other hand, may feel that his or her self-esteem is threatened by entering the healthcare system. The patient is expected to adapt to the routines and expectations of others. Some patients cannot accept this new role and may revert to using dysfunctional behaviors.

Optimally, "good" patients are consistently cooperative; comply with the nurse's instructions and agency rules; are pleasant, polite, and respectful; show improvement; and appreciate the nurse's help. These patients ensure that the nurse meets his or her own role expectations; that is, the nurse feels helpful, effective, and accepted and valued by both patients and colleagues. "Difficult" patients produce the opposite effect. The nurse can experience frustration, anxiety, feelings of incompetence, lowered self-esteem, and a sense of being out of control.

Nurses must objectively evaluate some common myths about these role expectations. A prevalent one is that nurses can control their patients' behavior to conform to expectations. They cannot. They can encourage, suggest, negotiate, and set limits. Only in very rare situations such as when a patient poses a threat of imminent danger to himself or herself or to the staff can the nurse force a patient into expected behaviors. A nurse who believes that he or she can control a patient's behavior is creating a set-up for failure.

Many nurses believe that only certain feelings toward patients are acceptable. Because nurses are human, they respond with a whole range of human emotions, including empathy, sympathy, disgust, love, hate, and, possibly, sexual feelings. Experiencing all feelings is acceptable. Displaying these feelings to patients may not be. The nurse must use professional judgment in determining which feelings are helpful to display to the patient and which are not. Responding genuinely to the patient with realistic concern is usually appropriate. If the nurse determines that it would not be appropriate to display other feelings, he or she may want to find suitable ways to express them. Often just acknowledging the feelings to a trusted colleague can be beneficial.

Once the nurse has learned to accept and tolerate a broader range of human responses within himself or herself, he or she will develop more tolerance for formerly forbidden feelings displayed by patients. The nurse will be less likely to blame or avoid patients who stir up disturbing feelings. Often, before engaging with patients to work on problems, the nurse needs to work with ways to accept and assimilate personal experiences. Throughout this book, common nurses' reactions are listed as a way to help the reader identify them.

The following recommendations are listed to assist nurses in maintaining professional distance while remaining available to patients:

- Listen to what the patient is really asking. People have a need to be heard. When a patient tells a nurse about his or her concerns and problems, he or she may simply need someone to listen and understand his or her feelings and suffering and to feel less alone. The nurse may erroneously believe that he or she has to do something or give advice.
- Assess the patient's ability to use comments or receive information about more negative emotions like anger before sharing them and risking alienating the patient. Occasionally, however, it may be therapeutic to share even very negative feelings if this is done in a calm, matter-of-fact tone without accusation. For example, when working with a very provocative patient, point out that this behavior elicits angry responses and pushes others away. The patient may not be aware of the cause and effect. Bringing it to his or her attention may lead to a fruitful discussion of the true fears underlying the behavior and ways of developing a realization of why others often react negatively.
- If a nurse determines that, even with the advice of specialists, he or she would not be able to work with the patient without bias, then alternate arrangements for patient care need to be made.

PATIENT ISSUES

COVERT COMMUNICATION

Consciously or unconsciously, patients often communicate their real needs and wishes indirectly, possibly because they may not even be aware of their fears. When their communication is not analyzed, the nurse may select ineffective interventions because he or she is dealing only with what the patient said, not what is really meant. Once the real concerns are identified, more effective interventions can be used. For example, the noncompliant patient may be indirectly expressing fear or a need for more reassurance or help. If fear is the underlying issue, interventions directed toward reassuring the patient will be the most successful.

TRANSFERENCE

This is a common issue with difficult-to-care-for patients. Sometimes even without being aware of it, the patient transfers early childhood perceptions, feelings, and experiences onto people with whom he or she is currently interacting. The patient may take positive or negative experiences with parents, teachers, siblings, or other significant people in his or her life and connect them to the nurse if there are superficial or substantial similarities between them. This usually occurs on an unconscious level, but the patient then feels, expects, and responds as if the nurse were that other person. For example, if the patient sees the nurse as his loving but somewhat controlling mother, he may respond with dependence tinged with resentment along with magical expectations of the nurse's effectiveness, reflecting earlier responses to his mother. If the nurse is viewed as a hostile, attacking parent, the patient may become hostile and defensive for self-protection.

Other examples of patient behaviors suggesting transference include a preoccupation with a particular nurse, a desire to be the nurse's only patient, jealousy if the nurse spends time with other patients, and recurrent attempts to provoke a specific emotion from the nurse. A common warning sign of transference is when a patient displays a strong attachment to a single staff member.

If you suspect that the patient is using transference, use the following guidelines:

- Find out if the patient is responding in similar ways to other staff members.
- Determine, if possible, whether the patient acts in similar ways toward other individuals in his or her personal life.
- Ask other staff members to provide support for the patient and a more balanced viewpoint.
- Avoid increasing the patient's dependency on you.
- Consult with a supervisor or specialist to determine the appropriateness of gently confronting the patient with these issues.
- Set limits on the patient's behavior. Do not allow the patient to obtain special privileges.
- Do not personalize any hostility.

NURSING ISSUES

Usually, not all nurses have the same amount of difficulty dealing with a patient who displays problematic behaviors. Each nurse responds to the behavior based on individual expectations of correct and proper patient behavior, previous experience working with a particular type of patient behavior, and the degree of success he or she has had in dealing with a similar situation. Personal value systems, coping mechanisms, styles of communication, conflicts, and "pet peeves" also play a role. The following issues may contribute to a deteriorating nurse-patient relationship.

IDENTIFICATION

The nurse may identify with a patient because of similarities such as age, gender, and social interests and then superimpose his or her own conflicts, values, and expectations onto the patient. So when the nurse seems to be responding to the patient, he or she is actually responding to himself or herself. A classic example of identification is a young female nurse who is caring for a critically ill woman her own age. The nurse sees herself in the patient and begins feeling intense sadness for all the things she (the nurse) has not yet accomplished in life. The nurse may do things for the patient that she would want done for herself, regardless of their significance for this patient.

COUNTERTRANSFERENCE

Countertransference is a conscious or unconscious emotional response to the patient based on the professional's own inner needs rather than the patient's. It occurs when the nurse transfers significant positive or negative early childhood figures and conflicts onto the patient. This may present problems if the nurse does not recognize what is happening and therefore chooses interventions based on faulty assessment findings. For example, a nurse whose father physically abused her may find herself reacting with fear or rage toward a particular male patient and initially may not understand why. If she does not recognize what is triggering her response, she may conclude that the problem is with the patient's behavior rather than her response to the patient.

For both countertransference and identification, the nurse must identify both personal feelings and the patient's behavior, speech, or attitudes that contribute to the discomfort and then determine whether the difficulty lies with the patient's behavior or stems from his or her own distorted or exaggerated response to it. It is always important for nurses to compare their own reactions to their usual way of responding and question other nurses to determine whether they have a similar reaction to the patient. If other staff members have not had the same reaction to the patient, the nurse may want to examine his or her own personal feelings more closely. Box 4–1 lists guidelines to identify countertransference.

JUDGMENTAL ATTITUDE

Judging another's behavior by personal values can significantly influence the nurse-patient relationship. Patients can usually sense these attitudes and may withhold important information for fear of being judged. The nurse may be unable or even unwilling to refrain from judging immediately but needs to be aware of these attitudes to diminish their impact on the patient.

RESCUE FEELINGS

The nurse may believe that he or she is the only person who really understands the patient and will be the one to save or cure a patient. This usually involves some internal needs of the nurse that are often reinforced by the patient. Secrets and secret alliances may result. Keep in mind, however, that the

---

BOX 4-1. Identifying Countertransference

- Repeatedly experiences affectionate feeling toward certain patients
- Experiences depressed or uneasy feelings during or after interactions with certain patients
- Permits or even encourages resistance in the form of acting out
- Persistently attempts to impress a patient
- Cultivates a patient's continued dependence on nurse
- Is sadistic or unnecessarily sharp with a particular patient
- Experiences a strong need to care for patient
- Experiences conscious satisfaction from patient's praise, appreciation, and evidence of affection
- Constantly argues with the patient
- Rigid about the structure of the nurse/patient relationship
- Has an intense reaction to the patient
- Instantly likes or dislikes patient
- Does not trust anyone else to care for patient
- Feels intimidated by or is angry with the patient

Source: Adapted from information from Lewis, A, and Levy, J: Psychiatric Liaison Nursing. Reston Publishing, Reston, VA, 1982; and Leach McMahon, A: The nurse-client relationship. In Haber, J, Miller, B, Leech McMahon, A, Price Hoskins, P (eds): Comprehensive Psychiatric Nursing (5th ed). Mosby, St. Louis, 1997.

nurse's becoming a rescuer undermines the patient's responsibility for his or her own health care.

LOSING CREDIBILITY

Stating facts such as "85 percent of patients have no complications with this type of surgery" is very different from telling a patient that he or she will not have any problems with upcoming surgery. In this example, if problems do occur after the nurse has stated that they would not, he or she will lose credibility, and the patient may stop sharing further concerns because the patient no longer feels confident in the nurse's opinions or information. Reassurance should be based on proper information and facts. Being evasive or dishonest destroys credibility.

LABELING

Labeling or referring to the patient by his or her diagnosis, problem ("he's just a junkie"), or even room number diminishes the value of the person. Almost without realizing it, once a label is used, nurses will begin to focus on the label and place less value on the patient's underlying needs and feelings. Optimal patient care requires that those needs and feelings be recognized and honored.

STRATEGIES FOR SURVIVAL

Some overall recommendations can help nurses to cope better with difficult patient behaviors. Table 4–2 offers some general guidelines for selecting effective interventions. Personal survival strategies also need to include strategies to maintain objectivity and prevent burnout. These can include using relaxation and stress management techniques and assertiveness training, as well as developing a professional support group to share concerns and help with problem solving. Developing a sense of team cooperation also lessens the chances of a single nurse's being called upon to meet everyone's needs. Attending classes and reading about managing commonly seen difficult patient behaviors gives the nurse more effective tools as well. Maintaining a satisfying personal life is also very important. Nurses tend to give of themselves as much in their personal life as they do at work. To prevent becoming burned out, you need to create a balance in life. Developing supportive relationships and participating in enjoyable activities can decrease the pressure to have patients behave in ways that meet personal needs. Adequate rest and exercise and good nutrition are also extremely important.

IDENTIFYING PSYCHOSOCIAL RESOURCE PERSONNEL

Many times outside assistance is needed in addition to the nurse's own personal strategies. A first step is to identify the sources of help that are available in your agency. Depending on the institution, any or all the following may be available:

TABLE 4–2. STAFF RESPONSES TO DIFFICULT-TO-CARE-FOR PATIENTS

Staff Responses	Intervention
Feeling inadequate to respond effectively to patient's symptoms	Lower emotional reactivity.
Feeling angry when patient gets angry	Maintain objectivity.
Fear of the patient who exhibits bizarre or unpredictable behavior or who is confused, psychotic, or exhibits other psychiatric symptoms	Provide staff education on identifying and handling patients.
Identifying with patients who are the same age or race or who share similar life experience	Use empathy rather than sympathy to protect self and yet not harm patient.
Frustrated because there is not enough time or energy to work with patient	Share workload evenly.
Concern over being manipulated by patient's demands	Schedule consistent staffing.
Labeling patients rather than their behavior in an attempt to achieve an emotional distance	Foster staff value system that precludes patients labeling.
Uncomfortable with certain personal topics related to family dynamics or personal history	Support staff through discussion and education.

Source: Reproduced with permission of Fincannon, JL: Analysis of Psychiatric Referrals and Interventions in an Oncology Population. Oncology Nursing Forum 22(1):87, 1995.

- Social workers
- Clinical nurse specialists, nurse managers, educators
- Psychiatric liaison staff
- Psychiatrists or psychologists, including those specializing in chemical dependency, rehabilitation, or pain
- Chaplains
- Psychotherapists or staff members from other agencies who are familiar with the patient and his or her problem and previous treatment

MENTAL HEALTH CONSULTATION

Sometimes agencies request outside consultation from mental health professionals for staff support and education, management of a crisis such as patient suicide, problem solving for difficult patient behaviors, or improving workplace communications. The consultant may be a mental health clinical nurse specialist, psychologist, psychiatrist, or social worker with consultation experience. This specialist needs to have experience and skill in providing consultation as well as some understanding of the type of problems the staff is encountering. The consultant may be from within or outside the agency. Staff attitudes can significantly influence whether this option can be used. Facilitative attitudes encourage use of these resources. These include:

- Feeling comfortable identifying problem areas and learning needs
- Recognizing that requesting assistance for areas outside personal knowledge or expertise is a sign of strength, not of weakness, and is necessary for professional development
- Approaching use of consultant as a resource and role model
- Anticipating the opportunity to gain insight

Hindering attitudes discourage or prevent use of resources. These include:

- Fearing exposure of inadequacies or embarrassment about not having all the answers
- Underestimating the specialized skill or knowledge needed to work with patients' problems
- Viewing patients' difficult-to-manage behaviors as deliberate or willful
- Calling the consultant too late and then challenging him or her to "fix" everything
- Harboring a prejudice against or fear of psychiatry
- Not maintaining confidentiality of group process

If the staff is meeting with the consultant as a group, the group leader will usually establish the ground rules for staff participation at the first meeting. If multiple sessions are planned, it will be necessary for all involved staff members to make a commitment to attend all the sessions. The administration needs to ensure adequate resources for coverage to ensure patient safety and reduce the level of staff discomfort about leaving their patients to attend the meetings. All members need to be aware of the objectives of these meetings. Hidden agendas, such as finding out who the troublemaker is, must be avoided.

Even though today's healthcare environment is facing tremendous economic pressures, mental health consultation has been recognized as providing a cost-effective way to enhance problem solving, reduce workplace stress, and, potentially, increase productivity. For example, anger in staff members that has been expressed by chronic lateness or increased sick time can be explored through consultation. This resource should therefore not be overlooked.

Crisis Intervention

LEARNING OBJECTIVES

➤ Identify variables that influence the response to a crisis.
➤ List interventions the nurse can use to reduce the impact of a crisis for a patient.
➤ Describe key questions to ask a patient experiencing a crisis.

All people experience crises. Crisis is a state of disequilibrium resulting from a stressful event or perceived threat to one's self when usual coping mechanisms are ineffective and lead to the individual's experiencing increased anxiety. Nurses see patients and families in a crisis state as part of their daily routine.

It is impossible to predict what events will trigger a crisis in an individual. A diagnosis of serious illness, a breakup of a relationship, or a minor car accident may cause a crisis situation for one person but not another. Certain events, such as the death of a spouse, trigger a crisis in everyone.

Many factors influence how an individual responds to a specific situation and whether or not a crisis will ensue. Unresolved losses, coping with other stressful events at the same time, or being excessively tired or in pain, which may reduce one's ability to cope, increase the risk of viewing the situation as a crisis. Personal issues, such as low self-esteem, difficulty with anger, or need to control, may also cause an event to become a crisis in a vulnerable individual. With or without intervention, a crisis usually resolves in 4 to 6 weeks because it is much too difficult for the individual to maintain the high level of tension and distress. The person develops some type of coping mechanism to get through the situation, changes the goal, or redefines the problem.

A crisis represents both danger and opportunity. A person is at risk for emotional breakdown, but the period of vulnerability can also stimulate personal growth and strength. Crisis intervention is short-term active support that focuses on immediate problem solving and reestablishing emotional equilibrium to facilitate a positive and adaptive resolution.

NURSES' REACTIONS TO PATIENT CRISIS

The ways in which a nurse responds to a patient in crisis are as varied as the ways in which the patient will respond because nurse and patient are influenced by the same factors. Some common responses may be:

- Feeling anxious or unsure about how to proceed
- Becoming overinvolved and attempting to take over for the patient, possibly causing the patient to become dependent on the nurse
- Viewing the patient's crisis as insignificant
- Taking on some of the patient's anxiety
- Setting unrealistic expectations or goals

ASSESSMENT

Aguilera (1998) identified three factors to determine the development of a crisis. They include:

Perception of the event: Successful resolution is more likely if the stressor is seen in a realistic rather than in a distorted way. For example, two students may get a C grade on an examination. One student may see this as an indication of the need to study harder and may realize that it is only a part of the final picture for the school year. The other student may view the grade as a personal failure, reflecting his low self-esteem and feelings of worthlessness.

Situational support: Lack of available resources or personal support systems, in addition to the specific situation, could be the factor that changes the situation into a crisis. In contrast, having someone to whom to turn to vent grief or frustration can increase one's ability to cope.

Adequate coping mechanisms: Having proven mechanisms to deal with anxiety can prevent the situation from escalating into a crisis. If the individual has never used effective coping mechanisms or the mechanisms are not currently available, the situation could escalate into a crisis. For example, an individual who uses smoking or running as a mechanism to reduce stress may have a crisis response to being hospitalized in an intensive care unit because he will not be able to smoke or run.

To effectively assess the patient's response, follow these guidelines for conducting a crisis interview:

- Identify the precipitating event and determine its meaning.
  - What has happened in the past few days or hours?
  - If the patient describes an ongoing problem, what is different about the problem today from yesterday? Be specific.
  - What does the event mean to the patient?
  - What is the patient most worried about in relation to the event?
  - What are some of the consequences of the event?
  - Does the patient see this event as influencing his or her future?
- Evaluate the patient's support system.
  - With whom does the patient have a close relationship?
  - To whom does the patient talk when he or she has a problem?
  - Are these people available now?
  - Have these resources helped in the past?
  - Whom does the patient trust?
  - Are any other resources available in the patient's life such as a clergy member or a counselor?
- Evaluate previously used effective coping mechanisms.
  - What does the patient normally do to cope with stress?
  - What is he or she doing now to cope with this situation?
  - If this has not helped, does the patient have any idea why not?
  - What has helped in the past in similar situations?

INTERVENTIONS

Crisis intervention is short-term problem-oriented support that ideally allows the individual to advance to a higher level of functioning as he or she develops new insights, strengths, and coping mechanisms. At the minimum, the individual will return to the precrisis level of functioning. The crisis is considered unresolved if the person functions at a lower level after the crisis, for example, by abusing substances, communicating ineffectively with family or loved ones, or exhibiting signs of depression or psychosis.

When facing a crisis, consider the following interventions:

- Make an accurate assessment of the precipitating event, the patient's perception of the event, and the available support systems and coping mechanisms. Also assess the patient's safety.
- Provide only small amounts of information at a time, and be prepared to repeat the information several times. Focus on concrete actions rather than vague ones.
- Communicate in a supportive, nonjudgmental way. Use gentle physical contact, as appropriate. Use calming hand gestures, a calm voice, and an unhurried manner.
- Help the patient to confront the reality of the event. This should be done slowly at first, such as gently bringing the patient back to a discussion of a

car accident. More concrete, specific wording may be needed. This process may need to be repeated.

- Help the patient focus on one "here-and-now" problem at a time rather than jumping from one possible problem to another. For example, a man who is frantic about his continuing pain may begin thinking about what will happen if the pain never stops. This will only escalate his anxiety. Rather, help him stay focused on dealing with the pain he is having now.
- In some situations, you may need to direct the person as to what to do next. His or her ability to make even the smallest decision may be compromised due to the overwhelming anxiety the crisis is producing.
- Encourage the patient to express his or her emotions in a socially acceptable manner.
- Assist with problem solving. This may include brainstorming all possible options and helping the patient narrow these down to the ones that can be used now. Focus on one or two possible options to give the patient a sense of control without overwhelming him or her with multiple options.
- Encourage the people in the patient's support system to become involved. Be sure to obtain the patient's permission before notifying family and friends to ensure that the patient maintains control of the situation. Be creative in identifying sources of support.
- Reinforce the patient's self-esteem by acknowledging how difficult the situation is and saying that you understand he or she is doing all that is possible to cope with it. Provide positive feedback.
- Reinforce effective coping mechanisms such as deep breathing, exercising, or making prioritized lists.
- Identify other resources in the agency that could provide assistance. Avoid being the only staff member assisting this patient.
- Assess the need for medications to reduce anxiety.

Occasionally, a patient's response to a crisis requires more intense intervention, including psychiatric treatment or hospitalization. The nurse needs to recognize signs of patient decompensation that go beyond the usual symptoms of a crisis. For example, suicidal behavior, evidence of psychotic thoughts, or violent behavior that could endanger others must be identified and resources for intervention obtained. If these signs occur, be sure to obtain a consultation for specialized assistance.

Cultural Considerations: Implications for Psychosocial Nursing Care

LEARNING OBJECTIVES

➢ Explain the concept of culturally sensitive psychosocial nursing care.
➢ Acknowledge differences and similarities in perspectives, values, and expectations on mental health and mental illness.
➢ Discuss factors to consider when assessing culture and ethnicity in patients and their families.
➢ Consider treatment approaches to patients in various cultural and ethnic groups.
➢ Describe guidelines for using interpreters and what to do when an interpreter is not available.

CULTURALLY COMPETENT NURSING CARE

Culture has many definitions. One definition is that it is a system of beliefs, behaviors, and symbols that are learned, shared, and passed on through generations of a social group. Culture influences what people perceive, guides their interactions, and changes over time. Culture describes a particular society's entire way of living. Ethnicity is a somewhat narrower term: it relates to people who identify with each other because of a shared heritage.

Culturally competent nursing care is defined as being sensitive to issues related to culture, race, religion, gender, sexual orientation, and social or economic class. Cultural competence implies not only awareness of cultural differences but also the ability to assess and intervene appropriately and effectively. Cultural competence in nursing care requires more than simply acquiring knowledge about other ethnic or cultural groups. It is a complex combination of attitudes and skills as well as knowledge. (Campinha-Bacote, 1994)

Cultural information by itself can interfere with care if nurses use it in a "cookbook" manner. Inappropriate use of cultural information can lead to stereotyping patients by making assumptions based on limited information. Because stereotyping comes from jumping to conclusions based on insufficient data or experience with a cultural group, it is important to suspend judgment as long as possible. (Lipson & Steiger, 1996)

Cultures can be compared using six phenomena that vary with application and use, yet are seen across all cultural groups. (Giger & Davidhizar, 1995) These phenomena are:

1. *Communication:* This refers to all verbal and nonverbal behavior in the presence of another. Communication has its roots in culture. Cultural mores, norms, ideas, and customs are all expressed through communication. The nurse who cares for diverse patients must have an understanding of the client's needs and expectations as expressed through their communication and culture.
2. *Space:* This element of culture refers to territoriality, density, and distance. It relates to how space is controlled, used, and defended. Three interpersonal dimensions of space in Western culture have been identified: the intimate zone (0–18 inches), the personal zone (18–36 inches), and the social zone (3–6 feet).
3. *Social organization:* Cultural behaviors are acquired through social interactions in groups such as families, religious groups, and ethnic groups. This process of learning cultural values is called acculturation.
4. *Time:* Awareness of time is learned gradually. Some cultures place great importance on punctuality and efficiency, whereas others ignore the clock. Time orientation, meaning present-, future-, or past-oriented perceptions, influences many aspects of a culture.
5. *Environmental control:* This element has to do with the degree to which individuals perceive they have control over their environment. Persons from various cultures have different beliefs about how much they can influence events in their lives, some being more fatalistic and others more active. To provide culturally appropriate care, nurses should respect the individual's unique beliefs while understanding how these beliefs can be used to promote health in the patient's environment.
6. *Biological variations:* This element refers to biological differences in people from various racial and ethnic groups, such as body size and shape, skin and hair color, physiologic responses to medications, susceptibility to disease, and nutritional preferences. A new field called ethnopharmacology is addressing different responses to medications.

Acknowledging that people from different cultures and ethnic groups perceive these phenomena in different ways can help the nurse understand variations in patients' behavior, values, and expectations. (Meleis et al., 1995)

A cultural assessment helps the nurse gather and use other information related to culture that is vital in providing culturally sensitive care. The nurse must be aware that beliefs about health and the causes of illness, appropriate care, and who should provide that care, can differ among cultures. It is important for the nurse to listen to what the patient believes, what has been done in the past, and even to consult with the patient's cultural healers (perhaps a spiritualist, curandero, shaman, or medicine man).

The nurse must realize that mental illness is unacceptable in some cultures. People who believe that expressing emotions is unacceptable present unique problems in a psychiatric setting. Nurses need to work slowly to establish trust and rapport with patients from other cultures. In some cases, it may be necessary to follow the health care practices that the client views as essential, as long as they do not harm the patient. For example, letting family members bring in special foods, inviting a folk healer to the hospital, or making time for a spiritual reading, serve as important acknowledgment of the patient's traditional medical care. (Townsend, 2000)

CULTURAL ASSESSMENT

A thorough cultural assessment may take several hours. The list of questions in Box 6–1 can provide a brief but helpful focus for a relevant cultural assessment. Answers to these questions do not guarantee culturally competent care, but nevertheless good care cannot be provided without specific cultural and ethnic information. (Lipson, Dibble & Minarik, 1996)

BOX 6–1. Cultural Assessment— Questions to Ask

- Where was the patient born? If an immigrant, how long in this country?
- What is the patient's ethnic affiliation, how strong is the ethnic identity?
- Who are the patient's major support people? Does patient live in an ethnic community?
- Who in the family takes responsibility for health concerns and decisions?
- Any activities in which the client may decline to participate because of culture, religious taboos?
- Any special food preferences, food refusals because of culture, religion?
- What are the primary and secondary languages, speaking and reading abilities?
- What is patient's religion, its importance in daily life, current practices?
- What is the patient's economic situation, is income adequate for needs?
- What are the patient's health beliefs and practices?
- What are patient's perceptions of health problem and expectations of health care?

CULTURAL INFLUENCE ON MENTAL HEALTH BELIEFS

Culture can significantly influence communication, particularly when the cultures of the nurse and patient are vastly different and not understood by each other. Culture is defined as a configuration of learned behaviors and beliefs that are shared and transmitted in a society and by a particular group of people. The values, beliefs, traditions, attitudes, and prejudices that each of us brings from our culture and past experiences influence all interactions with others. Ethnocentrism is defined as the belief that one's own cultural beliefs and healthcare practices are superior to those of other cultures. To provide quality care to all individuals, nurses must be sensitive to patients' cultural differences and as aware as possible of their own cultural beliefs and behaviors. (Spector, 1996)

Rather than stereotyping individuals into specific cultural classes, nurses should approach each patient as an individual who holds very personal attitudes, beliefs, and values that are influenced by his or her culture and environment. (See Box 6–2 for ways of enhancing cultural sensitivity.)

Culture often influences what a patient believes about his or her illness, its causes, and when and from whom to seek care. Although you may not be able to be aware of the specific beliefs of every culture, having some general information about the culture and ethnicity of patients for whom you care is frequently important. Incorporating some questions in the assessment on culture and observing for influences can help you become more familiar with these cultures. (Purnell & Paulanka, 1998)

Questions to be included in the assessment may include, "What do you believe caused your illness?" and "What other treatments for the illness have you pursued?" Recognize the impact of these beliefs on the patient's ability to accept the illness and his or her response to it. For example, in cultures that view males as always being strong, even a mild illness could contribute to depression. (Spector, 1996)

Be sensitive to each individual's beliefs about his or her illness and its causes, and design your care to incorporate these ideas. For example, in a culture in which the oldest woman plays a pivotal role in the family, the grand-

---

BOX 6–2. Enhancing Cultural Sensitivity

- Know your own attitudes, values, and beliefs.
- Be aware of your own ethnocentrism.
- Be aware of your own prejudices that may influence your assessment.
- Maintain an open mind and seek out more information about your patient's culture, beliefs, and values.
- Communicate your interest about the patient's beliefs and values.
- Approach each patient as an individual. Avoid assuming people from one cultural background all hold the same beliefs.

mother may be the one the patient consults on decisions about surgery, discharge planning, and follow-up care. She would need to be incorporated into the treatment planning in order for this patient to receive the best follow-up care. If a patient believes in folk healers or cures, don't ridicule or judge his or her beliefs. Rather, acknowledge the beliefs, and incorporate them into the treatment plan if possible. For example, if a Chinese patient is taking herbs to cure his diabetes, it is more beneficial to discuss the possible impact of these herbs on blood sugar than to ignore their use or forbid the patient to use them. (Lipson, Dibble & Minarik, 1996)

Respect the role of the family in the patient's treatment. In some cultures, the family is responsible for protecting the patient, especially when the patient is the parent. In their role, family members may want to protect the patient from bad news. This may be contrary to your own belief in patient autonomy and may therefore lead to conflicts between the healthcare providers and the family. Of course, the patient must be in agreement with involving the family. Also be aware that in psychiatric settings, different approaches may be used to preserve patient autonomy and confidentiality.

Psychiatric professionals have recognized that some symptoms commonly seen in mental illness, such as delusions or hallucinations, could represent a culturally appropriate behavior. For example, being possessed by an evil spirit could be a delusion or a culturally sanctioned experience of an altered state of consciousness. Be careful not to judge individual cultural variations as psychopathology. It is helpful to discuss these issues with other healthcare providers from diverse cultural or ethnic groups who can increase your understanding of behaviors and beliefs outside your own experiences. (Townsend, 2000)

CULTURAL AND ETHNIC INFLUENCE ON COMMUNICATION

Verbal and nonverbal communication patterns are closely tied to cultural beliefs and practices. Eye contact, hand gestures, facial expressions, and personal space, as well as how words or slang are used and what can be discussed, are defined by our culture and environment. For many people, eye contact indicates honesty, openness, and alertness. However, people in some cultures do not value eye contact and, in fact, even avoid it. For example, in some Asian cultures eye contact is viewed as impolite and an invasion of privacy. It is especially inappropriate with authority figures, such as doctors and nurses. Judging a patient's response based on eye contact without understanding this difference can lead to an invalid assessment finding. (Luckmann, 1999)

Some nonverbal behaviors such as facial expressions, hand gestures, and social distance vary among cultures. For example, it may be important to know that lack of facial expression in some Asian groups is not an indication of lack of feeling or that an Arab family member who stands very close is not threatening but rather standing at the distance considered appropriate in their culture. Addressing a patient, especially an elderly one, by his or her first name may suggest a lack of respect, or even seduction, in many Asian and Latin cultures. Also, some patients may be extremely uncomfortable when asked intimate, very personal questions, no matter how accepting and professional the nurse may be. If this information is vital to patient care, efforts need to be made to explain how the information will be used. (Schuster, 2000)

COMMUNICATING THROUGH AN INTERPRETER

Language differences pose a barrier to even the most basic communication and cultural assessment. Caring for a patient who does not speak the same language as you can cause anxiety, frustration, fear, and a sense of helplessness on your part as well as the patient's. It may cause resentment because of the extra time and work that are needed. Some nurses try to compensate for their perceived deficiency by concentrating on performing tasks rather than on the patient's concerns. Although it is not usually possible to learn the language of every potential patient, it would be beneficial to learn the language spoken by a majority of the patients you care for. If you cannot speak the language, use an interpreter as much as possible.

There may be a family member who can translate, and you may need to provide accommodations if this person needs to stay with the patient. When using a family member to translate, keep in mind that, because of the emotional ties or role conflicts and lack of medical vocabulary, the person may base messages to both patient and provider on his or her own perception of the situation and may withhold vital information because it may embarrass or overwhelm the patient. For example, if the family member does not want the patient to know about the seriousness of his or her condition, he or she may not relay all the information to the patient. In addition, patients may feel too embarrassed to disclose key information in the presence of their relatives, especially if it is of a sensitive nature. Using family members as interpreters is probably best when basic communication is needed rather than when critical conversations are needed for diagnosis, treatment, and psychosocial assessments. (Luckmann, 1999)

Check with your institution to see if an interpreter is available. The Civil Rights Act of 1964, the 1973 Rehabilitation Act, and the more recent Americans with Disabilities Act (ADA) have established the federal standards that ensure that communication does not interfere with equal access to health care for all people. Therefore, all healthcare institutions must establish systems for identifying available language interpreters, as well as interpreters trained in sign language, telecommunication device for the deaf (TDDs), closed-caption decoders for television, and amplifiers on the phones. Many institutions have access to telephone interpretation services, such as the AT&T Language Line. This nationwide, 24-hour service provides interpreters for about 140 languages. Although this service cannot take the place of a trained interpreter at the bedside, it does allow patients to communicate their history and symptoms to healthcare providers, especially in emergencies.

Interpreters can be professional interpreters or employees of the institution who have other duties. If you are using employees, evaluate their ability to understand the information you wish to have translated and how much time they have to provide the service. If the interpreter has limited medical knowledge or knowledge of the patient, it may be difficult to ensure effective communication.

In the home, family members and neighbors are usually the only resource unless nurses who speak the language are available. In addition to being aware of agency resources for interpreters, the nurse should become familiar with key words that can be useful in assessing patients who speak another language. A language board containing key words in the languages most frequently used in your agency can be a very effective, time-saving tool.

When using an interpreter, keep the following points in mind:

- Address the patient directly rather than speaking to the interpreter. Maintain eye contact with the patient to ensure the patient's involvement.
- Do not interrupt the patient and interpreter. At times their interaction may take longer because of the need to clarify, and descriptions may require more time because of dialect differences or the interpreter's awareness that the patient needs more preparation before being asked a particular question.
- Ask the interpreter to give you verbatim translations so that you can assess what the patient is thinking and understanding.
- Avoid using medical jargon that the interpreter or patient may not understand.
- Avoid talking or commenting to the interpreter at length; the patient may feel left out and distrustful.
- Be aware that asking intimate or emotionally laden questions may be difficult for both the patient and the interpreter. Lead up to these questions slowly. Always ask permission to discuss these topics first, and prepare the interpreter for the content of the interview.
- When possible, allow the patient and interpreter to meet each other ahead of time to establish some rapport. If possible, try to use the same interpreter for succeeding interviews with the patient.
- If possible, request an interpreter of the same gender as the patient and of similar age. To make good use of the interpreter's time, decide beforehand which questions you will ask. Meet with the interpreter briefly before going to see the patient so that you can let the interpreter know what you are planning to ask. During the session, face the patient and direct your questions to the patient, not the interpreter. After the session, review the questions and answers with the interpreter to check any remaining concerns. (Luckmann, 1999)

GUIDELINES FOR WORKING WITHOUT AN INTERPRETER

If an interpreter is not available, using picture charts or flash cards can help the patient communicate some basic questions such as degree of pain or needs like water and elimination. Some patients with limited English may tend to appear agreeable and nod yes even though they do not understand. Be sure to determine that the patient understands by asking questions that require more than a "yes" or "no" answer.

If the patient understands a little English, you may be able to gather useful information without an interpreter by following these suggestions:

- Greet the patient respectfully. Be polite and formal, especially with older patients.
- Identify the patient's primary language. If you can pronounce any words in the language, use them to show you are trying to communicate. A simple "buenos dias" or "bonjour" may help to reduce the patient's anxiety.
- Speak slowly, clearly, and quietly in English if this is your only option. Do not shout. Make an effort not to appear frustrated, irritated, or hurried.
- Ask one question, talk about one symptom at a time. Use simple sentences.
- Try to avoid medical terminology. For example use "bleeding, pus, or liquid" rather than "discharge."
- Use picture cards or a phrase chart if they are available to verify patient information.
- Be aware that some patients may act as if they have understood all your questions to avoid looking ignorant or rude. (Luckmann, 1999)

Problems with Anxiety

THE ANXIOUS PATIENT

LEARNING OBJECTIVES

➤ Differentiate among the cognitive, affective, behavioral, and physical symptoms of anxiety.
➤ Use the different manifestations of anxiety to assess the anxious patient.
➤ Select the most appropriate interventions for dealing with the patient with anxiety.
➤ Identify possible nurses' reactions to an anxious patient.

GLOSSARY

Acute stress disorder—A disorder characterized by a high level of anxiety immediately after a traumatic event.

Agoraphobia—Fear, anxiety, or avoidance of places or situations from which escape may be difficult or where help may not be available.

Anxiety—An unpleasant feeling of tension, apprehension, and uneasiness or a diffuse feeling of dread or unexplained discomfort; accompanied by physiological, psychological, and behavioral symptoms; may serve as an early warning that alerts the individual to impending real or symbolic threat to self, significant others, or way of life; motivates the individual to take corrective action to relieve the unpleasant feelings. The source of the anxiety is often nonspecific or unknown to the individual.

Anxiety disorder due to a general medical condition—Anxiety characterized by prominent symptoms directly related to the physiological consequences of a general medical condition (e.g., hyperthyroidism or hypothyroidism, hypoglycemia, chronic obstructive pulmonary disease).

Generalized anxiety disorder—A disorder characterized by at least 6 months of persistent and excessive anxiety and worry.

Obsessive-compulsive disorder (OCD)—Recurrent thoughts or ideas (obsessions) that an individual is unable to put out of his or her mind and actions that an individual is unable to refrain from performing (compulsions).

Panic attack—A discrete, sudden, unpredictable, intense episode of severe anxiety characterized by personality disorganization; a fear of losing one's mind, going crazy, being unable to control one's behavior; a sense of impending doom, helplessness, and being trapped.

Post-traumatic stress disorder (PTSD)—Anxiety and stress symptoms that occur after a massive traumatic event; often includes the feeling that the event is reoccurring, lasting for weeks, months, or years.

Post-traumatic stress response—A persistent, disorganizing, and distressing reaction to a catastrophic event that affects a person's emotional, cognitive, and behavioral dimensions and relationships and extends beyond the time of the immediate crisis.

Social anxiety disorder—Intense, persistent fear of social situations.

Specific phobias—Irrational fears characterized by clinically significant anxiety provoked by exposure to a specific feared object or situation, often leading to avoidance behavior.

Substance-induced anxiety disorder—A disorder characterized by prominent anxiety symptoms directly related to physiological consequences of drug abuse, medication use, or toxin exposure.

Anxiety is the primary emotion from which many other emotions, such as anger, guilt, shame, and grief, are generated. The term anxiety brings up images of someone pacing and wringing his or her hands with pounding heart and rapid breathing, perhaps before taking an important test in school or while waiting to hear from the doctor about a biopsy. Words such as worry, concern, fear, and uncertainty are often associated with the term anxiety.

Anxiety can also have a positive meaning, implying eagerness and readiness to face a challenge or perform some skill. Being mildly anxious can enhance experiences such as performing in a piano recital or completing a term paper. Anxiety is a healthy response to novel and unique experiences. In fact, being mildly anxious helps us to perform our best because perceptual, emotional, and physiological arousal can enhance learning, problem solving, satisfaction, and pleasure during and after an event. Just as pain serves as a cue and a response to potential or actual physical danger, anxiety can serve as a cue and response to emotional, social, or spiritual danger.

Anxiety is a universal emotion; everyone has experienced some level of anxiety associated with life events. Anxiety disorders are the most common psychiatric disorder in America. Between 10 and 25 percent of the U.S. population suffers from a diagnosable clinical anxiety disorder in any one year. People vary significantly in their ability to manage feelings of anxiety and in their styles and patterns of coping with anxiety-producing situations. Knowing the meaning of the subjective experience to a particular individual is essential in understanding how to intervene with that individual.

The DSM-IV-TR (2000) divides anxiety into these diagnostic categories: Panic Disorder with or without Agoraphobia, Social Phobia (also called social anxiety disorder), Specific Phobias, Obsessive-Compulsive Disorder, Post Traumatic Stress Disorder, Acute Stress Disorder, Anxiety Disorder due to a General Medical Condition, Generalized Anxiety Disorder, and Substance-Induced Anxiety Disorder. Panic attacks and Agoraphobia may occur alone or in the context of several of these disorders. For treatment purposes, anxiety is often categorized into four levels: mild, moderate, severe, and panic (Table 7–1).

Mild or moderate anxiety usually speeds up physiologic operations, whereas severe anxiety may slow them down. Prolonged panic can cause complete paralysis of functioning and occasionally result in death. Anxiety can also be classified as normal or abnormal. The same feelings and behaviors (uncertainties, helplessness, and an intense sense of personal discomfort) characterize both, and the level of anxiety may be equally intense.

Normal anxiety results from a realistic perception of the danger and prepares the person for defense or change in face of the threat. Normal anxiety can be motivating and useful (e.g., to motivate a student to study harder and therefore to do better on a test). Abnormal anxiety arises when the perception of danger is distorted, unrealistic, and out of proportion, resulting in maladaptive, defensive coping and inappropriate behavior.

ETIOLOGY

Theoretical approaches to anxiety are wide ranging. In the biological perspective, anxiety is the uneasy feeling aroused by a threat or danger and is accompanied by a physiological response. This response prepares the person for "fight or flight." The fight response (sympathetic stimulation) causes changes primarily in the cardiovascular and neuroendocrine systems. During the flight response (parasympathetic stimulation), which occurs in acute fear states, an effort is made to conserve body resources. Other evidence suggests a biological basis for anxiety. Research on the metabolism of monoamines and the function of the limbic system are central to the expression of emotions such as anxiety; the discovery of the benefits of benzodiazepines for chronic anxiety; and studies on sodium lactate in persons with panic attacks.

In psychoanalytical theory, anxiety represents a person's struggle with the demands and prohibitions in his or her environment, including the internal

TABLE 7–1. CHARACTERISTICS OF ANXIETY LEVELS

Level	Characteristics
Mild	• Enhanced ability to deal with stressors • Heightened awareness, problem-solving abilities; increased attention to details • Curiosity increased, asks questions • Alert, confident • Logical thinking intact
Moderate	• Hesitation and procrastination, blocking loss of train of thought • Narrowing of perceptual field • Change in voice pitch; speech rate accelerates • Selective inattention • Frequent change in topics • Repetitive questioning, joking • Increased respiratory rate, heart rate, muscle tension • Dry mouth • Palpitations • Changing body positions frequently, restlessness • Purposeless activity (wringing hands, pacing)
Severe	• Highly distorted perceptual and cognitive function • Focus on small or scattered detail, inability to see connections between events • Selective inattention, inability to concentrate • Fear of losing control • Purposeless activity (pacing, wringing hands) • Difficult and inappropriate verbalizations, inability to learn • Sense of impending doom • Sweating • Hyperventilation, tachycardia, frequency and urgency • Nausea, headache, dizziness • Gross motor tremors, trembling, shaking • Numbness or tingling sensations • Dilated pupils
Panic	• Dyspnea, choking feeling, chest pain • Extreme discomfort, emotional pain • Unrealistic, distorted perception of situation • Disruption of visual field, distortion and enlargement of detail • Inability to speak, unintelligible communication, incoherent speech • Vomiting, incontinence • Feeling of personality disintegration • Fear of losing mind, fear of dying

struggle among the person's instinctual drives (id), the realistic assessment of the possibility for need fulfillment (ego), and the conscience (superego). Anxiety is a signal from the ego that an unacceptable drive is pressing for conscious discharge. A conflict results between the drive, usually of a sexual or aggressive nature, and fear of punishment or disapproval. Phobias are fears that are disproportionate to the situation and cannot be explained or reasoned away. The significance and meaning of anxiety depend on the nature of the underlying conflict.

Interpersonal theorists believe that anxiety arises from experiences in relationships with significant others (SOs) throughout a person's development. If a child is treated malevolently, the foundation is laid for the child to become insecure and feel inferior and anxious in future situations. The child is forced to use coping strategies to allay anxiety; these become part of the personality when the child becomes an adult.

Learning and behavioral theorists explain anxiety as the result of a conditioning process in which a neutral stimulus has come to represent punishment, pain, or fear. The individual learns to reduce anxiety by avoiding a negative stimulus or by approaching a positive reinforcer. Extinction of behavior is a process of reducing response strength by nonreinforcement. An eclectic understanding of anxiety, incorporating components of all these theories, is most helpful. Anxiety can be understood as experienced at conscious, unconscious, or preconscious levels. Sources of anxiety fall into two major categories:

1. *Threats to biologic integrity:* Actual or impending interference with basic human needs such as food, drink, shelter, warmth, safety and health
2. *Threats to self-security or self-esteem:*
   ◦ Unmet expectations important to self-integrity
   ◦ Unmet needs for status and prestige
   ◦ Anticipated disapproval by SOs
   ◦ Inability to gain or reinforce self-respect or to gain recognition from others
   ◦ A severe, sudden, unexpected threat to sense of security, self-esteem, or well-being
   ◦ Guilt or discrepancies between self-perception and actual behavior

Experiences with anxiety in early life lead to the development of coping behaviors, personality traits, and defense mechanisms intended to reduce anxiety and increase a sense of security. Over time, the individual develops characteristic patterns of relief behaviors intended to provide comfort and protection in the face of anxiety. When these behaviors, traits, or mechanisms fail to relieve anxiety, the patient experiences intense emotional or physical discomfort.

Behavioral responses to anxiety can be constructive (problem solving, task-oriented) or destructive (defensive, aggressive, violent). When anxiety levels exceed a person's adaptive coping abilities, maladaptive behaviors may develop. Disturbed coping mechanisms are characterized by the inability to make choices, conflict, repetition and rigidity, and alienation. Frustration and anxiety can lead to anger, hostility, and violence.

Anxiety often increases when a person expects one thing and is suddenly confronted with something very different. The same stressor may not always lead to anxiety or the same level of anxiety in everyone or even in the same person at different times. Generally, the patient experiences anxiety as very painful and unbearable if it continues for any length of time. Behavior patterns used to cope with anxiety include:

> *Acting out:* Converting anxiety into anger, which is either overtly or covertly expressed
> *Paralysis or retreating:* Withdrawing or being immobilized by anxiety
> *Somatizing:* Converting anxiety into physical symptoms such as stomachache or headache

Avoidance: Evasive behaviors performed unconsciously to ward off or relieve anxiety before it is directly experienced (alcohol, sleeping, keeping busy)

Constructive action: Using anxiety to learn and problem solve (goal setting, learning new skills, seeking information)

Syndromes of abnormal anxiety frequently observed in patients include:

Panic attacks: Acute, intense attacks of anxiety associated with extreme changes in physical and emotional behavior that can last from minutes to hours, are severely debilitating, and are characterized by sudden, intense, and discrete periods of anxiety and fear that may occur without warning in previously calm and untroubled individuals. Recent research points to physical or organic causes for some patients.

Post-traumatic stress disorder (PTSD): Reexperience of the trauma of a previous traumatic event (e.g., rape, assault, military combat, flood, earthquake, major car accident, airplane crash, bombing, torture). The symptoms are usually more severe and last longer when the cause is a man-made rather than a natural disaster. Three subtypes of PTSD are recognized:

- *Acute:* Symptoms begin within 6 months of the event and do not last longer than 6 months.
- *Chronic:* Symptoms last for 6 months or more.
- *Delayed:* Symptoms begin after a latency period of 6 months or more.

Reexperiencing the trauma may include recurrent and intrusive recollections of the event, recurrent dreams or nightmares of the event, or sudden acting or feeling as if the event were recurring because of an association with an environmental or mental stimulus. Other behaviors and affect associated with the syndrome include decreased interest in usually significant activities, feelings of detachment or estrangement from others, and constricted affect. Symptoms not present before the trauma include hyperalertness or exaggerated startle response, sleep disturbance, guilt about surviving while others died or about behavior required for survival, memory impairment, difficulty concentrating, avoidance of activities that arouse recollection of the event, or intensification of symptoms by exposure to events that symbolize or resemble the traumatic event.

Phobia: An intense, irrational fear response to a specific external object or situation. Unlike an anxiety reaction, in which the anxiety is free floating and the person cannot easily identify the cause or source, a phobia is a persistent fear of specific places, things, or situations. The major dynamic mechanism of phobic behavior is the displacement of the original anxiety from its real source and the symbolization of the stressor in the phobia (e.g., fear of sex becomes a fear of snakes).

The hallmark of phobias is that they are irrational and persist even though the person recognizes that they are irrational. The unconscious operations involved in the phobia help the person to control anxiety by providing a specific object to attach it to. The phobic person can then control the intensity of the anxiety by avoiding the object or situation to which the anxiety has become attached. Some of the more common phobias include claustrophobia (fear of closed places), agoraphobia (fear of leaving home and of open spaces), acrophobia (fear of heights), xenophobia (fear of strangers), and zoophobia (fear of animals).

Obsessive-compulsive disorder (OCD): A paralyzing anxiety disorder associated with repetitive, compulsive thoughts (obsessions) and behaviors (compulsions). These patterns of thoughts and behaviors are senseless and distressing but help achieve the goal of avoiding anxiety. This disorder has been treated very effectively with some of the newer antidepressants, leading some investigators to think this disorder is related to serotonin reuptake.

RELATED CLINICAL CONCERNS

Anxiety is the most common complaint in medical practice. It presents in many ways and with great variation in intensity and duration; therefore treatment must be individualized and monitored very closely. Anxiety may be caused by many other medical and psychiatric problems such as cardiac and vascular disorders, sleep disorders, hyperthyroidism, anemia, depression with agitation, dementia, delirium, hypochondriasis, schizophrenia, mania, and personality disorders. Some medications, caffeine intoxication, and withdrawal from alcohol or sedatives may cause anxiety. Physical illness or underlying major psychiatric syndromes must be considered and ruled out before treatment for anxiety is undertaken.

LIFE SPAN ISSUES

CHILDREN

The anxiety most frequently experienced by children is separation anxiety. When a child is separated from those to whom he or she is attached, excessive anxiety to the point of panic may occur. Onset may be as early as preschool age. The child may refuse to go to sleep or go to school. Complaints of physical symptoms, such as headache, stomachache, and nausea and vomiting are also common.

ELDERLY PEOPLE

Anxiety in elderly people has not been systematically investigated. It is the consensus of clinical gerontologists that anxiety is a common response to the stresses of late life, including fear of dependency, illness, and dying, and multiple losses of friends, home, or lifestyle. A long-standing disposition to excessive anxiety can persist into late life and usually is not dysfunctional in the patient who has adapted to it. Anxiety in elderly persons may be the presenting symptom of a new illness, especially depression with agitation; of early dementia; or of low-grade or chronic toxic states caused by drugs, alcohol.

POSSIBLE NURSES' REACTIONS

- May be apprehensive and even fearful about caring for patients experiencing severe anxiety or a panic attack. Intense anxiety can be very contagious, not only to staff members but also with other patients.
- May try to determine the cause of patient's anxiety and do what is possible to reassure and assist patient to decrease it, then become frustrated when patient's anxiety continues.
- May find it too strenuous to work with patient for more than a day at a time if patient's anxiety does not subside as the nurse thinks it should.
- May interpret the anxiety as a weakness in the patient, who is seen as unable or unwilling to control it or may judge the anxiety as part of a more serious psychological problem and feel very uncomfortable caring for these patients.
- May prefer to keep patient sedated.
- May feel resentment and even hostility toward anxious patients who require more attention and time than their physical conditions alone warrant.
- May want to avoid family members or SOs who are also quite anxious and make unreasonable requests in a demanding or complaining manner. Most of these behaviors may be caused by the families' own frustration or apprehension in dealing with the patient's anxiety, and they are often unaware that their behavior is affecting the staff.

ASSESSMENT

Behavior and Appearance

See Table 7–1 for Characteristics of Anxiety Levels.

Mood and Emotions

- Dread, fear, apprehension
- Lack of control or self-confidence
- Guilt
- Anger
- Grief
- Sense of imminent catastrophe

Thoughts, Beliefs, and Perceptions

- Narrowed focus of attention
- Perceptual focus scattered or fixed
- Inability to focus on reality
- Inability to learn or remember, forgetfulness
- Inability to reason or problem solve

- Difficulty concentrating, lack of awareness of environment
- Distorted perceptions

Relationships and Interactions

- Withdrawal and isolation, avoidance behaviors
- Demanding, complaining, quarreling, attention-seeking behavior
- Defensive, uses denial
- Tense, strained relationships; others frustrated over dealing with patient's anxiety and maladaptive coping

Physical Responses

See Table 7–1 for physical responses to various anxiety levels.

Pertinent History

- Medical conditions that present with anxiety as a symptom
  - Thyroid, pituitary, and adrenocortical disorders
  - Low hemoglobin
  - Hypoglycemia
  - Impending heart attack
- Amphetamine usage
- Synergistic or idiosyncratic drug reactions
- Alcohol or sedative withdrawal
- Cerebrovascular disorders
- Pancreatic disorder
- Sequelae to head injury
- Chronic anxiety
- Recent loss of loved one, significant object, work, finances, or self-esteem
- Phobic behavior
- Recent reexposure to anxiety-causing situation
- Traumatic experience

COLLABORATIVE MANAGEMENT

Anxiety disorders are usually treated with some form of counseling or psychotherapy or pharmacotherapy, either alone or in combination. The milder forms may be effectively treated with cognitive or behavior therapy alone, but more severe and persistent symptoms may require pharmacotherapy.

Pharmacologic

The medications typically used to treat patients with anxiety are benzodiazepines and antidepressants. Benzodiazepines, such as diazepam, lorazepam, clonazepam, and alprazolam, are the medications commonly prescribed for treating most types of anxiety, including short-term (situational) anxiety and long-term (generalized) anxiety. Unfortunately, because they are so efficacious and safe, these medications are often prescribed without full appreciation of their potential problems. OCD and PTSD are more effectively treated by antidepressants, especially clomipramine, a tricyclic antidepressant. Five drugs in the selective serotonin reuptake inhibitors (SSRI) class of antidepressants, fluoxetine, sertraline, paroxetine, fluvoxamine, and citalopram, have emerged as the preferred type of antidepressant for treatment of anxiety disorders. Clonidine and beta-blockers such as propranolol and atenolol are also used. Herbal products include kava kava and valerian.

Psychological Treatments

During the past decade there has been increasing enthusiasm and demand for focused, time-limited therapies that address ways of coping with anxiety symptoms directly rather than exploring unconscious conflicts or other personal vulnerabilities. These therapies emphasize cognitive and behavioral assessments and interventions, such as relaxation training, biofeedback, systematic desensitization, reframing, thought stopping, aversion therapy, and social skills training.

The hallmarks of cognitive-behavioral therapies are evaluating cause and effect relationships among thoughts, feelings, and behaviors as well as using straightforward strategies to lessen symptoms and reduce avoidant behaviors. Therapeutic modalities such as guided imagery and muscle relaxation, exercise and rest programs, aromatherapy, and music and art therapy may be used as adjuncts to medication or alone. All mental health disciplines, including psychiatric mental health nurses, psychiatric social workers, psychologists, and psychiatrists, may use these anxiety reduction approaches in their collaborative treatment of clients with anxiety.

NURSING MANAGEMENT

ANXIETY MANIFESTED BY TENSION, DISTRESS, UNCERTAINTY
RELATED TO THREAT TO HEALTH, SELF-CONCEPT AND LIFESTYLE.

Patient Outcomes

- Demonstrates decreased level of anxiety
- Will report feeling less anxious after using coping strategies
- Will use coping strategies effectively when anxiety is recognized
- Demonstrates increased ability to prevent episodes of anxiety by problem solving

Interventions

- Speak in a calm, quiet voice; convey a sense of confidence and control and a tolerant, understanding attitude.
- Place patient in quiet environment; reduce distracting stimuli (e.g., noise, activity, light).

- Use discretion in conversations with patient and near patient's room.
- Recognize factors that may stimulate more anxiety.
- Reduce demands placed on patient until anxiety is reduced. Provide rest periods between tests, activities, and visitors.
- Provide diversional activity and exercise. Monitor changes in level of activity.
- Allow supportive others (clergy, social workers, volunteers) to visit patient. Explain tests and equipment to them so they can in turn be more relaxed around patient.
- Provide realistic feedback about patient's situation; do not give false reassurances. Help patient understand the anxiety by having him or her name the feeling.
- Encourage patient to express feelings (some crying and anger are appropriate).
- Have patient identify what happened just before the anxiety started and try to identify the causative event. Discuss the possible connection between the precipitating event and the meaning it has for the patient.
- Determine patient's usual coping mechanism in similar situations.
- Encourage patient to recall and think through similar instances of anxiety, what alternative behaviors could be used to cope more adaptively.
- Attempt to discuss what patient understands as cause of anxiety or panic once the anxiety level is reduced.
- Stay with patient but do not require explanations for the distress; individuals with severe or panic-level anxiety may become more agitated by attempts to communicate with them.
- Provide measures to relieve anxiety (e.g., warm bath, back rub, walk). Discuss other techniques for reducing anxiety (relaxation exercises, stress-reduction techniques) when patient is calmer and more rested. Encourage slow, deep breathing if patient is hyperventilating; breathing with patient to set pattern may be helpful.
- Assist patient in learning and problem solving when anxiety is diminished enough to allow concentration.
- Evaluate need for anti-anxiety medications; anxiolytics can be very effective in relieving panic; if none have been ordered, consult with physician for pharmacologic therapy.
- Assess for potential injury or violence to self or others.
- Give feedback about patient's current coping ability; reinforce any attempts to cope adaptively.
- Refer patients with recurrent anxiety and maladaptive coping mechanisms for further psychiatric/psychological evaluation and treatment.
- For patients with panic-level anxiety:
  - Take patient to a quiet area with minimal stimuli.
  - Administer anxiolytics as needed (ask what medications patient has used in past).
  - Remain with patient through the attack.
  - Give patient clear, honest feedback ("You are having a panic attack; I will stay with you").

INEFFECTIVE INDIVIDUAL COPING EVIDENCED BY ANXIETY/FEAR/ AVOIDANCE OF OBJECTS OR EVENTS, IRRATIONAL THOUGHTS RELATED TO PHOBIAS, EXTREME GUILT.

Patient Outcomes

- Demonstrate increased ability to think rationally and without undue guilt
- Identify thoughts and situations that evoke anxiety
- Show decreased anxiety related to improved thought processes and problem solving
- Demonstrate appropriate coping strategy for reducing anxiety related to phobia

Interventions

- Realize that phobic reactions are irrational and are not changed by rational, logical explanations; work around phobias (e.g., do not require a claustrophobic patient to use an elevator).
- Promote communication that reinforces rational thinking and decreases guilt.
- Verify your interpretation of what patient is experiencing (e.g., "I understand that you are afraid to go to the radiology department.")
- Use words familiar to patient when describing new events or expectations.
- Help patient to clarify thoughts and avoid misinterpretation; ask meaning of anything that you do not understand.
- Do not talk around or whisper near patient; include patient in conversation and check that he or she heard what you actually said by asking him or her to repeat it.
- Set limits on discussing irrational material; focus on topics based in reality that you can verify.
- Avoid belittling or derogating when patient misinterprets stimuli or is irrational; do not laugh or make fun of the individual.
- Assist patient to set limits on own behavior; suggest alternative ways to cope with anxiety (e.g., take a walk instead of crying).
- Be aware of potential for violence; observe for changes in behavior indicating increased anxiety, irrational thoughts, or any destructive behavior that requires attention.
- Anticipate difficulties in adjusting to return or transfer to home or other facility; discuss concerns with family or SO.
- Let patient have some control in anxiety-provoking situation; do not force patient to do anything that seems to be extremely frightening.
- Provide time to discuss anxiety or fear while continuing supportive verbal and behavioral interventions.
- Refer patients with phobias for more specific treatment (e.g., desensitization, behavioral modification) to a psychiatrist, psychologist, psychiatric

mental health nurse, or social worker if anxiety is not managed by previous interventions.

ALTERNATE NURSING DIAGNOSES

Altered Comfort
Altered Thought Processes
Disturbance in Self-Concept, Body Image, Self-Esteem
Altered Role Performance
Dysfunctional Grieving
Fear
Impaired Gas Exchange
Impaired Verbal Communication
Ineffective Individual Coping
High Risk for Violence: Directed at Self or Others
Post-trauma response
Sensory/Perceptual Alterations
Sleep Deprivation
Spiritual Distress (Distress of the Human Spirit)

WHEN TO CALL FOR HELP

- Increased anxiety leading to refusal of treatment or noncompliance
- Onset of paranoid psychotic thinking
- Onset of panic attack
- Staff conflict over management of patient behavior
- Increased staff anxiety over caring for patient

PATIENT AND FAMILY EDUCATION

- Teach patient and family or SO anxiety-reducing exercises such as muscle relaxation, guided imagery, music, or other activities for distraction.
- Discuss with patient and family or SO the causes and treatment of patient's anxiety.
- Review possible negative short-term and long-term effects of anxiety on physical and mental health.
- If patient is using anti-anxiety medications, review the need to monitor their use and potential problems when overused or discontinued without weaning.
- Educate on the use of appropriate medications to treat paralyzing symptoms such as OCD.

CHARTING TIPS

- Use objective assessment and nonjudgmental terms to describe behavior.
- Use patient's own words to describe amount and type of anxiety experienced.
- Note which interventions are most helpful in decreasing patient's anxiety and specific treatments that patient successfully learned to control own anxiety.
- Document family or SO responses to education about anxiety reduction methods.
- Document use of anti-anxiety medications and patient's response to them.

COMMUNITY-BASED CARE

- Discharge can be a particularly anxiety-provoking time for many patients. Begin discharge planning early and include all caretakers in planning for future care needs.
- Allow enough time to discuss alternatives and provide as much emotional support as possible during the transition time.
- Discuss available community resources: their functions, services, capabilities, and limitations.
- If transferring patient to another facility or agency for follow-up care, provide information about patient's progress in and successful interventions for dealing with anxiety.
- Refer to a psychiatrist or internist specializing in psychotropics if patient has frequent panic attacks or chronic, moderate to severe anxiety.
- Refer family for counseling early in patient's hospitalization so that therapeutic behaviors that will minimize patient's anxious behavior can be learned before patient returns home.
- To ensure consistency, record and communicate to family or others responsible for patient after discharge, those interventions that worked well.

Problems with Anger

THE ANGRY PATIENT

LEARNING OBJECTIVES

➤ Identify three positive functions of anger.
➤ Identify possible nurses' reactions to an angry patient.
➤ Differentiate among assertive, passive, and hostile expressions of anger.
➤ Select the most appropriate interventions for dealing with an angry patient.

GLOSSARY

Anger—A state of emotional excitement and tension induced by intense displeasure, frustration, and/or anxiety in response to a perceived threat.

Assertiveness training—Learning behavioral techniques that allow an individual to stand up for his or her own rights without infringing on the rights of others.

Assertiveness—Behavior directed toward claiming one's rights without denying the rights of others.

Frustration—Feelings generated from the inability to meet a goal.

Hostility—Feelings of anger and resentment that are destructive.

Passive-aggressive behavior—Behavior characterized by angry, hostile feelings that are expressed indirectly, leading to impaired communication and inappropriate expression. This behavior masks anger in such a way as to obstruct honesty in relationships. It may also be associated with obsessive-compulsive personality, borderline personality, and depression.

Rational anger—Anger expressed in a direct, socially acceptable manner.

Anger is a universal response to frustration, rejection, and fear. It can cause difficulty in our lives, especially when we have been taught that it is unacceptable to feel angry, have learned to display our anger inappropriately, or have developed a sense of fear that the anger can lead to abandonment. However, learning to deal with anger is an ongoing process, and when we learn how to deal with our anger and others' anger appropriately, we can gain a positive feeling of control, a sense of power and energy, and increased self-esteem. Some people fear anger because they think it could get out of control. Generally, though, anger tends to be of short duration and low intensity for most people. It does not necessarily lead to violence and aggression.

Anger can be viewed along a continuum. At one extreme is passive-aggressive behavior, in which a person avoids direct, open expression of anger but finds hidden ways to express it. At the other extreme is aggressive expression, in which a person inflicts pain on others when he or she expresses anger. Rational anger falls in the middle. When anger is rational, feelings are expressed in a direct, socially acceptable manner that allows the person to gain some control over the threat without causing harm to others.

ETIOLOGY

No single theory can explain the complex emotion of anger. Most likely, an intertwining of biological, psychologic, and sociocultural factors create each individual's unique response. Box 8–1 lists positive and negative functions of anger.

Biologic theories of anger focus mainly on neurotransmitters, such as dopamine, norepinephrine, and serotonin. The balance of these and other brain chemicals seem to influence or even aggravate response to anger and stress.

Psychologic theories look at the various dynamics and learned responses that cause anger. Anger occurs as a result of a buildup of frustration. Paquette (1998) points out that frustration and feelings of powerlessness precede expression of anger. Children often use inappropriate anger responses, such as temper tantrums, to deal with frustration and feelings of powerlessness. Positive reinforcement for this behavior can cause inappropriate anger responses to continue into adulthood. When the child's caregivers are demanding, hypercritical, and punitive, the child may develop coping mecha-

BOX 8–1. Positive and Negative Functions of Anger

Positive Functions	Negative functions
Energizes body for self-defense	Can lead to impulsive behavior
Can promote conflict resolution	Can lead to hostility and rage
Can increase self-esteem and sense of control	Can hurt others emotionally or physically

nisms aimed at avoiding expressing anger directly for fear of displeasing the caregiver and risking emotional abandonment or retaliation. These coping mechanisms often lead to a passive-aggressive anger response and resentment, which eventually erupt into inappropriate or destructive behavior. Anger can sometimes be a normal response to fear and help the person gain control of a perceived threat, or it can be part of the adaptive process in adjusting to a loss. In addition, suppressed anger can contribute to depression and low self-esteem (Townsend, 2000). Anger can also be a motivating factor to stimulate action that in turn can raise self-esteem.

Sociocultural factors also play an important role in the way an individual expresses anger. Social groups, including families, often display common patterns in the degree of acceptance of expressed anger. For example, in some families yelling and aggressive confrontation are acceptable means of dealing with anger and conflict, whereas in others any overt display of anger is not tolerated. Although both of these styles may work within individual families, they may not be the healthiest ways of dealing with anger.

Women are often socialized to deal with anger differently from men. They may tend to displace or suppress angry feelings and attempt to give in and compromise rather than deal with the conflict directly. This behavior can lead to passive-aggressive responses or resentment that may eventually become destructive. Such repression can also be detrimental and lead to misunderstanding when dealing with male colleagues.

CLINICAL CONCERNS

Medical conditions, such as chronic illness or loss of body function, may strain one's coping abilities and lead to an uncharacteristic display of anger. Illness often means facing feelings of powerlessness and frustration in meeting one's goals and contributes to angry responses such as irritability. Some conditions, including some brain tumors and different forms of dementia, may also directly contribute to inappropriate expressions of anger because of their influence on brain function. Studies have been inconclusive on the role of chronic anger in the development of heart disease and migraines.

Abuse of mind-altering substances may reduce inhibitions and negatively influence the anger response.

LIFE SPAN ISSUES

CHILDREN

Children normally respond with anger when faced with frustration. If they are raised in an environment where intense anger and violence are accepted, they can develop overly aggressive anger responses including cruelty to others, animal abuse, intolerance for frustration. Conversely, children who are taught that anger is unacceptable may tend to suppress or deny angry feelings and can develop extreme distress and guilt when faced with conflict. Children who learn appropriate ways to relieve tensions are more able to express anger rationally. Because children are vulnerable, they may be at increased risk of injury caused by inappropriate expressions of anger by caregivers.

ADOLESCENTS

Anger in adolescents is often seen as part of their developmental process of separation from parents and asserting their individuality. Hostility can also come from overstimulation from all they are dealing with. They may also have fears of being unable to control their impulses, leading to anxiety about anger.

ADULTS

Adults who must deal with difficult life experiences, such as a chronic illness or the onset of an acute illness compounding stressful life events, can become very angry. This anger can further complicate the disease by depleting coping skills and interfering with the recommended medical treatment.

ELDERLY PEOPLE

Uncharacteristic displays of anger in elderly people may be the result of frustration caused by a variety of physical, mental, and lifestyle changes such as dementia, altered sensory function (particularly hearing loss), altered mobility, changes in sleep-rest patterns, effects of medications, depression, loss of loved ones, and fear of dying. Inappropriate behavior may cause elderly persons to be alienated, further increasing their sense of fear, frustration, and possible confusion. Additionally, vulnerable elderly people are at risk of being victims of someone else's anger.

POSSIBLE NURSES' REACTIONS

- May take patient's anger personally, causing an unhealthy emotional response.
- May respond defensively by using an aggressive response or avoidance. This can accelerate the anger cycle.
- May attribute the patient's anger to a specific event, such as the quality of care provided, and respond by feeling unappreciated and resentful.

- May feel uncomfortable or fearful and respond by suppressing or denying the anger.
- May avoid confronting the patient for fear of emotional or physical retaliation.

ASSESSMENT

Behavior and Appearance

- Loud voice, change in pitch, or very soft voice, forcing other to strain to hear (Table 8–1)
- Intense eye contact or avoidance of eye contact
- Rapid, pacing movement
- Ruminating about an issue
- Passive-aggressive behavior, possibly including sarcastic humor; chronic complaining; socially annoying habits; pseudocompliance (agreeing to do something but not doing it)
- Possible physical violence

Mood and Emotions

- Annoyance, discomfort, frustration, continuous state of tension
- May be quick to anger, then let it go or take time to "stew" before expressing anger
- Guilt
- Powerlessness
- Vulnerability, easily offended
- Defensive response to criticism
- Passive-aggressive emotional response, possibly including being sullen, yet denying any concerns, or inappropriate cheerfulness for the situation

Thoughts, Beliefs, and Perceptions

- May believe that anger is normal and can be expressed without hurting others
- May take responsibility appropriately without blaming others
- May be angry at others but still care for them

TABLE 8–1. COMPARING BEHAVIORAL RESPONSES TO ANGER

Traits	Passive	Assertive	Aggressive
Speech content	Negative: "Can I, Should I" Puts self down	Positive: "I can, I will" "I" messages	Hostile: "You never . . . You always . . ." Derogatory
Voice	Whispers Whiny, weak	Firm, clear	Loud
Posture	Drooping	Erect, relaxed	Tense
Eye contact	Looks down	Appropriate	Invasive
Gestures	Fidgets	Appropriate	Threatening

- May lack ability to express true feelings
- May fear loss of love if anger is expressed directly
- May fear emotional or physical abandonment if anger is expressed
- May feel a sense of power when angry

Relationships and Interactions

- May communicate concerns clearly to avoid additional misunderstanding
- May avoid other hostile or angry persons
- May be catered to by others who fear patient's anger

Physical Responses

- Fight-or-flight response during confrontations, possibly including rapid pulse, increased blood pressure, rapid breathing, muscle tension, sweating, or intense feelings of wanting to attack or run
- Episodes of headaches, depression, sleep alterations, pain, or gastrointestinal symptoms associated with repressed anger

COLLABORATIVE MANAGEMENT

Pharmacologic

Antianxiety medications, including benzodiazepines, are sometimes used for short-term relief of feelings of tension and anger. However, they should not be used as a substitute for acknowledging and dealing with anger, and they should not interfere with pharmacologic actions of medications being taken for the underlying medical condition. In addition, antidepressants may be effective in controlling impulsive and aggressive behavior associated with mood swings. Beta blockers have also been used occasionally to control aggressive behaviors.

Common herbal products used for tension include St. John's wort, kava kava, and valerian.

NURSING MANAGEMENT

> **ANXIETY** EVIDENCED BY TENSION, DISTRESS, UNCERTAINTY, REST-
> LESSNESS, OR DISPLEASURE RELATED TO THREAT TO SELF-CONCEPT,
> FRUSTRATION, OR UNCONSCIOUS CONFLICT.

Patient Outcomes

- Verbalizes concerns and frustrations directly at an appropriate time
- Demonstrates reduced tension including lowered voice and more appropriate anger response
- Demonstrates problem-solving skills when faced with frustration
- Demonstrates behaviors to calm self when faced with frustration

Interventions

- Use therapeutic communication techniques including open-ended questions, appropriate eye contact, and supportive gestures to encourage patient to vent feelings and concerns. Avoid providing solutions before the patient has a chance to relieve tension.
- Listen with concern without being patronizing or condescending. Phrases such as "Tell me what happened next" or "That really sounds frustrating" allow the patient to feel accepted and understood. Avoid phrases that escalate feelings of powerlessness, such as "Calm down" or "It can't be that bad."
- If needed, direct the patient to a more private setting to express his or her feelings. Having others view the demonstration of anger can make it more difficult to back down and contribute to escalation of hostility or aggression.
- When the tension of the situation is reduced, focus on identifying the source of anger and validating the problem. Explore options on how to deal with the problem more constructively. Ask the patient which methods he or she has used successfully in the past when dealing with frustration. Teach problem-solving skills. Assist the patient to identify and use more effective coping mechanisms.
- Teach tension-reducing techniques, such as deep breathing, counting to 10, walking away, and talking to self about remaining in control.
- Encourage the patient to express angry feelings toward the appropriate person. Role playing before the confrontation may help the patient choose effective strategies.
- Recognize that an angry outburst may result from an accumulation of multiple stressors and cause the patient to overreact.
- If the patient is justifiably angry because of something you have done or not done, accept appropriate responsibility. Work with the patient or colleagues to resolve the problem. Accepting and validating the patient's feelings sends the message that you value his or her viewpoint.
- Encourage children to vent frustration by redirecting their activity, such as hitting a pillow or engaging in exercise.

INEFFECTIVE INDIVIDUAL COPING EVIDENCED BY INAPPROPRIATE EXPRESSION OF ANGER, DISTRESS, DESTRUCTIVE BEHAVIOR TO SELF OR OTHERS, AND RELATED TO THREAT TO SELF-ESTEEM OR UNCONSCIOUS CONFLICT.

Patient Outcomes

- Able to identify personal strength that may help to reduce stress
- Accepts personal limits in dealing with inappropriate demands
- Demonstrates effective skills for dealing with frustration

Interventions

- Identify ways to increase the person's self-esteem as part of expressing anger by treating him or her respectfully and acknowledging his or her skills or attributes. For example, when dealing with an angry daughter's confrontation about her parent's care, state, "Your father is lucky to have you as his advocate." Avoid a defensive response or ignoring complaints.
- Focus on the patient's strengths to deal with frustration. Help him or her identify which coping skills have been successful in the past.
- Teach the patient that anger is a normal response to loss. Some individuals are unable to accept this anger as normal and experience unneeded guilt.
- Encourage the patient to state the cause of the problem clearly to avoid erroneous assumptions.
- If the patient rejects or finds fault with all of your suggestions, place the responsibility for choosing the appropriate response on the patient. You might say, "We've discussed many options. Now it is up to you to consider which one is best for you."
- Set clear limits on the patient's expressions of anger toward the staff. Refuse to listen to extensive complaining if the patient is not willing to participate in determining an acceptable solution.
- Be assertive when explaining which types of behavior are not appropriate.
- Be consistent with the demands the patient can set on the staff.
- Be a role model for expressing negative emotions in a positive manner. Use "I messages," such as "I feel angry" rather than accusing the other person, which can lead to a defensive response. Speak firmly without yelling and avoid threatening gestures when confronting issues.

ALTERNATE NURSING DIAGNOSES

> Impaired Social Interaction
> Noncompliance
> Risk for Violence
> Self-Concept Disturbance

WHEN TO CALL FOR HELP

☐ Increased aggressiveness; violent behavior, including damaging property; increasing use of abusive language, threats made to patients or staff

☐ Onset of paranoid thinking or psychotic behavior

☐ Onset of extreme obsessive-compulsive behavior

☐ Increased staff conflict over management of patient behavior

☐ Increased staff anxiety over caring for patient

PATIENT AND FAMILY EDUCATION

- Teach assertiveness skills by role-modeling appropriate responses and helping the patient practice these skills.
- Review with the patient frequently encountered frustrations, and explain that giving up control of the outcome may be the most effective strategy for dealing with them.
- Review potential negative health effects of inappropriate anger expression.
- If the patient is using antianxiety medications, review the need to monitor their use and avoid using them in place of trying to resolve the cause of anger.

CHARTING TIPS

- Use objective, nonjudgmental terms to describe behavior.
- Document patient's response to frustration.
- Document the limits set on care plan or treatment plan for consistency.
- Document use of medications (including herbal products) and patient's response to them.

COMMUNITY-BASED CARE

- Communicate plan of care to all involved in discharge planning.
- Inform any appropriate agencies of patient behaviors to avoid miscommunication.
- Refer patient to counseling services or assertiveness training, if needed.
- Encourage patient's active participation in treatment plan.

THE AGGRESSIVE AND POTENTIALLY VIOLENT PATIENT

LEARNING OBJECTIVES

➤ Identify factors that precipitate aggressive behavior.
➤ Describe effective techniques for verbal deescalation of aggressive behavior.
➤ List possible nursing staff reactions to violent behavior in patients.
➤ List interventions a nurse could use in working with a violent patient.

GLOSSARY

Aggression—Any verbal or nonverbal, actual or attempted, forceful abuse of the self or another person or object.

Assaultive behavior—An intentional act that is designed to make another person fearful and produces harm.

Hostility—Anger that is destructive in nature and purpose as opposed to rational anger that is appropriate to the situation and is not destructive in intent.

Intimidation—The use of threats to frighten and control.

Physical restraint—Any physical method of restricting an individual's freedom of movement, activity, or normal access to his or her body.

Rage—Engulfing emotional experience of extreme anger.

Violent behavior—Exertion of extreme force or destructive acts with intent to hurt another and that can cause injury.

The presence of violence in our society has unfortunately become increasingly common. This increased violence is also reflected in the healthcare setting. High rates of violent, assaultive behavior have been reported in hospitals, emergency departments, nursing homes and home health care. U. S. Labor Department sta-

74

tistics report that 64 percent of nonfatal workplace assaults take place in hospitals and nursing homes. However, psychiatric nurses are at highest risk. Poster (1996) found that over 75 percent of psychiatric nurses had been assaulted at least once in their careers. Historically, nurses working with psychiatric patients have been taught to be alert to and manage violent, assaultive behavior; however, now all healthcare workers need to be alert to this problem. Healthcare facilities must institute security measures and policies to ensure the safety of staff and patients and to reduce the fear of impending violence among staff and visitors. Consistently being confronted with aggressive and potentially violent patients, families, and visitors can cause excessive fear, stress, job dissatisfaction, lost work time, poor morale, and possible injury. The Occupational Health and Safety Administration (OSHA) has developed voluntary guidelines for employers to address this problem. They created "Universal Precautions for Violence," which acknowledges that violence should be expected but can be avoided or mitigated by proper training, policies, and security measures.

Past history of violence is the greatest predictor of this behavior. In addition, a history of psychiatric illness, particularly schizophrenia, paranoia, borderline personality disorder, other personality disorders, post-traumatic stress disorder, and dementia is frequently associated with predicting an aggressive outburst. Other major risk factors include drug and alcohol use. Studies show that young men are by far the most frequent perpetrators of violent acts.

The causes of the increased violence in our society and, consequently, in health care are varied and complex. Some of these causes include:

- Attitudinal changes in society with increased acceptance of violent response to authority figures
- Increased prevalence of handguns among patients, families, and visitors
- Increased use of mind-altering drugs and alcohol
- Court decisions that give psychiatric patients the right to refuse treatment and medication
- Healthcare staff members inadequately prepared to respond to aggression or who deny the risk of violence and fail to report it
- Increasing frustrations in health care settings, including inadequate staffing and long waits
- Healthcare workers in isolated environments (e.g., examining rooms, in patient's home) with no backup, communication devices, or alarms
- Impersonal care, which may stress already frustrated patients
- Legal and ethical concerns about using chemical and physical restraints
- Media coverage of violence, which triggers additional crimes

Using restraints to manage potentially violent patients can create ethical dilemmas for the nurse concerning patient autonomy, human dignity, and informed consent. In 1993, the Joint Commission on Accreditation of Health Care Organizations (JCAHO) created standards for physical restraints, requiring each agency to provide clear policies and education on appropriate restraint use. They have continued to refine these because of ongoing problems (JCAHO, 2000). The aim is to reduce the incidence of injuries that can result from restraint use, such as loss of mobility, skin breakdown, and, possibly, death from strangulation. In 1999, Medicare and Medicaid developed new federal standards for the use of restraints. Restraints can be applied only with a physician's order for each occurrence. Continuous assessment of the patient while he or she is being restrained must be done, and alternatives to restraints must be tried.

ETIOLOGY

Aggressive, violent behavior has many causes. Most studies of the causes of aggression have been done on subjects with mental illness or prison populations, which may skew the results.

Biologic theories include genetics, which links chromosomal abnormalities to aggressive behavior, hormone imbalances, and neurotransmitter irregularities, specifically the abnormal secretions of dopamine and serotonin.

Psychologic theories on aggression are related to a person's view of the world as a source of anxiety. Individuals prone to violence often have low self-esteem and need to maintain control to enhance their own feelings of power and self-worth. Fear and anxiety can distort an individual's perception of the stimulus. The presence of alcohol or other drugs can further distort these and reduce inhibitions. Aggressive behavior temporarily reduces the anxiety and creates a temporary sense of power. In addition, individuals with poor impulse control or a personality disorder may use violence to intimidate others. Aggressive individuals may have limited ability to tolerate frustration and demand to have their needs met immediately. Individuals who have experienced emotional deprivation in childhood may be particularly vulnerable and respond with violent outbursts when they sense an attack on their self-esteem.

Social learning theory views aggression as a learned behavior. Individuals with a tendency toward aggressive, violent behavior may be more likely to respond to stressors such as illness, school or work pressures, or relationship problems with anger and hostility because they have learned that such behavior temporarily reduces their anxiety.

Sociocultural theories look at an aggressive individual's poor interpersonal skills. Exposure to aggression and violence as part of family life may also be a significantly influential factor. Children who are treated with violence may view violence as a normal way to deal with others. The cycle of family violence continues when children learn to use violence as their only coping mechanism instead of more socially acceptable ones. Poverty, deprivation, and hopelessness can also increase the risk of violent behavior.

RELATED CLINICAL CONCERNS

A wide variety of organic disorders may be associated with aggressive and violent behavior. These include:

INTRACRANIAL DISORDERS
Brain tumors
Head injury
Seizure disorders

Cerebrovascular accident
Dementia

SYSTEMIC DISORDERS
Endocrine disorders such as thyroid storm or Cushing's syndrome
Electrolyte imbalance
Oxygen deficiency
Septicemia
Hepatic encephalopathy

EXPOSURE TO SUBSTANCES
Alcohol use or withdrawal
Use of mind-altering substances such as phencyclidine and amphetamines
Withdrawal from barbiturates and sedatives
Use of aromatic hydrocarbons (glue, paint)
Use of medications such as steroids, central nervous system stimulants, and anti-Parkinsonian agents
Exposure to toxic chemicals, pesticides, lead

LIFE SPAN ISSUES

CHILDREN

Constant exposure to violence in childhood is a major factor contributing to the cycle of child abuse and family violence. Children who learn to use violent behavior to cope with frustrations and problems are likely to carry these behaviors into adulthood and may need to learn effective coping skills. Early signs of problems may include cruelty to animals and other children as well as difficulty controlling responses to frustration. The alarming presence of violence in schools and neighborhoods and in the media has increased the number of children who are exposed to seeing aggressive behavior and weapons used to resolve frustration in what may appear to them to be socially acceptable, normal behavior. Autism, mental retardation, learning disabilities, and attention deficit disorders may also cause aggressive and violent behavior in children.

ADOLESCENTS

Adolescents may act out aggressive feelings by participating in self-destructive behavior such as drug or alcohol use, smoking, or crime. Using mind-altering substances increases the risk of violent behavior. Homicide is the leading cause of death in the 15–24 age group (Dowd, 1998).

ADULTS

Aggressive behavior in adults often reflects lifelong learned patterns. For instance, persons who abuse their spouses have often witnessed abuse in their parents' relationship or been abused themselves as children.

ELDERLY PEOPLE

Like anger, violent behavior can be a lifelong pattern or be caused by physical illness or adverse reactions to medications. Aggressive behavior may also be a self-protective response related to confusion, fear, or sensory loss (particularly hearing loss). Most frequently, aggressive behavior in elderly persons is associated with Alzheimer's disease, senile dementia, cerebrovascular accidents, metabolic disorders, and hypoxia.

POSSIBLE NURSES' REACTIONS

- May fear being hurt by the violent or aggressive patient or one who uses intimidation with the threat of violence. This fear can cause the nurse to use poor judgment or totally deny feeling fearful. Other common fear responses include avoiding the patient or bending the rules in an attempt to appease the patient. All of these responses can affect continuity of patient care.
- May feel abused and unappreciated, leading to defensive responses such as attempting to punish the patient. Defensive responses and treating patient with less respect can escalate anger.
- May feel guilty for not being able to control the behavior or feel uncomfortable for participating in applying restraints.
- May feel offended or frustrated because the patient does not respond to care positively.
- A nurse who has been assaulted in the past may experience self-blame and question his or her competence, depression, anxiety, and hyperalertness to any situation that could lead to aggressiveness.

ASSESSMENT

Behavior and Appearance

- Pacing, restlessness
- Tense facial expression and body language
- Unpredictable behavior
- Loud voice, shouting, use of obscenities, argumentative
- Overreacting to stimuli such as noise
- Exhibiting poor impulse control evidenced by acting quickly before considering consequences of actions
- Grasping potential weapons and attempting to use them

Mood and Emotions

- Anger, resentment, rage, hostility
- Anxiety; fear of loss of control leading to panic
- Inappropriate affect for situation, labile emotions

Thoughts, Beliefs, and Perceptions

- Low self-esteem
- Low frustration tolerance
- Thoughts or plans to harm someone
- Inability to trust others to follow through without strong intimidation and suspiciousness
- Hallucinations, paranoid delusions
- Views others as out to hurt him or her
- Sense of being out of control

Relationships and Interactions

- Difficulty with close relationships; lack of trust, which causes person to fear closeness
- Others fearful of and avoid aggressive person, believing that they might be hurt or manipulated
- Family and friends have learned to meet person's demands to avoid aggressive response or exhibiting passive-aggressive behaviors in response to the person's demands

Physical Responses

- Increased muscle tension
- Increased heart rate and blood pressure
- Altered level of consciousness, confusion, lethargy
- Possible abnormal laboratory values including blood sugar, blood alcohol, drug screening
- Increased use of medications

Pertinent History

- History of violent behavior, particularly assault
- Psychiatric diagnosis
- Substance and/or alcohol abuse
- Physical, emotional, or sexual abuse in childhood

COLLABORATIVE MANAGEMENT

Pharmacologic

It is important to use appropriate medications in adequate doses as an alternative or adjunct to physical restraints to manage aggressive behavior.

Pharmacologic management of acute aggressive or violent behavior may require rapid neuroleptization (also known as *rapid tranquilization*), which involves regular, frequent administration of antipsychotic medications such as haloperidol (Haldol). Parenteral administration may be required if oral route is not feasible. If the patient is in physical restraints, parenteral administration reduces the risk of aspiration. For example, haloperidol, 5 mg, may be administered every 30 to 60 minutes until symptoms are under control. Dosage should be reduced in elderly people. When using this drug, monitor the patient closely for hypotension and signs of extrapyramidal symptoms including akathisias and dystonia (see Chapter 20).

Antianxiety medications and sedatives may also be useful. Anticonvulsants, such as carbamazepine (Tegretol), have been used with some success. Lithium and beta blockers, such as propranolol, are other alternatives. Antidepressants have also been used to treat impulsive, aggressive behavior. When using these drugs, evaluate how they may interfere with the medications ordered to treat the patient's underlying medical condition.

Convincing an aggressive, agitated patient to accept medication can be difficult and may lead the nurse to face an ethical dilemma of giving medication against a patient's will. Be aware of hospital or agency policies and state laws regarding patient rights (Box 8–2).

Herbal products, such as valerian, may be used to calm the person.

NURSING MANAGEMENT

RISK FOR VIOLENCE, DIRECTED TO OTHERS EVIDENCED BY OVERT HOSTILITY AND/OR AGGRESSION TO OTHERS, THREATENING OTHERS, POSSESSION OF POTENTIAL WEAPON, ASSAULTING OTHERS RELATED TO IMPAIRED JUDGMENT, FEELINGS OF POWERLESSNESS, IMPULSIVE BEHAVIOR, INABILITY TO EVALUATE REALITY SECONDARY TO NEUROLOGIC PROBLEMS, PSYCHOTIC THOUGHTS, AND/OR DRUG/ALCOHOL USE.

BOX 8–2. Encouraging an Uncooperative Patient to Take Medication

- Have the nurse who has the best relationship with patient offer the medication. Avoid power struggles and confrontations, which would most likely escalate the situation.
- Have the medication in hand so that it can be given quickly when the patient gives consent. The patient may change his or her mind suddenly.
- Be prepared for the patient to spit out the medication. This is especially common in elderly, aggressive patients.
- Use liquid oral medication if available. It is absorbed more quickly and is less likely to be "cheeked." If medication needs to be given by injection, work quickly. Have adequate staff available in case violence erupts.
- Review with the patient the benefits of medication and that it will help him or her gain control of his or her feelings.

Patient Outcomes

- Demonstrates increased self-control while in nurse's care
- Does not harm others or self while in nurse's care
- Demonstrates alternative coping mechanisms to reduce tension while in nurse's care
- Behavior does not escalate while in nurse's care

Interventions

- Help patient to verbalize angry feelings by reflecting and by clarifying your understanding of these feelings. Communicate your interest by appropriate eye contact, restating what patient has said, and asking questions. Help patient identify source of anger. Recognize that response to illness may make the person feel helpless with the need to strike out to gain a sense of control.
- Early recognition of problem behavior is essential so that staff members can develop a plan.
- If needed, allow patient to release tension physically on inanimate objects such as pillows or in prescribed exercise, as appropriate.
- Do not take patient's behavior personally. For example, if a patient calls you derogatory names, refrain from reacting emotionally. Rather, remind yourself that you represent an authority figure to the patient and he or she is reacting to you as such. Remember that patient may use derogatory remarks as a way to bolster his or her own self-esteem and seem to zero in on your sensitive, vulnerable points, such as weight or speech patterns. Avoid responding with sarcasm or ridicule.
- Do not ignore aggressive behavior in the hope that it will go away. It needs to be addressed. Minimization of behavior and ineffective limit setting are the most frequent factors contributing to escalation to violence.
- Set clear, consistent limits in a timely manner on what will and will not be tolerated. Clarify any specific consequences of patient behavior. For example, "If you attempt to hurt anyone, we will be compelled to control your behavior, which may mean using restraints"(Box 8–3).
- Identify one or two staff members who are comfortable with the patient to handle most of the care if possible to help provide consistent interventions. Evaluate whether a male or female staff member has a more calming influence. Sometimes a male's presence is too threatening and powerful. Other times it is reassuring to the patient that a male staff member is available. A male patient may be less likely to hurt a woman and may see her as nurturing and supportive. Conversely, male patients may view the female staff as less able to provide control or have other conflicted feelings toward women.
- Free patient's environment of extra stimulation, such as noise or an agitated roommate. Extra stimulation may reduce impulse control. Remove objects around patients that could be used as potential weapons such as portable IV poles or food trays and utensils. Consider providing plastic food dishes and utensils. Avoid startling patient. Call patient by name before walking into room. Avoid sudden movements that the patient may interpret as threatening.

BOX 8–3. Setting Limits

1. Explain exactly which behavior is inappropriate. Don't assume the individual knows which behavior is inappropriate.
2. Explain why the behavior is inappropriate. Don't assume the individual knows why the behavior is inappropriate.
3. Give the individual reasonable choices or consequences. Present them as choices, and always present the positive first.
4. Allow time—if you don't allow time to comply, it may be perceived as an ultimatum.
5. Enforce consequences—limits don't work unless you follow through with the consequences.

Source: Reprinted from the Art of Setting Limits Participant Manual, p. 8, with permission of the National Crisis Prevention Institute, Inc., © 1991.

- Remain calm and communicate that you are in control and can handle the situation. Use a moderate, firm voice and calming hand gestures. Avoid touching patient. Table 8–2 lists a summary of staff interventions.
- Place yourself between door and patient. Always have a quick exit available. Never turn your back on this type of patient. Keep door of room open.

TABLE 8–2. SUMMARY OF STAFF INTERVENTIONS

Patient	Staff
Anxiety	Verbal intervention: • Assess. • Use verbal calming techniques. • Attempt to calm patient. • Do not invade patient's personal space; avoid antagonizing.
Threatening	Set Limits: • Continue verbal calming techniques. • Set clear and definite limits. • Be directive and matter of fact. • Be prepared to enforce limits.
Acting out aggression	Physical management: • Recognize mounting tension. • Have a plan. • Designate team leader. • Use only after other measures fail.
Tension reduction	Emotional support: • Allow patient to express feelings. • Listen nonjudgmentally. • Show concern for patient, not anger. • Discuss events with colleagues. • Avoid blaming.

Source: Adapted from Haven and Piscitello, 1989, and Lewis, 1993.

Let other staff members know you are going in patient's room. Protect other patients who may get in the way of the violent individual.

- Never force an agitated patient to have a test or treatment. Power struggles will escalate aggression. Rather, prioritize care that must be given and focus only on that. Explain all procedures and ask patient's permission before beginning. Give patient choices as often as possible.
- If the patient is psychotic, he or she may be hearing voices. If so, ask what the voices are telling him or her to do. This gives you more information on what to expect. Hallucinations that command the patient to initiate aggression can be an extremely powerful force for the patient to overcome.
- A nurse who has been assaulted in the past and is now faced with a potentially violent patient may bring fears from this past experience, which could inhibit his or her response. Sharing these fears with colleagues may provide much needed support. Use agency resources for support including employee assistance or critical incident debriefing to help colleagues.
- If a patient makes threats to harm specific people, the nurse needs to notify his or her supervisor and follow protocol for notifying potential victims.
- A visitor who becomes aggressive or violent needs to be reported to the agency security staff immediately and removed from the patient care area.
- Ensure that measures and policies are in place to prevent workplace violence. See Box 8–4.
- In the patient's home setting, be aware of exits in case a problem develops. Never stay alone in a home with a patient or family who is threatening violence, drinking, or displaying firearms. Consider making home visits with a colleague when there is a known risk of violence. Leave the home immediately if there is any sign of out of control behavior. Have access to a cellular phone in case of emergency.

RISK FOR INJURY EVIDENCED BY FALLS, PAIN, TRAUMA, SKIN BREAKDOWN RELATED TO RESTRAINING PATIENT TO CONTROL VIOLENT BEHAVIOR.

BOX 8–4. Preventing Workplace Violence

- Be particularly vigilant during change of shifts and on night shift. Most events occur between 8:30 p.m. and 10:30 a.m.
- Minimize stress factors such as long waits, crowded, confined spaces, and inflexible policies for patients where possible.
- Avoid wearing jewelry or neckties that can be grabbed or tugged.
- Immediately report all assaults to your supervisor and security.
- Be aware that many agency security staffs have minimal training.
- Receive education on local gangs and gang violence.
- Participate in agency safety committees to ensure that adequate security measures are in place.

Patient Outcomes

- Remains free of injury and complications during restraint application
- Demonstrates control of behavior once restraints are removed

Interventions

- The decision to use restraints should be made only after other efforts to reduce tension have been tried and proven ineffective. A physician's order must be obtained each time restraints are to be used. Standing orders are not acceptable.
- Once decision is made to restrain patient, act quickly and decisively. Determine what appropriate type of restraint is to be applied before approaching patient. Restraints include cloth chest and limb restraints or leather (hard) locked restraints. (Note: When using hard restraints, make sure you have the key, and double-check that they are locked after applying them to patient.) Have equipment ready before approaching patient.
- Never attempt to restrain a patient by yourself. Have adequate staff members available (usually three to five persons) and a plan of action before attempting to physically control a patient. Recruit reliable help from all possible sources, such as security. Assess their experience in managing a violent patient and review the plan. Decide in advance who will grab which arm or leg if patient must be restrained. The presence of a number of staff members (show of force) alone may subdue a patient. Identify a leader before taking any action.
- Designate one person to talk with the patient and another to direct the other staff. Only one staff member should talk with patient, preferably someone who knows him or her. It is important to communicate in a firm manner, speaking slowly. Lack of leadership can cause confusing and contradictory messages and result in someone being hurt or the patient escaping. Remove other patients from the area.
- Maintain a firm base of support for balance if you are suddenly pushed. Remove name badge, eyeglasses, jewelry, and so on to avoid injury.
- If patient is resisting, he or she may need to be distracted. Each staff member should grab one of the patient's limbs when given the command by the coordinating person and take patient down to the floor or bed quickly. Attempt to cradle patient's head to prevent injury.
- Once restraints are applied to bed frame, take the time to talk with the patient in a calm, concerned manner to try to humanize situation. Call patient by his or her name.
- Make sure patient has no potential weapons within reach. Patient needs to be searched for sharp objects, matches, and so on.
- Administer medications as ordered.
- Be aware of agency policy regarding application of restraints. Requirements for monitoring patients while in restraints, reasons for restraints, doctor's orders, and the length of time each order remains valid should be clearly spelled out in agency policies. If you are not sure about using re-

straints on someone, discuss with your supervisor to weigh your obligations to protect the patient versus going against the patient's wishes.

- Monitor patient closely and document findings according to agency policy including vital signs, circulation extremities, and intake/output.
- Remove restraints and observe patient closely when the situation is under control. Consider removing restraints from one limb at a time so that patient has time to adjust. For the high-risk patient, keep one arm and one leg in restraints at all times until it is clear that patient can be released. Inform other staff members that patient has been released. Establish clear criteria for reapplying restraints with patient and staff. Prepare family for patient's condition, as appropriate.
- Once the patient has regained control, discuss with him or her why that intervention was used, and allow opportunity to express feelings. This increases his or her sense of control and decreases dehumanization.
- If patient has a gun or other weapon, never attempt to disarm him or her. Contact security and/or law enforcement agency as soon as possible. Focus on getting assistance and protecting patients and staff. Patients and staff should remain in a safe area until help arrives.
- Consider taking a specialized class on use of defensive techniques such as management of assaultive behavior. Proper training is essential to prevent injury to patients and staff. Staff members can practice with each other to demonstrate how they would handle a violent patient.
- Identify jobs at higher risk of exposure to violence and ensure that employees in these jobs have adequate training.

ALTERNATE NURSING DIAGNOSIS

Altered Thought Processes
Ineffective Individual Coping
Noncompliance
Anxiety
Self-Esteem Disturbance

WHEN TO CALL FOR HELP

Escalation of behavior from aggressive to violent
Patient in possession of a weapon
Inadequate staff members available to control behavior
Increased staff anxiety over caring for the patient
Staff members at risk for violence without adequate training/security

PATIENT AND FAMILY EDUCATION

- Review early warning signs of escalation of aggressive behavior with patient and his or her family.
- Instruct patient on role of alcohol and drugs in contributing to aggressive behavior.
- Instruct on use of prescribed medications to control tension. Instruct on when to ask for PRN medications.
- If patient is in restraints, review with him or her criteria for removal and reinstatement.

CHARTING TIPS

- Document all actions taken to prevent violent behavior.
- Document application of restraints including type, length of time in restraints, reasons for application, patient response, release of limbs, and care given while in restraints. (Document per agency policy.) Document vital sign monitoring.
- Document need for and response to medication given.
- Document any threats patient makes.
- Document all interventions and responses to them.

COMMUNITY-BASED CARE

- Provide information to patient's family and/or caregivers about emergency psychiatric services, if needed. Discuss potential for violence with family to share possible strategies from nursing care plan.
- Provide information on shelters and/or domestic violence services, if appropriate.
- If patient is being transferred to another facility, share concerns about patient's behavior and interventions and share any history of violent behavior.
- Provide information to family and caregivers on what to do if behavior is out of control. Encourage them to call for help immediately.
- Provide information and referrals on drug treatment if appropriate.

Problems with Affect and Mood

THE DEPRESSED PATIENT

LEARNING OBJECTIVES

➤ Differentiate feeling depressed from a depressive disorder.
➤ Describe common physical symptoms seen in depressive disorders.
➤ Describe interventions for the patient with low self-esteem.
➤ Describe possible nurses' reactions to the depressed patient

GLOSSARY

Anhedonia—Loss of pleasure in activities or interests that were previously enjoyed.

Depression—Primary psychiatric illness manifested by characteristic symptom clusters such as depressed mood, lowered self-esteem, pessimistic thoughts, and loss of pleasure or interest in former activities.

Dysthymic disorder—Mild to moderate chronic depression lasting at least 2 years.

Masked depression—Concealed depression in which patient is not aware of depressed mood or does not display obvious sadness. The depression is expressed through other means, such as physical complaints or diverse psychiatric symptoms such as phobias or compulsions.

Psychomotor agitation—Classic symptom cluster of depression including restlessness with rapid, agitated, purposeless movements like pacing or wringing hands.

Psychomotor retardation—Classic symptom cluster of depression including slow movements and speech.

Seasonal affective disorder (SAD)—Depression associated with shortened daylight in winter and fall. It disappears during spring and summer.

Feeling down, discouraged, and depressed is something all people experience at different times in their lives. Periods of emotional highs and lows are normal. Depressive illness, also known as major depression, however, is very different from simply feeling depressed. Major depression is a psychiatric illness characterized by a cluster of symptoms including prolonged depressed mood, lowered self-esteem, pessimistic thoughts, and loss of pleasure or interest in former activities for at least 2 weeks. It is a painful, debilitating illness. It needs to be differentiated from short-term depressed moods or grief reactions, which are normal. Although grief displays many of the signs and symptoms of depression, it is a time-limited condition in response to an obvious loss and does not cause lowered self-esteem. DSM-IV-TR also describes dysthymic disorder as a chronic depressed mood most of the day for more days than not during a period of 2 years. This is another form of depression.

Depression is the most common reason for seeking out mental health professionals. Because the symptoms of depression can be hidden, vague, or atypical, and may present as physical symptoms instead of a mood disturbance, primary care physicians may be the first to see the patient. Surveys consistently show that 6 to 8 percent of all outpatients in the primary care setting have major depressive disorders (DHHS, 1993). However, the symptoms of depression can often go unrecognized and are often misdiagnosed. Undiagnosed and untreated depression is considered a major national health concern, contributing to poor work performance, family disruption, substance abuse, and premature death as a result of suicide or lack of self-care. Family history, stressful life events, and a previous history of depression are major predictors (Li-Shiun, et al, 2000). Women are twice as likely to suffer from depression as men. It crosses all ethnic lines. In addition, depression can be part of a bipolar disorder (manic depression), psychosis, eating disorders, or dementia. Depression can also be secondary to a primary problem such as substance abuse or schizophrenia.

Once a person experiences a depressive episode, there is a high risk for recurrence. After one depressive episode, an individual has a 50 percent chance of another; after two episodes, there is a 70 to 80 percent risk of another; and after three episodes, the individual is at very high risk for chronic disability from depression (Kupfer, 1991). Depression is frequently underdiagnosed and undertreated. A major source of diagnosis is primary care providers who diagnose one-third to one-half of people identified as having depression (Improving Quality of Care for People with Depression, 2000).

ETIOLOGY

No single theory of depression is accepted by all theorists and clinicians. Different theories may apply to the divergent pathways that patients travel to arrive at the various types of depression.

Biological theories have focused on an insufficiency of neurotransmitters, especially norepinephrine and serotonin. These insufficiencies may be the result of inherited or environmental factors. The effectiveness of antidepressants may result from enhanced levels of these neurotransmitters. The most severe depressions are predominantly biologically determined. Hormonal factors, including abnormal melatonin metabolism, are associated with seasonal affective disorder (also called major depression with seasonal pattern).

Genetics may be a factor in more severe depressions. Relatives of people with depression have a higher incidence of this illness than those in the general population.

Psychologic theories about a predisposition to depression have focused on a personal history of deprivation, trauma, or significant loss during childhood. These patients may be more susceptible to depression as current losses revive memories of former losses. They are more likely to experience low self-esteem and powerlessness.

Depression can be viewed as forbidden anger that has been turned inward. Classic psychoanalytic theory identified depression as the reaction to the loss of a significant person who has been both hated and loved. The patient handles this ambivalence by turning the hatred inward, resulting in depression and low self-esteem, whereas the memory of the departed person remains beloved and idealized.

Certain predominant issues of low self-esteem and helplessness are major contributors. For instance, low self-esteem may be based on the faulty development of an adequate, competent sense of self during childhood. As a child, the patient may have received attention and approval only when meeting parental needs and expectations. In adulthood, the absence of external support and praise and especially the loss of a supportive person may make the patient vulnerable to loss of self-esteem, which triggers depression.

Learned helplessness is displayed by a lack of adequate effort based on the belief that a person cannot be effective in getting needs met or making an impact. This person grew up in an environment that did not respond to any actions or initiative that he or she took (Seligman, 1975).

Distorted thinking can generate depression. Typically, the patient has negative expectations about himself or herself, the world, and the future. If he or she consistently overgeneralizes any mistake into the conclusion "I can't do anything right" and judges himself or herself as deficient, these negative beliefs can build toward depression. Negative expectations of the world, such as receiving no help from others or expecting only criticism, reinforce helplessness and lead to hopelessness (Beck, 1979).

RELATED CLINICAL CONCERNS

Clinically significant depressive symptoms are detectable in about 12 to 36 percent of the medically ill population (DHHS, 1993). Valente and Saunders (1997) report that 20 to 25 percent of people with cancer experience depression that often goes untreated. Untreated depression in the medically ill can contribute to longer hospital stays, poor compliance, poorer quality of life, and increased doctor visits. The patient's response to a medical illness could cause depression, and in some cases physiologic problems could contribute to it. In some medical disorders, depression is a symptom. Symptoms of these illnesses can also mask depressive symptoms such as fatigue or changes in appetite or bowel habits. These disorders include:

- Stroke (especially frontal lesions)
- Myocardial infarction
- Adrenal disorders
- Dementia
- Diabetes
- Cancer
- Hypothyroidism
- Some brain tumors

In addition, some medications can trigger depression (Box 9–1).

BOX 9–1. Drugs that Cause Depression

- Antihypertensive agents
  - Reserpine
  - Beta blockers
  - Methyldopa
- Oral contraceptives
- Steroids
- Benzodiazepines

- Cancer chemotherapeutic agents
  - Vincristine
  - Vinblastine
  - Interferon
  - Procarbazine
- Psychoactive agents
  - Alcohol
  - Amphetamine or cocaine withdrawal
  - Opioids

Sources: L Rouchell, AM, Pounds, R, and Tierney JG: Depression. In Rundell, JR and Wise, MG (eds): Textbook of Consultation-Liaison Psychiatry. Washington, DC: American Psychiatric Press, 1996, and Akiskal, HS: Mood Disorders: Clinical features. In Sadock, BJ and Sadock, VA (eds.): Kaplan & Sadock's Comprehensive Textbook of Psychiatry (7th ed.), Philadelphia: Lippincott Williams & Wilkins, 2000.

LIFE SPAN ISSUES

CHILDREN

Experts do not agree on the prevalence of depression in children; however, there is consensus that it does occur, even in young children. Depression could be the aftermath of emotional deprivation, abuse, or separation. Because the child may be unable to express feelings or worries, other signs need to be analyzed, including acting-out behaviors, conduct disorders, inappropriate aggression, not meeting developmental tasks, sleep disorders, inability to experience joy (anhedonia), and self-destructive behaviors. There is a higher risk of depression in children when one or both parents suffer from major depression. Depression can also be a secondary reaction to other problems such as learning disorders and substance abuse. Children have been treated successfully with antidepressants in conjunction with psychotherapeutic interventions. Maternal depression while a child is young puts him or her at particularly high risk.

ADOLESCENTS

Adolescents often do not express feelings of depression verbally because they may fear exhibiting feelings of vulnerability and dependency. Rather, their feelings of depression are often expressed in self-destructive or antisocial behaviors including sexual promiscuity, school truancy, threats, or petty crime. Some experts believe that substance abuse and eating disorders in adolescence may be masking or related to depression. A depression-prone adolescent with low self-esteem will have greater difficulty achieving a positive sense of self as an adult. Adolescent victims of abuse are particularly vulnerable to depression.

POSTPARTUM

Debate continues as to whether the cause of postpartum depression is solely hormonal or represents an intermingling of psychologic and physiologic stressors. Although postpartum "blues" (a few days of labile mood after the birth of a baby) are extremely common, more severe reactions are relatively rare. Postpartum depression can include psychotic symptoms including delusions that often concern the newborn infant. Bonding with the infant is disrupted. Women with a history of prenatal depression and bipolar disorder are at higher risk. Once a woman experiences a major postpartum depression with psychotic features, the risk of recurrence in subsequent deliveries is between 30 and 50 percent (DSM-IV, 1994).

ELDERLY PEOPLE

Depression is the most common emotional disorder of later life. Elderly people are at higher risk because they experience more multiple losses and medical illnesses than the rest of the population. However, in geriatric patients depression is more likely to be masked rather than exhibited by typical depression symptoms such as sadness, so it is often not diagnosed. Symptoms are often more physical or expressed as personality changes, including irritability. Depression can also be superimposed on dementia or confused with pseudodementia because common depressive symptoms in elderly persons include confusion, distractibility, and memory loss. In addition, some of the physical symptoms of depression such as fatigue, anorexia, constipation, and psychomotor retardation can be confused with physical illness, medication interactions, substance abuse, or "signs of old age." Treatment with antidepressants must be very closely supervised because of the possibility of severe side effects, but it can be very helpful. Electroshock treatments may also be tried in an elderly patient who is unresponsive to antidepressants.

POSSIBLE NURSES' REACTIONS

- May feel depressed when working with these patients. A patient's despair and unhappiness can be very painful to be around and could lead to the nurse's avoidance of the patient.
- May reject the patient because of own perception of the patient's dependency. Or may become overinvolved because of patient's needs and inadvertently create more dependency.
- May resent patient because of the longer time it takes to provide care.
- May feel angry or frustrated with depressed patient who isn't "helping himself or herself" or can't just "snap out of it."
- May feel inadequate when unable to make a quick impact on a patient's depression. Nurse may create unrealistic expectations of patient's recovery.
- Staff members may have inaccurate beliefs about the cause of depression, which may lead to their minimizing the degree of the patient's suffering.
- Because of the high prevalence of depression in our society, the nurse may have personally experienced it or may have witnessed a family member's struggle with depression. This can cause the nurse to identify with the depressed patient and reexperience these feelings.
- Reaction may depend on whether the nurse believes that the expression of sadness is an acceptable behavior; for example, the nurse may believe sadness is acceptable in women but not in men.

ASSESSMENT

Behavior and Appearance

- Persistently sad, anguished, or apathetic facial expression
- Dejected appearance: Head down, poor eye contact, posture slumped as if bearing a heavy weight
- Psychomotor agitation and/or retardation
- Decreased interest in grooming and self-care
- Decreased sexual interest
- Makes statements like "I don't care any more"
- May have difficulty with even simple tasks
- Anhedonia

Mood and Emotions

- Dysphoric mood: Verbalizes feelings of sadness and depression
- Inability to enjoy activities that were enjoyed previously
- Low self-esteem with feelings of worthlessness and inadequacy
- Feeling ineffective, powerless, and helpless
- Pessimistic: May appear brooding and express feelings of futility and despair
- Feelings of great heaviness
- Mild to high levels of anxiety, possibly including panic attacks and irritability
- Unexpressed anger, turned inward against self
- May express generalized anger
- Ambivalence: may feel two opposing ways at the same time

Thoughts, Beliefs, and Perceptions

- Thoughts slowed
- Poor concentration with possible temporary impairment of recent memory
- Self-doubt with relentless rumination and obsessions
- Lack of self-worth: Believes self undeserving of good experiences
- Indecisiveness
- Preoccupation with body changes
- Loss of perspective: May reject positive comments from others; gives self no credit for achievements
- Excessive guilt: condemns self; feels deserving of punishment
- Narrowing of interest to self
- Possible suicidal thoughts
- Confusion
- In severe depression: delusions; hallucinations that express feelings of worthlessness; guilt
- Believes life has no meaning and that there is no future

Relationships and Interactions

- Withdrawal from social interactions
- Deterioration of relationships because of preoccupation with self, anger, and anxiety
- Increasing dependence on others because of inability to make decisions or care for self

Physical Responses

- Slowed physiologic functioning evidenced by:
  - Lethargy and fatigue, especially in the morning
  - Constipation
  - Decreased appetite with weight loss or increased appetite with weight gain
  - Sleep problems including early morning awakening, frequent awakenings, waking up feeling tired, sleeping all the time

○ Body aches; pains such as headaches; indigestion; dizziness
- Thyroid function tests may be ordered to rule out hypothyroidism

Pertinent History

- Past history of depression, bipolar disorder, panic attacks, suicide attempts
- Family history of depression
- History of substance abuse
- History of stroke or myocardial infarction (particularly high rate of depression)

COLLABORATIVE MANAGEMENT

Pharmacologic

The advent of so many new antidepressants has provided many more opportunities for successful treatment. Because there are so many on the market, the specific medication choice is based on side effects, patient profile, history of previous response, type of depression, concurrent medical or psychiatric illnesses, and other medications the patient is taking. See Chapter 20 for a detailed discussion of antidepressants, their side effects, and nursing implications. Most antidepressants require at least 3 to 4 weeks of use before full benefits are obtained. Often, relief of other symptoms occurs before a change in the patient's subjective sense of feeling better. Side effects must be monitored closely. The patient may need to remain on a maintenance dose of antidepressant for many years.

Monoamine oxidase inhibitors (MAOIs) are less used today but may be a second-line treatment for depressions that do not respond to the more commonly used antidepressants. If the patient is experiencing anxiety, panic attacks, hallucinations, or delusions, other medications may need to be added.

Herbal products that are used for depression include stimulants such as ma huang, which contains ephedra. SAM-e is sometimes used for depression. The most common herbal product for this use is St. John's wort. As with most herbal products, there are potential side effects and drug interactions. St. John's wort is known to interact with some HIV medications and can inhibit effectiveness. An alternative, nonpharmacologic approach is light therapy, particularly useful in seasonal affective disorders.

Psychotherapy

Psychotherapy is recommended for mild to moderate major depression and in conjunction with antidepressants in more severe depressions. The federal guidelines on depression (DHHS, 1993) recommend a short-term trial of 6 to 12 weeks of psychotherapy to determine symptom response. If there is no significant improvement after 12 weeks, antidepressants should be added or changed. One short-term psychotherapy approach is cognitive therapy. This method is brief, structured, directive treatment designed to alter the negative thoughts so common in depression. Group therapy can also be helpful to enhance the patient's socialization.

Electroconvulsive Therapy

Electroconvulsive therapy (ECT) is a first-line treatment option only for patients with more severe or psychotic forms of depression. It may also be used for those who have failed to respond to other therapies or those with medical conditions that preclude the use of antidepressants.

NURSING MANAGEMENT

SELF-CARE DEFICIT EVIDENCED BY DECREASED ABILITY TO MANAGE OWN HYGIENE, GROOMING, FEEDING, AND DAILY ACTIVITIES RELATED TO LOSS OF ENERGY, INHIBITION OF MOTIVATION, ANXIETY, AND/OR DEPENDENCY.

Patient Outcomes

- Increased participation in self-care, daily activities
- Improved grooming and hygiene

Interventions

- Determine patient's level of self-care before onset of depressive symptoms to set realistic goals.
- Assess whether the patient is expressing certain psychologic needs such as dependency or rebellion by not performing self-care. Observe whether patient acts more independently when unaware of being watched.
- Encourage as much independence as possible. Take the time to allow patient to do things for himself or herself. Assign care to staff member who may have more time or is especially patient. Make sure all staff members reinforce patient's participation. Encourage patient's participation in decisions about timing, sequence, and approaches to self-care.
- Create a positive attitude that patient can learn and progress with practice. Avoid taking over for the patient if he or she has trouble.
- Break down tasks into small steps so patient can experience some success. For instance, have the patient focus on washing his or her face rather than completing the whole bath.
- Create an environment to ease patient's participation, such as having proper utensils available at mealtime or having the walker available in room if patient is ambulating to bathroom.
- Provide reassurance and encouragement. Avoid minimizing patient's problems or infantilizing him or her.
- At times, a nurse may need to make all decisions for a very depressed patient such as when to eat. Then, as the patient begins to improve, limited

options can be presented. With further improvement, the patient should take on increasing decision making.

> **SELF-ESTEEM DISTURBANCE** EVIDENCED BY STATEMENTS OF LOW SELF-ESTEEM, MISINTERPRETING POSITIVE OR PLEASURABLE EXPERIENCES, EXPRESSIONS OF SHAME AND GUILT RELATED TO FEELINGS, THOUGHTS OF WORTHLESSNESS, FAILURES, AND NEGATIVE REINFORCEMENT.

Patient Outcomes

- Identifies positive aspects of self
- Modifies unrealistic expectations for self
- Demonstrates reduced symptoms of depression

Interventions

- Provide emotional nurturing through empathetic listening and supportive encouragement. Treating the patient as a valued individual will enhance his or her self-esteem.
- Avoid blanket reassurances like "things will get better soon." These tend to alienate the patient, who may feel that you don't understand his or her pain.
- Encourage patient to share feelings, especially negative ones. If this is too difficult, consider alternative means of expression such as writing about feelings or drawing pictures.
- Point out any specific improvement, no matter how small. Depressed people often do not see improvement because they are so focused on the negative. Consider keeping a progress chart at the bedside to record concrete accomplishments such as the number of times the patient ambulates or the percentage of food he or she eats.
- Encourage patient to speak up if he or she disagrees or feels his or her rights are being violated. Reinforce assertive response.
- Recognize and point out manifestations of self-destructive or self-undermining thinking or behavior:
  - Requiring self to be perfect or setting unattainable goals
  - Assuming responsibility for and feeling guilt about failures and events that are outside the patient's control
  - Basing entire feeling of self-worth on one achievement or attribute, a single relationship, or obtaining approval from others
  - Projecting own feelings of self-hate onto family, staff, or friends, such as "All the nurses hate me." "My family blames me for my illness."
  - Expressing self-hate directly via suicidal thoughts and behavior
  - Expressing self-hate indirectly with repeated accidents, noncompliance, provoking or being antagonistic to others, thereby unwittingly creating rejection
  - Covering poor self-esteem with anger, blaming, or other maneuvers that displace responsibility onto others

- Suggest that the patient identify a few achievements from the past.
- Discuss and practice with patient alternative ways to respond to stress and to ask for what he or she wants.

> **POWERLESSNESS** EVIDENCED BY LACK OF INITIATIVE, NONACHIEVEMENT OF REALISTIC GOALS, PASSIVITY; NONPARTICIPATION IN DECISION MAKING RELATED TO DECREASED MOTIVATION, DECREASED ENERGY, HOPELESSNESS, PERFECTIONISTIC EXPECTATIONS OR SADNESS.

Patient Outcomes

- Identifies factors that he or she can control
- Participates in decisions about his or her care

Interventions

- Encourage the patient to describe feelings or the experience of powerlessness. Let the patient know that you are interested and you understand his or her pain. For instance, you may state, "You believe there is no hope for you to ever feel better."
- Once the patient indicates that he or she feels understood, suggest alternative viewpoints. Work with patient to identify times in life when he or she felt better or felt more in control.
- Work with the patient to identify realistic goals to work toward. Encourage having patience and accepting current limitations. Break down goals into small steps and recognize progress as each is achieved.
- Allow the patient to maintain reasonable control over some of the daily routine if able.
- Have the patient list specific situations in which he or she felt powerless. Correct distorted assumptions, discuss alternative ways to handle situations, and identify helpful resources.
- Direct the patient to other topics if he or she obsesses on unrealistic goals or things that cannot be changed.

ALTERNATE NURSING DIAGNOSES

Altered Nutrition
Anxiety
Dysfunctional Grieving
Hopelessness
Impaired Social Interaction
Altered Thought Processes
Ineffective Individual Coping
Risk for Injury
Sleep Pattern Disturbance
Social isolation

WHEN TO CALL FOR HELP

☐ Extreme self-care deficit to point of not being able to care for basic needs

☐ Suicidal thoughts, threats, or attempts

☐ Hallucinations or delusions

☐ Severe side effects from antidepressants, including severe urinary retention, dramatic fluctuations in blood pressure, cardiac complications, seizures

PATIENT AND FAMILY EDUCATION

- Teach the patient that depression can generate feelings of helplessness, powerlessness, and pessimism. Encourage the patient to delay major decisions and actions based on those feelings, and reinforce the idea that the severe symptoms will abate with treatment and time.
- Reinforce the idea that depression is a treatable illness. Even though the patient may feel hopeless, the illness is not.
- For patients on antidepressants, review potential side effects and importance of taking the medication even when they start feeling better. Patient should know which side effects to report to physician.
- Inform the patient that other medications are available if the side effects from the current one are too uncomfortable.
- Encourage the patient to maintain a schedule of activity.
- Explain to the family the symptoms of depression, medication management, and interventions and what the family can do to assist and encourage the patient.
- Teach the patient and family to report signs of increasing depression or suicidal thoughts.
- Teach the patient that long-term, enduring self-esteem comes from beliefs about self as a valuable human being and is expressed through achievements, relationships, and healthful living.
- Inform the patient that the negative assumptions about himself or herself are not necessarily true.

CHARTING TIPS

- Document patient activity, intake, sleep patterns, and bowel patterns.
- Document any expressed suicide thoughts, plans, or attempts.
- Document side effects of medication.
- Document patient response to encouragement or support.

COMMUNITY-BASED CARE

- Strongly encourage patient to seek counseling. Give appropriate referrals. If patient is too depressed to have the energy to follow through, involve family or friends in seeking help.
- If patient is unable to care for himself or herself or is potentially suicidal, work with other members of the team as well as family to determine discharge options. Patient may need psychiatric hospitalization or temporary placement in a board and care or convalescent facility.
- Refer patient for psychiatric home health care for follow-up on medication compliance and self-care activities.
- Encourage patient to maintain follow-up with physician and compliance with treatment plan.

THE SUICIDAL PATIENT

LEARNING OBJECTIVES

➤ Identify risk factors for suicide.
➤ Differentiate between a suicide attempt and a suicide gesture.
➤ Describe effective interventions to protect the high-risk patient in the hospital.
➤ Describe common nurses' reactions to the suicidal patient.

GLOSSARY

Completed suicide—Suicide attempt resulting in death.

Lethality—The level of risk in suicide method chosen to cause death. The more lethal methods include guns, jumping, and hanging. Lower lethality methods include superficially slashing wrists, inhaling house gas, and ingesting pills because death is not immediate and there is more of a chance of being found and treated.

Suicidal ideation—Thoughts about harming one's self.

Suicide—A broad range of behaviors in which a person causes his or her own death.

Suicide attempt—Any act intended to end in suicide.

Suicide gesture—Any action that appears to be a suicide attempt but that is actually contrived or manipulative and that results in only minimal harm, such as superficial cuts on the wrist or a small overdose of sleeping pills.

Suicide threat—Verbal threat to commit suicide.

Some nurses mistakenly believe suicidal patients are found only in psychiatric settings. However, patients with suicidal tendencies are not always easily identified, and they can be the same patients you care for in an intensive care unit, medical unit, nursing home, or in their own homes.

Many people have experienced momentary self-destructive thoughts. But obsessive preoccupation with these thoughts and acting on them is another matter. Thinking about suicide does not mean that the individual will act on those thoughts; however, anyone who talks about, threatens, or attempts suicide must be taken seriously. In approximately 70 percent of suicides, the individual has one or more active or chronic medical illnesses at the time of death (DHHS, 1993). See Table 9–1 for key risk factors.

There are approximately seven suicide attempts for every completed suicide. Women make more attempts than men, but men are more likely to complete the suicide because they tend to use more lethal methods, particularly firearms. Generally, the risk of suicide is greater when the plan is more detailed and the method more lethal and accessible.

Statistics show that suicide is the eleventh leading cause of death in this country. (Moscicki, 1997) However, it may be higher because hidden suicides such

TABLE 9–1. SUICIDE: INTENSITY OF RISK

Behaviors or Symptoms	Intensity of Risk		
	Low	Moderate	High
Anxiety	Mild	Moderate	High or panic state
Depression	Mild	Moderate	Severe
Isolation or withdrawal	Some feelings of isolation; no withdrawal	Some feelings of helplessness, hopelessness, or withdrawal	Hopeless, helpless, withdrawn, self-deprecating
Daily functioning	Fairly good in most activities	Moderately good in some activities	Not good in any activities
Resources	Several	Some	Few or none
Coping strategies being used	Generally constructive	Some are constructive	Predominantly destructive
Significant others	Several available	Few or only one available	Only one or none available
Previous psychiatric help	None, or positive attitude toward	Yes, and moderately satisfied with	Negative view of help received
Lifestyle	Stable	Moderately stable	Unstable
Alcohol or drug use	Infrequently to excess	Frequently to excess	Continual use
Previous suicide attempts	None or low lethality	One or more; moderate lethality	Multiple attempts; high lethality
Disorientation or disorganization	None	Some	Marked
Depression	Some feeling	Some feelings	Negative view of self
Hostility	Little or none	Some	Marked
Suicide plan	Vague fleeting thoughts but no plan	Frequent thoughts; occasional ideas about a plan	Frequent or constant thought with a specific plan

Source: Adapted with permission from Suicide: Assessment and Interventions, by Hatton, C, and Valente S, Appleton-Century-Crofts, Norwalk, CT, 1984.

as "accidental" overdoses, auto accidents, noncompliance with medical regimens, or not seeking medical care for symptoms are not reported as suicides.

Because suicide is basically not accepted by our culture, it generates anxiety that has led to a number of myths (Box 9–2).

Surviving family and friends of the suicide victim often experience complicated grief reactions that may affect them for the rest of their lives. They are faced with the stigma of this form of death as well as many unresolved feelings of anger and guilt. Unfortunately, they may receive less support from others because of the discomfort surrounding the cause of death. In addition, many life insurance policies do not cover self-inflicted death, so the surviving family may be economically devastated.

BOX 9–2. Clearing Up the Myths About Suicide

Myth	Truth
Asking people about their suicidal thoughts will make them more likely to act on them.	Most patients are not afraid to talk about their thoughts of committing suicide and are usually grateful that someone is available and cares. Talking can reduce the sense of isolation.
All people who attempt suicide have a psychiatric disorder.	People can become overwhelmed with life circumstances without having a psychiatric disorder.
A person who talks about suicide won't do it.	Approximately 80 percent of individuals who attempt or complete suicide give some definite verbal or indirect clues. As many as 50 percent have seen their physician within the previous month, often with vague somatic complaints.
A person who attempts suicide won't try again.	Almost 75 percent of those individuals who complete suicide have attempted it at least once before.
People who attempt suicide are always determined to die.	Many individuals are ambivalent and are using the suicide as a cry for help.
People who attempt suicide just want attention.	Even if the suicide attempt is manipulative, the individual may go on to complete the suicide.
As the person becomes less depressed, the risk of suicide decreases.	As the depression lifts, the individual's energy level can increase before feelings of hopelessness are relieved. Once the individual makes the decision that suicide is an effective solution to the problems, his or her mood may even elevate.

ETIOLOGY

Suicide is not a disease in itself but a symptom of some underlying problem. *Biologic and genetic* theories are closely tied to those causing depression. It is believed that low levels of the neurotransmitters, serotonin and norepinephrine, are a factor in the decision to commit suicide. There is also a strong link to alcohol and substance abuse. Suicidal behavior also runs in families. This may be related to genetics or to psychological factors in which suicide is viewed as an acceptable way to cope. The risk of suicide in family members of individuals who have committed suicide is 15 times greater than in the general population.

Psychologic theory focuses on a number of motivating forces. Suicide can be a way to escape deep psychologic pain or atone for past sins. Intense feelings of hopelessness and helplessness are key factors. It can be related to unacceptable feelings of aggression, which the individual turns inward. The individual could believe that he or she is reuniting with a loved one. The wish to instill guilt in a significant person who is perceived as abandoning or rejecting could motivate the suicidal person. Individuals with limited coping reserves who become overwhelmed with stress may seek self-destructive acts as a way to escape these feelings. Because the suicidal person may be severely depressed, the theories on etiology of depression and substance abuse may also relate to suicide.

Suicidal behavior can also be a symptom of psychosis as the person acts out hallucinations or delusions. Command hallucinations, in which voices tell the patient to kill himself or herself, create a very high risk. Severe anxiety and distress regarding psychotic symptoms as well as lack of judgment or reality testing may lead to suicide as a way to escape overwhelming anxiety or disturbed thoughts.

Suicidal gestures with nonlethal self-mutilation may occur in individuals who have poor impulse control or a high need for the attention or control of others. An individual with a history of multiple threats and gestures may have a borderline or other personality disorder.

Sociologic views look at a person who may feel alienated from others. A susceptible individual who no longer feels part of his or her culture or social group could be at an increased risk, especially if cultural or religious taboos against suicide are not very strong. For some, suicide is a way of expressing political beliefs. Economic losses or unemployment could also play a role as a person feels trapped and powerless to change. Suicide is an increasing problem in minority and economically deprived groups. It can also be associated with substance abuse.

RELATED CLINICAL CONCERNS

Physical illness is a frequent contributor to suicidal behavior. Illnesses associated with suffering and dependency, such as advanced cancer and AIDS, can be associated with higher suicide rates. Uncontrolled pain and delirium are the key variables with these illnesses. Controversy over the terminal patient's "right" to commit suicide has recently received much attention. Right-to-die groups have supported initiatives in several states seeking physician-assisted suicide for terminal patients. The patient's ability to remain in control until death is a key motivation for this action. Other illnesses, such as multiple sclerosis and Huntington's disease, that may not be terminal but are chronic and debilitating may also be associated with increased suicide risk. Suicidal patients with physical illnesses should be carefully evaluated and treated for depression. In addition, every effort to identify and control any uncomfortable symptoms will enhance quality of life.

Medications that contribute to depressive or psychotic symptoms could also precipitate a suicide attempt. See Box 9–1 and Box 11–3 for lists of medications that contribute to these symptoms. Patients with suicidal tendencies who are taking prescribed analgesics, tranquilizers, or sleeping pills may be at risk for saving up medications to use later for a possible suicide attempt.

LIFE SPAN ISSUES

CHILDREN

Although the rate of suicide in children is low, it is rising and is cause for great concern and analysis. Young children have tried to kill themselves by jumping out of windows, hanging themselves, or running in front of moving cars. These actions are generally impulsive and in response to intense emotion. A suicidal act may be an attempt to gain power, punish a parent, or escape stressful situations. It could also be a response to parental neglect, rejection, or abuse. A young child who does not understand the finality of death may not understand the consequences of his or her action. Children could also be imitating parental behaviors. Suicidal behavior can also be related to substance abuse and school problems.

ADOLESCENTS

Suicidal behavior in adolescents is considered a serious health problem. It is the second leading cause of death in teens, accidents being the first. And some accidents could be concealed suicide attempts. Teens who are depressed, socially isolated, or using drugs and alcohol are at highest risk. Low self-esteem, history of abuse, not fitting in with peers, and school pressures may be other risk factors. As with adults, girls make more attempts but boys are more likely to use more lethal methods such as firearms. The availability of firearms in our society is believed to contribute to the increase in teenage suicides. Carbon monoxide poisoning and ingestion of pills are other common methods used by adolescents. High-risk behaviors like drug use, drag racing, and gang activity could be masking suicidal thoughts.

"Cluster" suicide, in which adolescents copy an episode of suicide of an acquaintance or celebrity, is a recent and alarming trend. To some teens the suicide of an idol can be romanticized.

ELDERLY PEOPLE

Elderly people commit suicide more often than any other age group in the United States. Elderly white men over age 80 are at highest risk (Moscicki, 1999). Guns remain the most frequent method. Suicide statistics in elderly persons are probably even higher because of the prevalence of passive suicides. Elderly people are more likely to use noncompliance with medical regimens or refusal to eat as a way to hasten their death. Risk factors include living alone, widowhood, lack of financial resources, poor health, and social isolation. In addition, misuse of alcohol and antianxiety medications may contribute.

POSSIBLE NURSES' REACTIONS

- May see a suicidal patient as weak or bad because of personal religious or moral beliefs.
- May experience feelings of anxiety with these patients, which prevent recognition of warning signs.
- May avoid dealing with suicidal patients for fear of saying the wrong thing or contributing to their suicide because of lack of adequate training. May believe talking to patient about suicide would increase risk.
- May believe he or she is rescuing patient and then experience intense guilt if patient does attempt or complete suicide. May take patient's behavior as a personal rejection.
- May feel angry with patient for creating chaos, especially if the nurse perceives that the patient has much to live for, such as children and a good job. The nurse's anger may conflict with his or her mission of promoting health and saving lives.
- May deny or minimize suicidal behavior as a defense against anxiety and helplessness.
- Patient's behavior could stir up personal feelings of depression. Nurses have six times the suicide rate of the general population and much higher lethality because of their knowledge and access to drugs.

ASSESSMENT

Behavior and Appearance

- Direct verbal statements (e.g., "I wish I were dead")
- Indirect verbal statements (e.g.,"You won't see me when you come back to work" or asking about specific suicide methods)
- Giving away possessions
- Agitation
- Sudden changes in eating, sleeping, or usual activities
- Neglecting appearance or hygiene
- Drawing up a will
- Refusing medications

Mood and Emotions

- Depression or despair
- Sudden lifting of depression, sudden elevation in mood
- Apathy
- Hopelessness
- Helplessness
- Anxiety
- Bitter anger

Thoughts, Beliefs, and Perceptions

- Disorganized, chaotic, irrational thinking
- Tunnel vision—unable to see options other than death
- Poor judgment
- Persecutory delusions and hallucinations, especially commands
- Excessive guilt or self-blame
- Low self-esteem

Relationships and Interactions

- Social isolation; withdrawn; feels alone and abandoned
- Recent loss of significant person through death or separation
- Recent tumultuous termination or interruption of psychiatric treatment

Physical Responses

- Chronic debilitating illness
- Unrelieved pain
- Terminal illness
- Recent, catastrophic loss of physical abilities

Pertinent History

- History of suicide attempts
- Self-destructive behavior, such as drug abuse, reckless acts, or self-mutilation
- Family history of suicide attempts or depression
- Psychiatric illness
- Recent significant loss

COLLABORATIVE INTERVENTIONS

Pharmacologic

Suicidal patients may benefit from taking antianxiety medication, such as lorazepam, to reduce feelings of intense anxiety or distress. In addition, antipsychotic and antimanic medication may be prescribed as needed. If antidepressants are being started, it is important to remember that it will take a number of weeks to lift depression, so other interventions must be used in the interim to prevent suicide. Antidepressants could actually increase suicide risk if the patient gets a sudden burst of energy to act out the plan before the depression lifts. Overdosing on antidepressants is an increasingly frequent method of suicide.

Adequate symptom management for pain and other distressing symptoms must be provided to the patient with a serious or terminal illness. A patient's belief that his or her symptoms cannot be controlled could be a contributing factor in suicide.

Patients at high risk for suicide may need to have medications administered in liquid or parenteral form to avoid "cheeking" and hoarding pills. Outpatients should be given only a few days' supply of any medication that could potentially be used in a suicide attempt.

NURSING MANAGEMENT

RISK FOR VIOLENCE TO SELF EVIDENCED BY SUICIDE ATTEMPTS, SELF-MUTILATION, SUICIDE PLAN RELATED TO SUICIDE IDEATION, POOR IMPULSE CONTROL, DEPRESSION.

Patient Outcomes

- Remains free from injury
- Verbalizes intent not to harm self
- Expresses more optimistic view of future in specific terms

Interventions

- Determine if patient has a plan and how potentially lethal and available that plan is. (Box 9–3). A patient in the hospital who talks about using a gun to kill himself or herself would be at lower risk (until discharge) as long as he or she does not have a gun available. A patient who has a stash of medication would be at higher risk. Seek input from other professionals to participate in this assessment. If your agency has mental health professionals on staff, it is essential to involve them in the assessment. See high risk interventions in subsequent text.
- Make a thorough assessment of patient's risk of suicide (see Table 9–1). Note: research is being conducted to develop assessment rating scales to better predict suicide potential.
- Talk openly with patient about your concern that he or she is suicidal. Let the patient know you are concerned and available to help and that confidentiality is shared among the entire healthcare team for optimum care. Encouraging the patient to talk about this does not increase risk for suicide. Do not promise to keep secrets from the team. Notify all members of the healthcare team of the patient's risk of suicide. Staff members must be supportive, empathetic, and familiar with treatment plan.

BOX 9–3. Assessing Current Suicide Lethality

1. Do you think about hurting or killing yourself? If yes:
2. Do you have a plan? How have you considered doing it? If yes:
3. Do you think you may or will do something to act on your thoughts? If yes, where and when? Do you feel you have control over your own behavior?
4. Do you have the means available (such as rope, rolled-up sheet, gun, saved-up pills [note lethality of plan])?
5. Have you ever tried to harm yourself in the past? If yes, how? Did you expect to survive?
6. Are you willing to contract or notify staff whenever you feel you may act on these thoughts? Our side of the contract is to be available and actively help you during these times.

If patient denies having a suicide plan, ask about other plans for the future and support systems.

1. What do you see yourself doing in a week, in a month, and in a year from now?
2. Do you feel optimistic or pessimistic about the future?
3. Do you have family members or friends with whom you can freely discuss your problems?

- If the patient has attempted suicide, see Box 9–4.
- Talk to patient about making a no-suicide contract with you. Ask him or her to wait or postpone action so that you and other professionals have time to help. Point out that depression is not permanent (with time, medication, and therapy there is hope for a change) but that death is permanent and cuts off other options. Renew the contract each shift and as needed between patient and main caregiver.

BOX 9–4. Assessing the Suicide Attempt

1. Did the patient expect to die? (yes, no, uncertain). Did the patient think his or her chance of dying was high, medium, or low? Did he or she underestimate?
2. How does the patient feel about surviving? If the patient regrets surviving, question him or her about any current plan to attempt suicide.
3. If the patient's objective in suicide attempt or gesture was to manipulate a significant other to behave differently, have the sought-after changes occurred? Does the patient have alternative, more adaptive methods for coping?
4. Is the support system present (helpful, unhelpful)?
5. Does the patient have any hope for the future? How optimistic or pessimistic is he or she?
6. Is the patient willing to make a no-suicide contract?

- Never attempt to work with a suicidal patient by yourself. Involve all members of the team. Seek additional resources such as social workers; notify supervisory staff.

For patients assessed to be at high risk for suicide:

- Follow agency policy for need for continuous supervision. Discourage use of family for this purpose.
- If patient is in the hospital, arrange for a room close to the nurses' station or in an ICU for closer monitoring.
- Avoid checking on patient at predictable intervals; check more frequently during danger times (changes of shift) when patient may think staff will be preoccupied.
- Remove objects with self-harm potential (such as glasses, razors, belts, or lighters) from the room. Be aware of agency policy regarding need to search personal belongings or do a body search.
- Make sure windows cannot be opened.
- If all other interventions have been ineffective, use physical restraints for brief periods to prevent patient self-harm.
- Make sure family and friends are not bringing in potentially dangerous items such as medications, alcohol, or razors.
- Arrange (per physician) to transfer the suicidal patient to a psychiatric unit as soon as medically stable.
- If patient is not hospitalized, make sure family and friends are aware of the possible suicide risk. The patient probably should not be left alone. Give him or her a list of resources such as hotlines, therapists' phone numbers, or support people he or she can call. Call MD/Psychiatric Assessment Team if you believe the patient is still at risk of suicide.

HOPELESSNESS EVIDENCED BY EXPECTATIONS THAT THERE WILL BE NO IMPROVEMENT IN SITUATION RELATED TO DEPRESSION; OVERWHELMED BY LIFE CIRCUMSTANCES.

Patient Outcomes

- Verbalizes more optimistic expectations for the future
- Initiates realistic plans for the immediate future
- Demonstrates initiative in decision making

Interventions

- Recognize that extreme hopelessness is a strong indicator of suicide; assess thoroughly.
- Listen to patient's concerns and issues. Convey empathy to promote verbalizing about doubts and fears. Reflect back patient's despair without agreeing with it. For instance, you might say "You describe a world that seems empty."
- Encourage patient to discuss recent events or stresses that have contributed

to the hopeless view. Offer alternative analysis viewing the event without arguing or minimizing patient's concerns. Minimizing or joking about the patient's feelings will increase the patient's sense of isolation and lack of trust.

- Emphasize the patient's strengths and problem-solving abilities. Describe a recent situation in which you observed the patient being successful. Have him or her describe a past success. Point out obstacles or negative thinking that get in the way of effective problem solving.
- Provide a balanced point of view to counteract patient's tendency to judge himself or herself harshly. Point out unrealistic, perfectionistic thinking. Offer more constructive interpretations to open real options for the future.
- Acknowledge that you understand that the patient feels that everything is useless and nothing will help, but also that you believe something helpful can be done.

INEFFECTIVE INDIVIDUAL COPING EVIDENCED BY REPEATED SUICIDE THREATS/GESTURES, RELATED TO STUNTED AREAS OF PERSONALITY DEVELOPMENT WITH INTERMITTENT SELF-DESTRUCTIVE IMPULSES.

Patient Outcomes

- Decrease in self-destructive behaviors
- Demonstrates more adaptive means of communicating thoughts, feelings, and needs

Interventions

- Determine if self-destructive behavior is a pattern.
- Remain calm and neutral; treat patient's suicide threats and gestures in matter-of-fact manner. Treat any physical injury without excessive emotion. Avoid creating a sense of alarm about the patient's behavior. *Caution:* Do not dismiss any threat or gesture as manipulative or not serious. Any self-destructive threat or gesture should be taken seriously and not ignored.
- Ask the patient to identify any disturbing thoughts or feelings that occurred just before the threat or action. Encourage him or her to put thoughts and feelings into words rather than acting them out impulsively and destructively. Teach that anger can hide more painful feelings such as sadness and rejection.
- Teach alternate coping: talking, relaxation, distraction, exercise, music, and so forth.
- Confront the patient who wants to commit suicide for revenge and retaliation. These patients may state, "They'll be sorry when I'm dead." Remind patient this is not a solution because he or she won't be there to see the results.
- Encourage the patient to alert staff members if feeling out of control or when having thoughts of self-harm. Consider discussing a no-suicide contract and including guidelines for behavior.
- Establish limits with patient on amount of time staff will spend listening to patient's concerns. Set limits on the patient's use of verbal abuse and demands.

- Review with the patient possible causes for self-destructive behavior that could include an attempt to get others to assume responsibility for patient's life. The patient needs to be encouraged to take more self-responsibility. See Chapter 12, The Manipulative Patient, for additional interventions.

ALTERNATE NURSING DIAGNOSES

Altered Thought Processes
Anxiety
Dysfunctional Grieving
Risk for Self-Mutilation
Self-Concept Disturbance
Spiritual Distress (Distress of the Human Spirit)

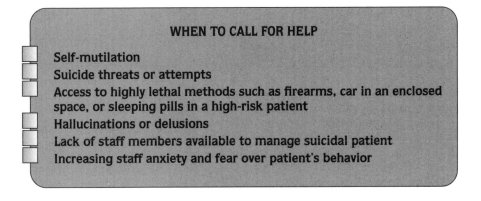

WHEN TO CALL FOR HELP

Self-mutilation

Suicide threats or attempts

Access to highly lethal methods such as firearms, car in an enclosed space, or sleeping pills in a high-risk patient

Hallucinations or delusions

Lack of staff members available to manage suicidal patient

Increasing staff anxiety and fear over patient's behavior

PATIENT AND FAMILY EDUCATION

- Teach patient that his or her view of the options available becomes narrowed when he or she is depressed or suicidal. Review alternative ways of viewing problems.
- Review with the patient the idea that he or she needs to reach out to others for support and assistance. Teach the patient to reach out immediately when feeling the urge for self-harm.
- Encourage the patient to report and seek out adequate treatment for uncomfortable symptoms of physical illness, possibly including analgesics, to reduce suffering.
- Teach alternative outlets for anger rather than self-destructive ones. (See Coping Interventions.)
- Make sure that patient and family understand the purpose of close observation by staff members if patient is actively suicidal.
- Make sure that the family knows signs of increasing suicide risk and interventions.

- If a patient does commit suicide, prepare the family for the complex grief reaction that may follow (Box 9–5).

CHARTING TIPS

- Document all behaviors that could be considered a suicide thought, threat, or action, and who was notified about them.
- Note patient's response to suicide assessment.
- Document all measures in place to prevent suicide.
- Document patient's response to a no-suicide contract and teaching.
- Document any information from others on availability of potential methods for suicide available to the patient and interventions to protect patient.

COMMUNITY-BASED CARE

- Make sure that patient and family have information on referrals for follow-up counseling. They should also have emergency numbers such as suicide hotlines. Provide written information and education.
- Determine if psychiatric evaluation needs to be made before the patient leaves the agency/institution.
- Determine the appropriate quantities of prescribed medications to send home with the patient.
- Refer for home health follow-up and make sure that the agency is aware of the patient's suicide risk. Refer for psychiatric home care if available.
- If patient is high suicide risk, transfer to a psychiatric hospital.

BOX 9–5. Information for Survivors of Suicide

- Recognize that their grief may have an added burden of guilt, shame, and anger.
- Sharing their grief with others about the cause of death will put the tragedy out in the open and provide added support.
- Recognize that factors contributing to the suicide may be out of the family's control.
- Provide information on dynamics of suicide.
- Encourage attendance at bereavement support groups specific for survivors of suicide.

THE GRIEVING PATIENT

LEARNING OBJECTIVES

➤ Describe the variables that contribute to the intensity of the grief response.
➤ Describe some common behavioral responses to grief in children.
➤ Identify dysfunctional grief reactions.
➤ Describe effective nursing interventions to assist the grieving family.
➤ Describe common nursing staff reactions to the grieving patient.

GLOSSARY

Absent grief—In an effort to avoid aspects of the loss and avoid relinquishing the lost object, no grief is experienced.

Anticipatory grief—Grief response before and in preparation for a significant actual or potential loss.

Bereavement—State of having suffered a loss.

Delayed grief—The absence of grief behavior when it would be normally expected.

Distorted grief—Abnormal extension or overelaboration of grief behavior.

Dysfunctional or complicated grief—Grief reaction that does not follow the usual pattern and may include delayed and/or distorted grief.

Grief—Subjective, emotional response to a loss.

Loss—Situation, real or potential, in which a valued object is rendered inaccessible or is altered in such a way that it no longer has the valued qualities.

Mourning—The process by which grief is resolved.

Prolonged grief—Continued grief behavior lasting much longer than would be expected.

Experiencing loss, such as friends' moving away, loss of a job, loss of functional abilities or physical health, or the death of a loved one, is a normal part of life. Grief is the normal human response that usually follows these experiences. As things change in our lives, we must adapt. This process of adaptation is called grieving. The purpose of grief is to begin to face the loss, work through the emotions, and eventually let go or adapt with renewed energy to focus on new relationships and goals. Because all individuals respond to loss differently, the process of adapting varies widely and can take days, months, or years depending on many variables. Grief does not decline in a linear, predictable fashion over time. Rather, it can fluctuate over time and be affected by many factors. Variables that can influence the sense of loss include:

- The meaning of the lost object to the person (Generally, the more important the loss is to the person, the more intense the reaction.)
- The degree of preparation and past unresolved losses
- Physical health
- The degree of conflict or dependency in the relationship
- Support system
- Concurrent stressors

Culture also influences the way an individual responds to loss. Most cultures have specific rituals and traditions that provide support and reassurance during the grieving process. Grief caused by a death can be influenced by the cause of death. Unexpected deaths, deaths viewed as preventable, and the death of a child all create additional distress. Death resulting from a cause with a social stigma, such as suicide or AIDS, can be particularly difficult. With suicide, death is unexpected, violent, and possibly preventable. Survivors may experience intense anger, guilt, and self-blame. Those who lose a loved one from AIDS may have had time to prepare for the death, but many complicated feelings may still need to be resolved before grieving can be accomplished. Society's reactions to deaths caused by problems such as these may affect the type of support the mourners receive.

ETIOLOGY

There is no one comprehensive theory that explains normal grief. Research has shown that grief occurs in a sequence of phases or stages with predictable symptoms that change over time, and that these stages do not necessarily progress in an orderly, set fashion.

Acute grief symptoms were first described in Lindemann's classic study of 1944 after the Coconut Grove Night Club fire in Boston. Symptoms include sighing, sobbing, hyperventilating, and a sense of unreality or shock as the first reactions to facing a major loss. Elisabeth Kubler-Ross (1969) and Theresa Rando (1993) both describe stages through which individuals advance in their progression toward resolution (Table 9–2). These stages give us guides for expected behaviors, but each individual goes through the process in his or her own way and time. During the initial period of shock, the mourner may experience denial or avoidance as a protective mechanism from the over-

TABLE 9–2. ADAPTING TO LOSS

Stage	Purpose	Behavior
Rando's Stages of Adapting to Loss		
Avoidance phase	• Recognize the loss	• Acknowledge loss (intellectually first, then emotionally)
Confirmation phase	• React to separation	• Experience pain of loss—it will impact all areas of functioning
	• Recollect and re-experience the deceased	• Make changes in one's life to adapt to life without person
	• Relinquish old attachments to deceased and old assumptive world	• Change old habits, find new support systems
Accommodation phase	• Readjust to move adaptively into new world without forgetting old	• New relationship with deceased
		• Form new identity
	• Reinvest	• Emotional energy into new things
Kübler-Ross's Stages: Adapting to a Loss of Self		
Denial	• Unconscious avoidance to protect self from painful reality	• "No, not me."
		• Lack of expected reaction; using unproved treatment methods; doctor shopping to avoid confronting diagnosis
Anger	• Attempt to take control when feeling out of control by attacking, blaming others	• "Why me?"
		• Irrational demands; criticizing staff; hostile behavior
Bargaining	• Attempting to change reality by making agreement, bargains for more time	• "It's me, but . . ."
		• "I want to live til my son's wedding, then I'll accept death."
	• Indicates beginning acceptance	• Making bargains with God to change if can have more time, change reality
Depression	• Work of grief as realization hits	• "It's me."
	• Involves despair, the pain of experiencing loss	• Sad, tearful, life review
Acceptance	• Resolution of feelings about death	• Comforting others to accept impending death; remembering the past with fondness but without fighting to hang on to life
	• Neither happy nor sad	
	• Acceptance of reality, sense of peace and letting go	

Source: Adapted from Rando, 1993, and Kübler-Ross, 1969.

whelming stress to block out the pain. As denial and shock fade, the mourner begins to face the sadness of the loss. In addition to depression, there may be periods of anger and guilt. Anger can be directed at the lost person for leaving or the person responsible for the situation (if applicable), or it can be displaced onto others. Guilt feelings, possibly evidenced by self-reproach for real or imagined acts of negligence or omissions, can be especially painful. All of these behaviors force the individual to confront the pain over and over again.

However, not all reactions cause the individual to feel discomfort. Some can provide comfort, such as a sense of being watched over by the lost person.

The ability to tolerate intense emotions, increasing periods of stability, taking on new roles and relationships, and having the energy to invest oneself in new endeavors may indicate that the individual is recovering. Remembering both the positives and negatives of the lost person or object can indicate successful completion of grieving. However, brief periods of intense feelings may still occur at significant times, such as anniversaries and holidays. Because each individual is unique, the extent of a grief reaction may vary. People may grieve as deeply over the loss of a pet or a longed-for goal as over the death of a family member. In addition, the length of time to resolution is individual, not necessarily fitting the 1-year tradition. Also, grief may be delayed because of extreme situations, such as multiple losses, in which the mourner must deal with many responsibilities before taking time to experience the loss.

RELATED CLINICAL CONCERNS

The physical stress of grief can place the mourner at risk for health problems. Lack of sleep, poor eating, and changes in routine can predispose the individual to illness. Loss of a spouse in elderly people is associated with higher morbidity and mortality rates. Two months after a death, bereaved elderly persons report more illness, greater use of medications, and poor health ratings.

LIFE SPAN ISSUES

CHILDREN

Often adults try to protect children by not including them in the crisis or expressions of grief for other family members. However, they need to be included in the process, based on their level of development, so that they do not feel abandoned and left to face their fear and loss alone. Children generally display grief differently from adults, and it is important not to misinterpret their behaviors to mean that they are not grieving or that they are unaware of what is happening. Children often use symbolic or nonverbal language to communicate their awareness of loss and may even feel ashamed of their loss because they feel differently from their peers. Because they may also need more time to really assimilate what has happened, grief reactions may be delayed (Table 9–3).

ELDERLY PEOPLE

Elderly people face multiple changes, often including the loss of a spouse, friends, job, financial status, health, and mobility. In spite of the extent of these losses, most elderly persons seem able to adapt, probably because of their past experience. However, the death of a spouse or partner still remains

TABLE 9-3. CHILDREN'S UNDERSTANDING OF DEATH

Age	Understanding of Death	Common Behaviors in Response to Death
Infant to toddler	• Unable to comprehend death • Fears separation and abandonment	• Frightened, difficulty separating
3–5 years	• Views illness as punishment for real or imagined wrongdoings • May view death as sleep; cannot comprehend death • Magical thinking; may think they caused the event by their thoughts or actions	• Sadness • Clinging to parent • Nightmares, sleep disruption • Regression in toilet habits • Complaints of stomachache and headaches • Temper tantrums
School age	• Associates death with punishment, mutilation, violence • May feel responsible for event • By age 9, understands that death is final	• School phobia, diminished school performance • Aggressive behavior • Preoccupation with parent's health • Loss of appetite • Change in relationship with friends
Adolescence	• Understands own mortality • May seem to have adult view of death but not emotional view	• Acting out; substance abuse • Increased time with peers • Withdrawal from family • Depression

one of the major losses in life. This loss requires multiple life changes that become more difficult with increasing age. Grief can be masked by symptoms of dementia, depression, suicidal ideation, and substance abuse.

POSSIBLE NURSES' REACTIONS

- May feel helpless and uncomfortable, not knowing what to say. This could lead to avoidance or inappropriate hopefulness.
- May fear saying the wrong thing that will cause the patient or family to feel more pain.
- May fear losing control of emotions, crying.
- May make judgments regarding the degree of intensity of grief behavior, such as thinking that a family is "not upset enough."
- May feel guilty for "causing" client to cry when discussing the loss.
- May become detached from the situation and attempt to minimize the loss to the patient with phrases like "This was for the best" or "At least you can have more children."
- May expect all people to experience the stages of grief in the same way.
- May relive past and unresolved personal losses, causing intense emotions.

ASSESSMENT

Behavior and Appearance

- Crying, agitation
- Extreme change from usual behavior patterns
- Unable to concentrate, distractible
- Taking on behavior traits of lost person
- No apparent reaction when one would be expected
- Unkempt, not caring for self

Mood and Emotions

- Shock, numbness
- Depression (Table 9–4)
- Anxiety, panic
- Mood swings
- No obvious emotional reaction or one that is inappropriate to situation
- Anger
- Guilt, remorse
- Relief that ordeal is over

TABLE 9–4. DIFFERENTIATING GRIEF FROM DEPRESSION

	Uncomplicated Grief	**Major Depression**
Reactions	• Labile • Heightened when thinking of loss	• Mood consistently low • Prolonged, severe symptoms lasting over 2 months
Behavior	• Variable, shifts from sharing pain to being alone • Variable restriction of pleasure	• Completely withdrawn or fear of being alone • Persistent restriction of pleasure
Sleep patterns	• Periodic episodes of inability to sleep	• Wakes early morning
Anger	• Often expressed	• Turned inward
Sadness	• Varying periods	• Consistently sad
Cognition	• Preoccupied with loss • Self-esteem not as affected	• Focused on self • Feels worthless; has negative self-image
History	• Generally no history of depression	• History of depression or other psychiatric illness
Responsiveness	• Responds to warmth and support	• Hopelessness • Limited response to support
Loss	• Recognizable, current	• Often not related to an identified loss

Source: Adapted with permission. Schneider, J M: Clinically significant differences between grief, pathological grief, and depression. Patient Counselling and Health Education, 4th quarter, p 276, 1980.

Thoughts, Beliefs, and Perceptions

- Self-blame
- Idealizing lost person
- Remembering only positive aspects of lost person
- Ruminating over events leading to the loss
- Obsession with lost person
- Illusory phenomena in which mourner thinks lost person is present
- Preoccupied with thoughts that can bring only pain
- Imagining that lost person is watching over mourner
- Difficulty making decisions

Relationships and Interactions

- Seeking support from others, may become more dependent
- Fear of being alone
- Unable to participate in conversation because of preoccupation with loss
- Feeling that others do not understand the pain ("How can they have a good time when I hurt so much?")
- Projection of anger onto others

Physical Responses

- Initial symptoms that may include hyperventilating, sighing, sobbing, muscle tension, chest pain, fainting
- Gastrointestinal distress
- Loss of appetite
- Change in bowel habits
- Insomnia, constant fatigue
- Dehydration

Pertinent History

- Unresolved or multiple past losses
- Ambivalent relationship with lost person
- History of psychiatric disorder or substance abuse
- Tendency to isolate self

COLLABORATIVE INTERVENTIONS

Pharmacologic

Sedatives and tranquilizers are often used in the early stages of grief to reduce the impact of the intense emotions and promote rest and sleep. However, these medications suppress the intense emotions and interfere with the purpose of the grief process. Antidepressants may be useful, along with psychotherapy, when depressive symptoms are prolonged.

Spiritual

As people face loss and grief, they may be more likely to reach out for spiritual support. They may question their beliefs, talk about an afterlife, and face past wrongdoing. Allow the patient to express feelings and, as needed, seek out clergy available within the agency or ask the patient's or family's own clergy to assist. Churches and temples may also offer special support programs. If the patient requests, provide information on important religious rituals such as the Sacrament of the Sick and prayer, and provide religious articles such as Bibles, prayer books, medals, rosaries, candles, and special clothing. Clergy may also provide important support for staff members who may be struggling with helping patient or family with spiritual issues.

NURSING MANAGEMENT

GRIEF EVIDENCED BY DENIAL, ANGER, DEPRESSION, SORROW RELATED TO SIGNIFICANT PERSONAL LOSS (ACTUAL OR POTENTIAL) INCLUDING CHANGE IN RELATIONSHIP, UNEXPECTED OUTCOME, ILLNESS, DEATH.

Patient Outcomes

- Acknowledges loss
- Expresses concerns, feelings of grief
- Verbalizes feeling of being supported in the grieving process
- Identifies potential coping mechanisms, support systems

Interventions

- Accept all grieving behavior. Recognize that responses to grief are highly individual.
- Provide private environment for person to acknowledge loss and express grief.
- Recognize your role as listener. Providing an accepting, supportive environment to share feelings is extremely important. Recognize that words are often less important than just being present at these times.
- Support grief rituals used by individual from his or her culture. These can provide reassurance and comfort to the bereaved.
- Accept feelings, tolerate mourner's expressions of extreme emotions such as sobbing, wailing.
- Provide privacy for the mourner.
- Recognize that it is not only acceptable but preferable to talk about the loss and express feelings. Not talking or not expressing feelings is a greater concern.
- If you are helping someone who just heard about the death or other loss, provide needed information such as mortuary, support groups in small amounts. Information may need to be repeated several times. Focus assis-

tance on helping to get other family members or friends to assist so that mourner will not be alone. Assist with making phone calls. Provide concrete written information whenever possible.

- Seek assistance from colleagues if possible. Dealing with acute grief can be very draining.
- Use touch; holding the mourner can be very supportive. Recognize that waves of emotions will come and go. Be prepared for more intensity as the person relives events leading to the death or other loss.

> **DYSFUNCTIONAL GRIEVING** EVIDENCED BY INHIBITION, SUPPRESSION, ABSENCE, PROLONGATION, OR DISTORTED GRIEF REACTIONS RELATED TO SIGNIFICANT LOSS, MULTIPLE LOSSES, UNRESOLVED GUILT, LACK OF SUPPORT SYSTEM, DIFFICULTY EXPRESSING FEELINGS.

Patient Outcomes

- Acknowledges the loss
- Demonstrates absence of abnormal, prolonged, excessive reactions to loss
- Resumes or develops social relationships.
- Expresses feelings expected with the loss

Interventions

- Recognize that the individual needs to confront the loss slowly and accept it into his or her reality at the individual's own pace. Part of this process will include talking about the loss, reliving memories, talking about events leading to the loss, and expressing feelings.
- Use supportive phrases such as "It must be hard for you now" or "I'm so sorry to hear of your loss." These phrases acknowledge the loss and encourage the person to tell his or her story. Avoid phrases such as "At least you had him for 20 years." These statements diminish the loss to the mourner and can lead to feeling isolated and misunderstood.
- Monitor for signs of dysfunctional grieving, including prolonged denial, lack of emotional response, living in the past, or self-destructive behavior. If the mourner exhibits these behaviors, monitor closely and talk with him or her about your concerns. Point out feelings or reactions that the individual might be experiencing, for example, "You might be feeling like you're in a dream right now" to encourage expressing feelings.
- Encourage involvement in new activities and meeting new people. Help the person to set small goals to begin these activities very slowly, and identify realistic expectations.
- Assist the mourner to redefine the relationship with the lost person or object. This includes remembering the positives and negatives and acknowledging possible angry feelings.
- If the mourner does not acknowledge the loss, bring up the subject. You might say "I notice you never mention your deceased husband. How has it been for you?"

- Provide spiritual support as requested. Encourage involvement of clergy.
- Recognize that patients with histories of psychiatric disorders or substance abuse may need additional support to maintain their past improvements during these times.

ALTERNATE NURSING DIAGNOSES

> Anxiety
> Ineffective Family Coping: Compromised
> Ineffective Individual Coping
> Knowledge Deficit
> Powerlessness
> Self-Esteem Disturbance
> Sleep Pattern Disturbance
> Social Isolation
> Spiritual Distress (Distress of the Human Spirit)

WHEN TO CALL FOR HELP

Disturbing behavior including hallucinating, delusions, obsessions

Evidence of intense prolonged preoccupation with the loss

Recurrence of psychiatric symptoms, substance abuse

Dwelling on detailed events leading to loss or death long after the event

Long periods of depression, possibly including suicidal thoughts or gestures

Living in the past many months or years after loss occurred

No emotional reaction to loss for a prolonged period of time

Or if the staff exhibits:

Intense emotional reaction to death of patient

Difficulty in dealing with personal grief to the extent that it impacts on patient care

---

PATIENT AND FAMILY EDUCATION

- Prepare patient and family for the normal stages of grieving.
- Inform them that anticipatory grief does not necessarily reduce the emotional impact of the loss. Mourners still may expect an intense reaction.
- Tell the family the signs of dysfunctional grief and encourage them to seek help if they begin to experience them.
- Tell the patient that feelings of anger and guilt may be normal. Encourage

seeking professional help if he or she is having difficulty resolving these feelings.
- Encourage mourner to be very patient through this process. Time is needed to slowly face the grief. Discourage making major decisions early on in grieving.
- Discourage use of tranquilizers as a way to avoid intense emotions.
- Let the mourner know that his or her feelings may be intensified at key times such as holidays and anniversaries and that they may last for a few days.
- Encourage good nutrition and good health habits, especially for elderly people. Encourage seeking medical attention, as needed, during the bereavement period because the mourner is at an increased risk of illness.
- Prepare mourner and family for delayed grief reaction when intense feelings may occur in response to future loss.

CHARTING TIPS

- Document grieving behaviors.
- Document use of medications such as tranquilizers and analgesics.
- Avoid documenting judgments about patient behavior.
- Document available resources identified to support grieving individual.

COMMUNITY-BASED CARE

- Provide information on bereavement counseling and support groups. Provide the information in writing because mourners may be unable to concentrate.
- Inform referring agencies and home health agencies about patients' recent losses and grief reactions.
- Identify opportunities for socialization. Encourage involvement in activities when appropriate.
- Encourage involvement of family and friends to expand mourner's support system.
- Provide follow-up phone calls to mourner to reinforce information given.

THE HYPERACTIVE OR MANIC PATIENT

LEARNING OBJECTIVES

➢ List the outstanding characteristics of mania.
➢ List possible contributing factors to manic episodes.
➢ Describe effective nursing interventions for a manic episode.
➢ Describe possible nurses' reactions to manic behavior.

GLOSSARY

Cyclothymic disorder—A chronic mood disturbance lasting at least 2 years that can be thought of as a muted version of bipolar disorder

Hypomanic episode—A distinct period that is similar to a manic episode but with less severe symptoms. There is impairment of social or occupational functioning, mood is clearly different from usual non-depressed mood, but psychotic features may not be present.

Manic episode—A distinct period during which there is an abnormally and persistently elated, expansive, or irritable mood possibly accompanied by inflated self-esteem or grandiosity, decreased need for sleep, pressured speech, flight of ideas, or subjective experience that thoughts are racing, distractibility, increased involvement in goal-directed activities or psychomotor agitation, and excessive involvement in pleasurable activities with a high potential for painful consequences. Marked changes in social or occupational functioning or need for hospitalization or psychotic features must be present.

Mixed episode—A period during which the criteria for both a manic and a major depressive episode are met nearly every day.

Rapid cycling—At least 4 episodes of a mood disturbance in the previous 12 months that meet criteria for a major expressive episode or a manic, mixed, or hypomanic episode.

Schizoaffective disorder—An uninterrupted period of illness during which, at some time, there is a major depressive, manic, or mixed episode concurrent with the characteristic symptoms of schizophrenia.

In the early phase of a manic episode an individual can become engaging, outgoing, and charming, presenting as one who is achieving and successful with excessive energy and optimism. During the hypomanic episode, the person accelerates to an "abnormally and persistently elevated, expansive or irritable mood lasting at least 4 days." (APA: DSM-IV-TR 2000, p 365). Mania can continue to accelerate to a continuously frenzied, out-of-control pace, leading to seriously impaired decision making and potentially very hazardous activity. An increasing manic episode can be viewed as a series of stages during which the symptoms become more intense and severe. For example, an initial overestimation of abilities ("I can earn more money than any other salesman in the United States") can balloon to grandiose delusions ("I am Jesus Christ") and hallucinations. What begins as pressured, rapid, but still organized speaking can escalate to constant loose flitting verbalizations from topic to topic with little or no connections and, eventually, incoherence. Irritability, especially when demands are not met, can escalate into belligerent explosiveness and combativeness. Restlessness can peak into a state of continuous motion. A patient in an escalated manic phase frequently denies the seriousness or even the existence of illness, both medical and psychiatric. This individual could walk endless miles for days, expecting cars to clear a path for him or her, ignores the need for any food and sleep, and disregards any physical impairment. Without medication, a manic episode can last months.

Interestingly, descriptions of manic episodes reflect a mirror image of depression. Depression is characterized by an insidious slowing down of movement, thought, self-esteem, and initiative, accompanied by dejected, constricting, pessimistic, and even despairing mood. Internally focused guilt abounds, and anger is usually self-directed. In mania, everything seems to speed up, including: thought, speech, decisions, activity, mood, self-esteem and a belief that all desires and dreams can be fulfilled. Externally focused anger and blame are directed outward: guilt is noticeably absent. In the extreme forms of both depression and mania, there is a psychotic break with reality, including delusions and/or hallucinations.

Bipolar disorder, formerly called "manic depression," is best viewed as a recurrent illness in which there are symptom-free periods. More than 90 percent of patients who experience a first manic episode go on to have future episodes. The majority of individuals with bipolar disorders return to a fully functional level between episodes. Many patients with bipolar I disorder (see next paragraph) return to work when properly medicated. Manic and hypomanic episodes often precede or follow major depressive episodes in a characteristic pattern for a particular person. The frequency of manic episodes varies. Some have periodic episodes separated by years, and some have close repetition. Long-term, even lifelong medication may be necessary. (Medication-free trials should be tried only under physician supervision.)

DSM-IV-TR further defines two types of bipolar disorders: bipolar I and bipolar II.

> *Bipolar I disorder:* Characterized by the occurrence of one or more manic episodes or mixed episodes. Often, but not always, individuals with this disorder also have one or more major depressive episodes.

Bipolar II disorder: Characterized by the occurrence of one or more major depressive episodes with the presence (or history) of at least one hypomanic episode.

ETIOLOGY

Bipolar disorder is a complex phenomenon in which a variety of factors converge.

Biologic theory predominates. Studies indicate that this disorder is caused by an imbalance in neurotransmitters, particularly norepinephrine and serotonin. Increased levels are believed to be present in manic episodes and decreased in depressive ones. Impaired interrelationships of the hormonal and endocrine systems are currently being explored. Investigation of brain electrical activity is also being studied because valproate, carbamazepine, and other anticonvulsants have been successfully used with lithium-resistant manic episodes. Electroencephalographic changes have been linked to mood disturbances as well. Disruptions in circadian rhythms and exposure to light, as in light therapy for depression with seasonal pattern, can contribute to manic episodes.

A genetic link has also been demonstrated through family studies. Bipolar patients have a significantly greater percentage of relatives with bipolar and depressive disorders than the general population. Studies done on twins and adopted individuals provide strong evidence of a genetic influence for bipolar I disorder.

Sociologically, there are no reports of differential incidence of bipolar I disorder based on race, ethnicity or sex. Mania is more often the initial episode in men and depression in women. Bipolar II disorder may be somewhat more common in women.

Psychologic theory views mania as a defensive flight from an underlying extreme depression with its attendant painful feelings of hopelessness, worthlessness, and emptiness. It is suggested that the individual uses denial as a defense mechanism. Hypotheses requiring further investigation are that the patient uses manic symptoms to covertly get dependency needs met; approval from others maintains self-esteem while manic symptoms prevent others from setting limits and containing out-of-control behavior.

RELATED CLINICAL CONCERNS

Hyperactive symptoms caused by substance abuse, medication use, or a general medical condition are not considered to be a bipolar disease. Under these circumstances, the diagnoses would be substance-induced mood disorder or mood disorder caused by a general medical condition (Box 9–6).

Manic episodes can be induced by other somatic treatments for depression, such as electroconvulsive (ECT or "shock") therapy or light therapy for depression with seasonal pattern (exposure to increased amount of bright visible-spectrum light during seasons of the year with diminished daylight).

BOX 9–6. Drugs and Physical Illnesses That Can Cause Manic States

Drug-Related
Steroids
Levodopa
Amphetamines
Tricyclic antidepressants
Monoamine oxidase inhibitors
Methylphenidate
Cocaine
Thyroid hormone

Infections
Influenza
Q fever
St. Louis encephalitis
Other Illnesses
Hyperthyroidism
Multiple sclerosis
Systemic lupus erythemotosus
Brain tumors
Stroke

Sources: Stuart, GW: Emotional responses and mood disorders. In Stuart, GW and Laraies, (eds.): Stuart and Sundeen's Principles and Practices of Psychiatric Nursing (6th ed.), St. Louis, Mosby, 1998; and Goodwin, FK and Jameson, KR: Manic Depressive Illness. New York, Oxford University Press, 1990.

Sleep disturbance is both a symptom of manic episodes and an irritant that can exacerbate manic episodes and worsen the overall condition.

LIFE SPAN ISSUES

CHILDREN

Studies indicate that 20 to 30 percent of bipolar disorders have their onset before age 20. The true diagnosis may need to be clarified in observing the patterns and manifestations of future episodes. The possibility of manic episode(s) occurring in young children is controversial. Because the incidence of manic episodes in children before the age of 12 years is extremely rare, there is a danger of a child with this disorder being labeled a "problem child" or misdiagnosed as attention-deficit disordered with hyperactivity.

ADOLESCENTS

Manic episodes in adolescents are more likely to include psychotic features and can be misdiagnosed as schizophrenia. Behavioral problems can lead to the misdiagnosis of conduct disorder. Approximately 10 to 15 percent of adolescents with recurrent major depressive episodes will go on to develop bipolar I disorder (DSM-IV-TR, 2000). Assessments should include a family history of mood disorders.

In adolescents, manic and hypomanic episodes may be associated with school truancy, antisocial behavior, school failure, or substance abuse. A significant minority of adolescents appear to have a history of long-standing behavior problems preceding a frank manic episode. It is unclear whether these problems represent a prolonged prodrome to bipolar disorder or an independent disorder.

Antimanic medications can be used in adjusted doses along with psychotherapeutic interventions in this age group.

ADULTS

The majority of first manic episodes in bipolar disorder occur between the ages of 20 and 30 years with preponderance in the early 20s. If the onset of a first manic episode occurs in a patient 40 years or older who has no previous psychiatric illness, medical conditions and drug-inducing manic symptoms should be ruled out.

In the adult years, uncontrolled symptoms can result in job losses, marital and other relationship breakups, grave financial problems, or serious legal repercussions from violating laws. During manic episodes parents may be unable to care for and provide safety for a child. Child abuse, spousal abuse, or other violent behaviors may occur during severe manic episodes or during those with psychotic features.

POSTPARTUM

"Postpartum onset" is applied to manic, depressive, or mixed episodes that occur within 4 weeks after delivery of a child. The symptomatology remains the same. If delusions are present, they often concern the newborn child. If a manic episode develops in the postpartum period, risk for recurrence in subsequent postpartum periods may be increased.

ELDERLY PEOPLE

The intervals between episodes tend to decrease in bipolar I disorder and to increase in bipolar II disorder as an individual ages. Medical conditions and drug reactions as causative factors in manic episodes need to be carefully evaluated particularly when initial episodes occur in elderly people. Managing patients with bipolar disorder in long-term care settings can create major challenges for staff members.

POSSIBLE NURSES' REACTIONS

- May be entertained or amused by the initial exuberance and acting out and not set limits
- May become irritable, anxious, or angry when patient is noncompliant with healthcare regimen or routine
- May be embarrassed or sense lowered self-esteem if the nurse believes that a "good" nurse should be able to control patients or prevent them from behaving strangely
- May feel verbally abused and unrecognized by the patient

- May feel manipulated, outsmarted, and defensive, needing to justify actions and motives
- May feel frightened if patient becomes violent

ASSESSMENT

Behavior and Appearance

- Excessive in all areas: bizarre, garish, flamboyant, eccentric
- Pressured speech (profuse, rapid, as if generated by an engine)
- Poor personal grooming and excessive and bizarre clothing or make-up changes
- Restlessness, hyperactivity with constant moving and pacing
- Flitting attempts to participate in multiple activities, unable to complete things, impulsive
- Poor judgment in decision making; undertakes risky or dangerous endeavors without awareness of consequences, including buying sprees, foolish business investments, reckless driving, hypersexuality
- Behavior inappropriate to situation
- Complaints, hostile comments, and angry tirades; may be violent

Mood and Emotions

- Elation; heightened sense of pleasure; unrealistic optimism
- Lack of shame or guilt
- Anger escalating to rage, especially when wishes are thwarted
- Labile mood swings including depression, irritability, and anger

Thoughts, Beliefs, and Perceptions

- Distracted; unable to concentrate on task at hand; overly attuned and responsive to stimulation from people and events
- Grandiose overestimation of own abilities, talents; exaggeration of past achievements; inflated self-esteem; impaired judgment
- Complicated plans to acquire unlimited fame, fortune, and/or power
- Poor insight; unaware of his or her distortion and negative effect on others
- Makes puns, plays on words, and jokes
- Flight of ideas (continuously jumps rapidly from one topic to another)
- Suspicious; escalates to delusions and/or hallucinations of grandiosity or persecution

Relationships and Interactions

- Excessively gregarious; can be charming; lacks true concern for others
- Forms superficial relationships quickly but becomes manipulative, demanding, intrusive, taunting
- Attempts to engage everyone into his or her plans and activities; constantly demands attention

- Manipulates self-esteem of others by flattery
- Irresponsible; gives quick, deceptively plausible excuses for own actions; puts responsibility on others
- Intimidating

Physical Responses

- Sometimes initial overeating; weight gain, even food hoarding
- As mania escalates, inadequate nutritional intake leading to weight loss and even dehydration
- Physical exhaustion with insomnia
- May exhibit side effects of drug abuse and symptoms of general medical conditions that can cause mania

Pertinent History

- Earlier episodes or family history of depressive and/or manic episodes
- Dramatic changes in personality during manic phases
- Psychiatric diagnosis and treatment of schizophrenia or schizoaffective disorder may occur; differential diagnosis is often confused because extremes of manic episodes have similar symptoms
- History of substance abuse

COLLABORATIVE MANAGEMENT

Pharmacologic

Patients may need to take antimanic medications for the rest of their lives; therefore education and compliance are very important.

Lithium carbonate is the most common first-line medication used in typical manic episodes of bipolar disorder. Lower maintenance doses are often continued in the intervals between episodes. Blood levels and side effects need to be monitored because lithium can reach a toxic range, possibly causing seizures, coma, and even death. Therapeutic lithium levels are between 0.8 and 1.2 mEq/L for most patients. Blood lithium levels can be elevated when there is significant lowering of body fluids as in such conditions as limited fluid intake, profuse sweating, or chronic diarrhea. It is essential to constantly monitor for adverse drug reactions because some individuals can become toxic at blood levels considered normal for most people. Onset of sedation, nausea, and vomiting are early warning signs of lithium toxicity. As toxicity increases, tremors and muscle twitching may occur.

Lithium can take 7 to 10 days to reach the desired effect. If psychotic symptoms are present, antipsychotics can be used on a regular or as-needed basis. The need should diminish as lithium or other antimanic medications reach therapeutic levels.

Antimanic drugs are available only in oral forms. If the patient is unable to take oral medications, other medications may be used, such as antipsychotics or antianxiety drugs, which can be given parenterally.

Anticonvulsants, such as carbamazepine and divalproex, are also used. Carbamazepine can cause agranulocytosis with lethal implications. The incidence of this adverse effect is low; however, it is important to monitor the patient continually for changes in white blood cell and granulocyte count and any signs of infection. Agranulocytosis subsides promptly when the drug is discontinued.

Herbal products such as valerian root and chamomile may be used to calm the person. During depressive periods the individual may use stimulants to recreate some of the feelings of the hypomanic period.

Dietary

A patient in an escalated manic phase may be too restless to sit down and eat. Patients may need "finger foods" that can be carried, such as sandwiches and milkshakes. A high-calorie diet should be provided if patient is in constant movement.

Psychotherapy

To gain the patient's acceptance of maintaining the medication regimen, the nurse must help him or her to accept the reality of having a bipolar disorder. This requires that the patient have the time to work through the denial and, later, anger over having an incurable condition. Medications can control the frequency and intensity of manic episodes, but exacerbations can still happen. The patient may need assistance in dealing with shame over behavior during manic episodes. He or she may also need to learn how to discriminate normal from abnormal moods and will probably need help in learning to tolerate more dysphoric feelings and moods.

As life becomes flatter and less colorful without mania, the patient may need to grieve for the losses associated with giving up mania, such as fantasies, high or euphoric states, increased level of energy and sexuality, decreased need for sleep, and possibly decreased degree of productivity and creativity.

Developmental tasks may have been overshadowed by the illness. For example, the adolescent tasks of establishing a separate identity and learning about relationships may have been disrupted. Once the patient is stabilized, these issues will need to be addressed. If the patient has an alcohol or drug abuse dependency, this needs to be acknowledged as a problem, especially because the patient usually denies the problem. Mood disorders can mask substance abuse just as substance abuse often masks mood disorders. Effective substance abuse treatment should be used concurrently with approaches for bipolar disorder (Goodwin and Jamison, 1990).

NURSING MANAGEMENT

ANXIETY EVIDENCED BY HYPERACTIVITY, DISTRACTIBILITY, DISORGANIZED AND UNREALISTIC THOUGHTS RELATED TO MANIC PHASE OF BIPOLAR DISORDER.

Patient Outcomes

- Slower and more controlled speech and behavior
- No evidence of delusions or hallucinations
- Demonstrates an increased ability to concentrate
- Demonstrates more realistic decision making
- Complies with medication regime

Interventions

- Determine psychiatric care provider for treatment of mania. If none, strongly encourage immediate referral and assessment. Make sure that physician and other staff members are aware of the patient's history.
- Provide firm, clear limits. Describe exactly what is expected and what is not allowed. Be realistic. For instance, patient may need to have a designated area in which to pace without being disruptive.
- Administer ordered antimanic medications; monitor blood levels, adverse effects, and signs of possible toxicity.
- Assess for psychotic symptoms; evaluate for need to administer PRN antipsychotic medications.
- Do not reinforce patient's delusional beliefs. Present reality without arguing with the patient.
- Be consistent even if the patient produces seemingly plausible reasons and excuses. Do not participate in verbal battles—just repeat the rules. Avoid power struggles. Keep directions simple and specific.
- Use a calm, relaxed approach.
- Provide a focus to conversation if patient jumps from one topic to another. Interrupt to slow him/her down. Refocus on the chosen topic. Phrase questions so that they require a brief answer. If the patient's thoughts are speeding to the point of confusion, do not encourage continued speaking, and, if possible, arrange for someone to sit quietly with patient. Supervise other caregivers who are unfamiliar with manic patients.
- Explain to staff, patients, and visitors who complain about patient's constant need for attention that the patient will feel better in a quiet atmosphere. Encourage them to limit interactions with the patient without abandoning him or her.
- Remove patient from external stimulation. If possible, place patient in a room in a quiet area and use dim lighting. A private room is preferable. Calming music may help.
- Assess whether patient should be allowed to verbalize anger or fear. If patient becomes overly agitated, change or redirect the topic of conversation. As the mania decreases, the patient may be better able to tolerate more processing of emotion.
- Limit the patient's choices. Attempt to limit the number of objects patient has in the room. Encourage family and/or friends to take home unnecessary possessions.
- Remove hazardous objects from patient's room.
- Provide brief activities because of short attention span. Tasks can be more complex as mania decreases.

- If the patient's behavior is unacceptable, distract with more productive activities. Do not reinforce inappropriate behaviors by giving them a lot of attention.
- Assess for activities patient can do in his or her room, such as writing or drawing.
- Provide an outlet for excessive energy. Assess whether a stationary bike or other equipment can safely be placed in the patient's room. Supervise any physical activity. Consider physical and/or occupational therapy evaluation.
- Support and encourage the patient's ideas that are realistic and consistent with the healthcare regimen.
- Assess for any injuries, bruises, and signs of infection.
- Assess for substance abuse.
- Assist the family in dealing with any negative feelings they may have toward the patient so that they can interact more constructively with him or her.
- Obtain support from peers and other resources if patient's manipulations begin to erode the nurses' abilities to maintain an effective approach.

> **SLEEP PATTERN DISTURBANCE** EVIDENCED BY INABILITY TO LIE DOWN AT NIGHT, SLEEPING ONLY BRIEF PERIODS, AND ERRATIC SLEEP PATTERNS RELATED TO MANIC/UNCONTROLLED ACTIVITY.

Patient Outcomes

- Remains alert and awake during the day without daytime fatigue
- Sleeps at least 5 hours per night
- Does not require naps during the day

Interventions

- Monitor sleep patterns and assess for signs of fatigue.
- Use calming techniques just before bedtime: warm milk, soothing music, or warm bath. Avoid stimulants such as caffeine.
- Decrease stimulation at bedtime: lights out, curtains drawn, phone unplugged. Avoid loud noises nearby and loud talking. Some patients may respond well to having someone sit quietly just outside the room until he or she is asleep. Encourage the patient to remain in bed long enough to fall asleep.
- Provide ordered sleep medication if patient is unable to sleep.
- Encourage the patient to go to bed at the same time each night.
- If naps are needed during the day, encourage taking them at the same time each day.

ALTERNATE NURSING DIAGNOSES

Altered Nutrition: Less Than or More Than Body Requirements
Altered Thought Processes
Fluid Volume Deficit
Impaired Social Interaction

Ineffective Individual Coping
Ineffective Management of Therapeutic Regimen: Individuals
Noncompliance
Risk for Injury
Risk for Violence: Directed at Others or Self-Directed

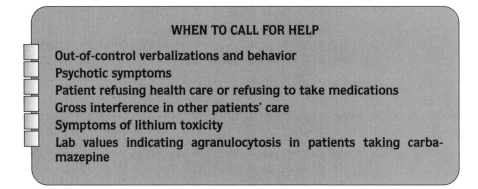

WHEN TO CALL FOR HELP

- Out-of-control verbalizations and behavior
- Psychotic symptoms
- Patient refusing health care or refusing to take medications
- Gross interference in other patients' care
- Symptoms of lithium toxicity
- Lab values indicating agranulocytosis in patients taking carbamazepine

PATIENT AND FAMILY EDUCATION

- Avoid health teaching until patient displays significant reduction in psychiatric symptoms and demonstrates good awareness of reality.
- Teach the family the symptoms of a manic episode so they can recognize what is occurring and not personalize the patient's interactions with them.
- Teach the patient and family the importance of continuing psychiatric medications and treatment, monitoring signs of medication adverse effects and toxicity, and noting early signs and symptoms of recurrent episodes.
- Teach patients, especially those on lithium, to maintain normal diet, fluid, and salt intake.
- Teach patients on lithium to check with their physician about withholding drug if excessive diarrhea, vomiting, or diaphoresis occurs.
- Teach the patient to make a contract with a family member or a trusted significant other to encourage and assist the patient to make contact with psychiatrist or counselor if there is a resurgence of symptoms. Often family members are the first to notice behavioral changes.
- Help the family to make plans for hospitalization so they will be able to act quickly if an emergency situation arises.
- Teach patient about the process of realistic decision-making and the effect of one's decisions on others.
- Teach patient that life includes accepting periods of sadness, disappointment, and uncomfortable feelings.
- Teach patient about his or her effect on others.
- Explain to the patient and family that alcohol or drug abuse can undermine bipolar treatment.

CHARTING TIPS

- Note the presence or absence of adverse effects of lithium.
- Document the amount of PRN antipsychotics given and the results if used.
- Document any factors that could lead to dehydration.
- Document percentage of food eaten and weight changes.
- Note changes in patient's behavior and thoughts expressed.
- Document patient's compliance or lack of compliance with healthcare regimen.

COMMUNITY-BASED CARE

- Reinforce the idea that it is essential that the patient continue in medical and psychiatric treatment and take prescribed medications after discharge.
- Make sure that patient has appointments for required blood level tests and follow-up referrals.
- Social service referrals may be helpful for patients who may have alienated friends, family, or associates before hospitalization. Financial and legal issues may be pending because of unwise actions such as excessive spending sprees.
- Recommend assessing the need for transfer to psychiatric facility if patient's behavior and thought processes are not sufficiently stabilized.
- Recommend that the patient attend community support groups for bipolar disorder such as the Manic Depressive and Depressive Association; refer for alcohol or drug problems if indicated.
- Recommend that the family attend support groups such as those sponsored by the National Alliance for the Mentally Ill (NAMI).

Problems with Confusion

THE CONFUSED PATIENT

LEARNING OBJECTIVES

➢ Differentiate between dementia and delirium.
➢ List the most common types of dementia.
➢ Describe common nurses' reactions to the confused patient.
➢ Describe effective nursing interventions for the confused patient with the following: memory deficits, unable to verbalize his or her needs, and at risk for falling.

GLOSSARY

Catastrophic reactions—Extreme overreaction in Alzheimer's patients to a seemingly neutral situation that requires the patient to process more information or decision making than is possible.

Delirium—Rapid fluctuations in mental status, memory deficits, disorientation, and perceptual disturbances over a short period of time.

Dementia—Multiple cognitive deficits: aphasia, apraxia, agnosia, or disturbance in executive function such as organizing or abstracting.

Dementia of the Alzheimer's type (Alzheimer's disease)—Progressive deterioration of memory, and intellectual functioning, often leading to complete loss of functioning and personality. Autopsy reveals brain atrophy, senile plaques, and neurofibrillary tangles.

Nocturnal delirium (Sundowning syndrome)—Increased confusion and agitation at dusk.

Prompts—Staff actions used to help dementia patient initiate self-care or other desired behaviors after loss of verbal comprehension.

Pseudodementia—Depression in elderly people that appears similar to dementia.

Substance-induced persisting dementia—Dementia caused by intoxication or withdrawal from a substance such as alcohol or drugs.

Vascular dementia—Dementia caused by multiple strokes that have usually occurred at different times and involve the cortex and underlying white matter.

Confusion is not just a state of the mind seen in elderly people. It has many causes and can occur at any age. It significantly influences a patient's dignity, independence, personality, and support system and can complicate the diagnosis and treatment of a patient's illness. Confused patients are experiencing an alteration in higher-level brain functioning such as comprehension or abstract thinking caused by delirium or dementia (Boxes 10–1 and 10–2). These patients have difficulty remembering, learning, following directions, and communicating needs and pains. Nursing care must be modified to help these patients to retain and regain the mental abilities that can be recovered and to compensate for those that cannot.

BOX 10–1. Factors That Contribute to Misdiagnosis in Dementia and Delirium

- The symptoms of dementia and delirium are similar.
- Several causes may occur simultaneously to bring about dementia.
- Delirium occurring in a patient with a dementia can exacerbate already existing symptoms.
- Healthcare personnel may harbor unfounded beliefs that serious memory deficits, confusion, and other progressive intellectual deficits are a normal part of the aging process.
- Healthcare personnel may harbor unfounded beliefs that confusion always indicates Alzheimer's disease in an older patient.
- Confusion and behavioral changes may be the first sign of medical illness in the elderly.
- Head injuries and other conditions causing brain tissue trauma may present with symptoms similar to those of dementia.
- Confusion is an adverse reaction to many medications.

Source: Gorman, L, Sultan, D, and Luna-Raines, M, 1989.

BOX 10–2. Characteristics of Delirium and Dementia

Delirium	Dementia
• Fluctuating levels of awareness and symptoms	• Slow, insidious onset with less fluctuation of symptoms
• Sudden onset	• Deterioration of cognitive abilities
• Clouding of consciousness	• Impaired long- and short-term memory (memory impairment always present)
• Perceptual disturbances (hallucinations, illusions)	
• Memory disturbance, more often for recent events	• Personality changes
• Highly distractible	• May focus on one thing for a long time
• Reversibility possible with treatment	• Often irreversible

Delirium is a reaction to underlying physiologic (illness, drug reaction, or exposure to a toxin) or psychologic stress. Nurses in the ICU often see delirium induced by the disorienting and confusing environment, sensory deprivation, or sensory overload. It may also occur postoperatively. Delirium is caused by a temporary malfunction of the brain. When the underlying causative condition is resolved, the delirium generally resolves. It is a medical emergency. If left untreated, it could progress to dementia, coma, or death depending on the underlying cause.

Dementia is generally a permanent condition caused by a variety of factors that lead to cellular brain changes or malformations. It is characterized by slow, insidious onset affecting memory (impaired ability to learn new information or to recall previously learned information), intellectual functioning, and the ability to problem solve. Types of dementia include Alzheimer's disease, vascular dementia, substance-induced dementia, and dementia caused by other medical conditions.

Alzheimer's disease is the most frequently seen type of dementia, affecting over 4 million Americans. (Surgeon General's Report, 2000) Initial changes occur so slowly that they may not be recognized. The person may be regarded as absentminded. Changes in communication, personality, and social skills occur gradually. In later stages, the individual may develop gait and motor disturbances and eventually become mute, bedridden, and incontinent. Death often occurs from severe debilitation, malnutrition, and dehydration. The average duration of the illness from onset of symptoms to death is 8 to 10 years.

Vascular dementia, the second most common form, is caused by multiple strokes. Symptoms are variable depending on the extent, location, and timing of the strokes. Impairment is limited and distinct depending on the area of the brain affected. This contrasts with more global intellectual impairment in Alzheimer's disease. Evidence of strokes, such as one-sided weakness, sudden onset of loss of speech, and focal neurologic signs, such as hyperactive deep tendon reflexes, occur with vascular dementia. Treatment of underlying hypertension and vascular disease may prevent further progression.

ETIOLOGY

Delirium can have biologic and psychologic causes. *Biologic* causes include a variety of medical conditions, exposure to toxins, and drugs. The onset of symptoms is related to exacerbation of a medical condition or introduction of a new medication for example, and contributes to the diagnosis. *Psychologic* causes include sensory deprivation or overload, relocation or sudden changes, sleep deprivation, and immobilization.

Dementia can be caused by a variety of *biologic* factors including the direct physiologic effects of a medical condition, the persisting effects of a substance (drug of abuse, medication, or toxin), or multiple etiologies such as the combined effects of a stroke and Alzheimer's disease. The etiology of Alzheimer's disease remains the focus of much research. Current theories under investigation include decrease in the activity of the neurotransmitter acetylcholine and presence in the brain of the protein beta-amyloid. Thus far, theories of environmental toxins, poisons, or a slow-acting virus are unsupported. Genetic factors may also be present. There is a greater incidence of Alzheimer's disease in the family members of patients who acquire the disease before age 50.

RELATED CLINICAL CONCERNS

DELIRIUM

Medical conditions that can generate delirium include systemic infections, hypoxia, hypercapnia, hypoglycemia, fluid or electrolyte imbalances, hepatic or renal disease, thiamine deficiency, sequelae of head trauma, postictal states, postoperative states, and complications of cancer. There is an up to 80 percent rate of delirium in the final stages of terminal illness. The presence of delirium increases the risk of complications associated with a medical illness and increases the risk of mortality.

Substance intoxication delirium can occur from ingestion of alcohol, amphetamines, cannabis, cocaine, hallucinogens, phencyclidine (PCP), opioids, hypnotics, and sedatives. Substance withdrawal delirium can occur from abruptly stopping significant abuse of alcohol (formerly called "delirium tremens"), hypnotics, antianxiety medications, and corticosteroids.

Many prescribed medications can contribute to delirium, including analgesics, anesthetics, anticonvulsants, antihistamines, antiparkinson drugs, corticosteroids, gastrointestinal medications, and psychotropic medications with anticholinergic side effects (see Box 11–3).

DEMENTIA

Medical conditions that contribute to development of dementia include stroke, Parkinson's disease, Huntington's disease, AIDS, Creutzfeldt-Jakob disease, hypothyroidism, multiple sclerosis, traumatic brain injury, brain tumors, anoxia, lupus, and hepatic failure. Substance-induced persisting dementia can also occur with a long history of alcohol or substance abuse.

LIFE SPAN ISSUES

CHILDREN TO ADOLESCENTS

Children may be more susceptible to delirium than adults, particularly in the presence of febrile episodes and in response to some medications such as anticholinergics. Assessment may be complicated by difficulty in eliciting the signs of problems in thinking, memory, and orientation. In fact, delirium can be mistaken for uncooperative behavior. One indication of delirium may be the inability of familiar figures to soothe the child.

Dementia is rare in children and adolescents but can occur as a result of medical conditions including AIDS, brain tumors, and head injury. As with delirium, dementia can be difficult to identify in young children. It may present as a deterioration in function, as in adults, or as a significant delay or deviation in normal development. Deterioration in school performance may be an early sign.

ELDERLY PEOPLE

Delirium is extremely common in medically ill elderly people. Ten to 15 percent of hospitalized elderly persons exhibit delirium on admission (DSM-IV-TR, 2000); 15 to 30 percent of hospitalized medically ill older people may develop it at some time while they are in the hospital. Multiple medications, multiple chronic illnesses, use of over-the-counter medications, and impaired kidney and liver function contribute to the development of delirium. A masked depression can appear as confusion (pseudodementia). Acutely confused elderly persons are often inappropriately labeled "demented" while potentially reversible conditions go undiagnosed and untreated.

Dementia in general is most common after age 85 and is often seen in residents of nursing homes. It occurs with increasing frequency after age 65 but is not a normal or expected part of the aging process.

POSSIBLE NURSES' REACTIONS

- May have a more positive attitude and take more active measures in care of patients if they believe the confusion is reversible.
- May feel very frustrated and helpless because of lack of improvement, constant need to repeat instructions or break tasks down step by step, repetition of the same question, and time requirements for care of patients with irreversible dementia.
- To avoid feeling hopeless and helpless, may become emotionally detached and give only impersonal care.
- May find themselves bored, unfocused, or confused if patients have considerable problems in communicating verbally.

- May be angry with patient's pathology; may believe patient can control own behavior.
- May become impatient with negative, hostile, impulsive patients who are very slow to respond.
- May feel repulsed by poor hygiene, messy eating behaviors, incontinence, or inappropriate behaviors.

ASSESSMENT

Behavior and Appearance

- Disheveled, inappropriate clothing; poor grooming
- Restless, agitated, impulsive, aggressive
- Wandering
- Impaired movement including:
  - Perseveration (involuntary repetitive movements, speech [most common] or activity)
  - Apraxia (inability to carry out motor activities despite intact comprehension and motor abilities)
  - Loss of coordination; stiff awkward movements; impairment of learned skilled movements
  - Unsteady, shuffling gait; stooped, leaning posture
  - Difficulty writing
  - Loss of ability to perform activities of daily living (ADLs)
- Types of aphasia including:
  - Echolalia (repetition of word, phrase, or syllable just said by someone else)
  - Repetitive questions
  - Palilalia (repeating sounds or words over and over)
  - Anomia (difficulty finding wanted words) leading to paraphasia (using similar-sounding words) and circumlocution (using many words in place of the one word that is wanted)
  - Slurred speech
  - In late stages may remember only a few key words used inappropriately in all situations (such as no)
  - May become mute
- Hypersexual behavior such as obsessive masturbation
- Hyperoral symptoms including increased appetite
- Inappropriate eating and toileting behavior
- Sleep disturbance including nocturnal delirium (sundown syndrome)
- Overreaction to neutral stimuli (catastrophic reactions)
- Inability to tolerate stress and change

Mood and Emotions

- Emotional lability
- Depression
- Suspicion, paranoia, hostility
- Anxiety

Thoughts, Beliefs, and Perceptions

- Loss of recent or remote memory or both
- Disorientation, first to time, then place, then person
- Impaired concentration
- Loss of abstract thinking ability
- Loss of ability to calculate
- Inability to learn and use new information
- Loss of ability to plan, initiate, sequence, monitor, and stop complex behavior
- Agnosia (failure to recognize or identify objects despite intact sensory function)
- Ability to read words without knowing what they mean
- Loss of ability to read
- Confabulation
- Loss of awareness of spatial relationships; loss of awareness of own body parts and how they are organized in relation to each other
- Illusions
- Delusions, hallucinations
- Impaired insight and judgment

Relationships and Interactions

- Personality changes: accentuation or alteration of premorbid traits that affects previous relationships (e.g., caretaker role reversals); family unsure how to interact with patient
- Loss of social skills; social withdrawal
- Clinging, demanding
- Inability to sustain real relationships as memory gaps eliminate continuity; in later phases, may not recognize family or friends
- Negative, belligerent, briefly combative at times; hostility caused by brain damage or by misinterpreting events; not necessarily by the behavior of others

Physical Responses

- The patient may not verbalize or demonstrate common physical signs of pain or other symptoms such as bladder distention, constipation, dehydration, injuries, or urinary tract infections.
- Laboratory data, medication history, and possibly drug screening should be performed to evaluate patient at the onset of confusion.

Pertinent History

- Complex medical history
- Chronic illness
- Substance abuse
- Head trauma

COLLABORATIVE MANAGEMENT

Pharmacologic

A great many medications cause confusion. Confused patients who are taking multiple medications may need to have the medications withdrawn one at a time to determine their impact on the symptoms and the underlying illness. Any medications used to treat confusion should be started at lower dosages.

Confused patients often become disruptive and may need to be controlled to protect the patient and environment. Haloperidol (Haldol) is frequently used to treat agitation and aggression. Side effects such as orthostatic hypotension must be closely monitored because the patient may not be able to verbalize how he or she is feeling.

Buspirone (Buspar) has been used successfully in patient's with Alzheimer's disease, although it may take several weeks to take effect fully. Hypnotics, antidepressants (particularly the selective serotonin reuptake inhibitors used for irritability), and anticonvulsants (used for rage) are also useful. However, using medications to control agitation should not replace other interventions. There can be a tendency to use medications to sedate the patient rather than pursue behavioral techniques. Some new medications such as donepezil hydrochloride (Aricept) have been used to temporarily improve cognitive function in patients with Alzheimer's disease. Current research also suggests that use of nonsteroidal anti-inflammatory drugs and estrogen may also provide some protection against developing this condition.

Rehabilitation

A multidisciplinary approach for the patient with dementia is essential. Physical and occupational therapy, nutritional support, speech therapy, psychiatry, social work, nursing, and medicine all need to be part of the long-term management of this patient. It is important that families use all available resources to reduce their isolation and stress.

NURSING MANAGEMENT

IMPAIRED VERBAL COMMUNICATION EVIDENCED BY INABILITY TO NAME OBJECTS OR SENSATIONS SUCH AS PAIN; INABILITY TO COMPREHEND VERBAL INSTRUCTIONS; INABILITY TO COMMUNICATE NEEDS; INAPPROPRIATE, DRAMATIC REACTIONS OR ACCUSATIONS, CATASTROPHIC REACTIONS RELATED TO CONFUSION, DISORIENTATION, MEMORY LOSS.

Patient Outcomes

- Demonstrates understanding of nurses and communication
- Able to communicate thoughts and needs
- Responds appropriately

Interventions

- Look directly at patient when speaking. Call patient by name frequently. Identify yourself by name before each conversation and refer to others by their names rather than "he" or "she."
- Keep interactions simple. Use short words and simple sentences that express one thought or question at a time.
- Ask specific questions such as "Does your stomach hurt?" rather than general ones like "How are you?"
- Reinforce speech with nonverbal techniques. For example, point, touch, or demonstrate an action while talking about it. For instance, if the patient is trying to tell you about his or her body, point as well as ask "Is this where it hurts?"
- Note in the chart or on the care plan the phrases, key words, and techniques that the patient responds to so that others can use them as well.
- If patient keeps repeating a question, try distraction and give reassurance that he or she will be cared for. Repetitive questions may indicate anxiety, and you want to be reassuring.
- If patient is searching for a particular word or trying to communicate something, guess at what it is, and ask if your guess is correct. If you are unable to determine what he or she is trying to say, focus on the feelings possibly being communicated. Always ask patient to confirm whether your determination is correct.
- If patient is reacting inappropriately, remain calm and reassure him or her that you are there to help. Avoid arguing or trying to convince patient that he or she is overreacting. Clarify any information or instructions. Assist patient with the next step of a task that is the source of frustration. Try to distract patient by removing him or her from disturbing situation.
- If patient makes inappropriate accusations, such as accusing the staff of stealing his or her glasses, help look for the missing item. Remember that patient may accuse you of stealing because of memory loss. Also, routinely check wastebaskets for missing items.

> **IMPAIRED MEMORY** EVIDENCED BY CONFUSION, DECREASED ABILITY TO PERFORM ACTIVITIES OF DAILY LIVING (ADLS), OR INABILITY TO FOLLOW THERAPEUTIC REGIMEN; INAPPROPRIATE EMOTIONAL OR BEHAVIORAL RESPONSES RELATED TO DELIRIUM, DEMENTIA, OR OTHER COGNITIVE DEFICITS.

Patient Outcomes

- Demonstrates improved orientation to person, place, and time
- Demonstrates improved ability to perform ADLs
- Displays less emotional or behavioral agitation

Interventions

- Establish a baseline assessment of patient's mental status and functioning:
  - Observe ability to perform ADLs.
  - Use a standardized method of mental status assessment such as that found in Table 3–1.
  - Ask the patient orientation questions. For example, ask patient personal questions such as names of his or her children or home address. Make sure that you can verify the answers from the chart or family.
- Assess if patient is willing to discuss memory lapses. Determine emotional responses to these lapses. Do not push the discussion if the patient becomes agitated or defensive.
- Be aware that patient may try to disguise memory loss by confabulation, avoiding responding, or by speaking in a rambling style to hide the fact that no thought or information is being expressed.
- Be aware that when social skills and personality are still intact, patient may mistakenly appear stubborn and resistant rather than unable to remember.
- Do not argue with patient about what he or she remembers. Rather, focus on immediate and specific tasks to be completed. Give patient step-by-step instructions on what needs to be done. Be directive without being domineering.
- Do not make demands that the patient cannot handle or focus on topics that clearly cause distress. Such demands will only add to the confusion and/or agitation.
- Break down complex tasks into individual steps. The seemingly simple act of brushing one's teeth can take over 10 steps. Be aware of the steps the patient can handle himself or herself and those requiring assistance.
- Establish a regular and predictable routine. Try to do things at the same time and in the same order each day, such as shave, bathe, and then eat breakfast. Communicate routines to the staff to coordinate patient's care and ensure that the same techniques are used. Obtain input from the family on patient's usual routine. Use prompts such as consistent cue words or signs to remind patient of the routine.
- Attempt to arrange for consistent staff to care for patient.
- Keep surroundings simple. Reduce clutter. Do not leave equipment in the patient's room if possible.
- Personalize patient's room. Have the family bring in photos and favorite objects.
- Place a large, visible clock and calendar in the patient's room. Cross each day off calendar daily. Place large signs on the wall noting where patient is and special events such as when the family is coming and the next upcoming holiday.
- Write lists of daily activities or tasks patient needs to do if still able to read and comprehend. Put labels on possessions and patient's name on his or her door in large letters.
- Avoid an overstimulating environment. In the hospital, patient's room should be close enough to nurses' station to monitor safety yet far enough away to avoid noise. Restrict the number of people visiting at one time.

- If patient tends to wander, make sure all staff are aware of this problem and can bring him or her back to the unit. Consider using alarms, if available, if patient is at high risk to leave the area. Monitor all exits. Draw a large red octagon-shaped stop sign and hang it by the exit. At home, make sure exits are monitored. Have the family notify neighbors of the problem and elicit their assistance to monitor for wandering. Make sure the patient always has some form of identification stating that he or she is confused, e.g., identification bracelet. Maintain photos of the patient to be shown if he or she is missing.
- Provide some form of night light. If the bathroom is connected to patient's room, leave the bathroom light on. Otherwise, use reflective tape in the shape of arrows to direct the patient to the bathroom door. Encourage the use of a bedside commode.

> **RISK FOR INJURY** EVIDENCED BY FALLS AND BUMPING INTO OBJECTS. RELATED TO PROBLEMS IN GAIT, VISION, HEARING, LACK OF COORDI-NATION, CONFUSION, OR LACK OF UNDERSTANDING OF ENVIRONMEN-TAL HAZARDS.

Patient Outcomes

- Remains free of injury
- Demonstrates appropriate actions to avoid injury

Interventions

- Be aware of factors that increase risk for falls (Box 10–3).
- Keep side rails up and bed in lowest position at all times.
- Even with side rails up, be aware that patient may get out of bed. Keep area around bed free from clutter. Make sure that there is always a clear path to the bathroom because that is the place where the patient will most often attempt to go. Make sure that patient uses the bathroom before going to bed at night. Plan administration of medications such as laxatives and diuretics so that they are not given in the evening. Recognize that the patient with dementia may have sleep pattern disturbances and become more confused at night.
- Make rounds frequently for patients at high risk for falling. Keep the patient's door open, and make sure all staff members know that this patient is at risk.
- Use restraints only after all other methods are ineffective. In some instances, restraints can increase confusion in elderly patients.
- If the patient has an unsteady gait, have him or her take your arm instead of the reverse while walking. Make sure the patient has access to any needed equipment such as walkers or wheelchairs. Provide instruction as appropriate within the patient's ability to understand. Ensure that any furniture or objects the patient leans on for support are sturdy and well balanced. Railings in hallways and bathrooms are very helpful. The patient may need prompts to perform simple actions, such as walking.

BOX 10–3. Causes of Increased Risk of Falls and Injury

- Stiff, awkward movements caused by damage to areas of brain that control muscle movement:
  - Difficulty getting out of bed
  - Stooped or leaning posture and shuffling gait as disease progresses
  - Apraxia, with inability to make or coordinate movements
- Overmedication: Changes in drowsiness, walking, posture, stiffness, agitation, falling, increased postural hypertension
- Visual problems:
  - Cataracts
  - Increased near- or farsightedness
  - Inability to distinguish between similar color intensities (may have difficulty identifying railings that are same color as walls; may stumble into walls of color intensity similar to that of floor)
  - Poor depth perception
  - Blurred vision (may be side effect of medication, anticholinergic action)
- Hearing problems: May not hear approaching machinery or people
- Agnosia: May bump into furniture, not recognizing what it is
- Diminished or absent pain perception:
  - Inability to recognize or communicate injury (for example, patient may try to walk on broken leg)
  - Only manifestation may be change in behavior
  - May burn self while smoking
- Sundowning syndrome (increased confusion at night) with night restlessness, wandering
- Any factor, including concurrent delirium, that increases confusion and disorientation

---

Source: Gorman, L, Sultan, D, and Luna-Raines, M, 1989.

- Make sure the patient receives adequate exercise within the limitations of his or her abilities and condition.
- If the patient wears glasses or a hearing aid, make sure that these are in place before any activity. Be sure to check that the hearing aid battery is good.
- Ensure that the room is adequately lighted for any activity and that the call light is within reach when patient is in bed, in bathroom, or sitting in chair.
- Check the patient routinely for bruises, cuts, or burns.
- Use colored waterproof tape along the area of the bathtub where patient is to stop filling with water. Decorative markers that stick to the bottom of the shower or tub can compensate for spatial disorientation.
- Use brightly colored materials in the room, if possible.
- Be aware that the patient may try to pull out catheters or intravenous tubing. Try to reduce risk of the patient's pulling out the tubes by reducing the discomfort associated with tubes. For instance, use the smallest-size nasogastric tube or cover the IV site with a large bandage to avoid the patient's pulling on the tubes. Wrist restraints or monitoring by a family member may be required to avoid injury.

- Be aware of medication interactions that could add to confusion and the risk for falls.

   SELF-CARE DEFICITS, ALTERED NUTRITION: LESS THAN BODY RE-QUIREMENTS, AND FLUID VOLUME DEFICIT EVIDENCED BY WEIGHT LOSS, ELECTROLYTE IMBALANCE, INCREASED CONFUSION, OR OTHER SIGNS OF DEHYDRATION. RELATED TO IMPAIRED RECOGNITION OF HUNGER AND THIRST, MEMORY LOSS, IMPAIRED MOVEMENTS.

Patient Outcomes

- Receives adequate nutritional and fluid intake
- Displays ability to recognize signs of hunger and thirst
- Demonstrates ability to feed self

Interventions

- Assess the patient's ability to feed and care for self (Fig. 10–1).
- Provide assistance, as needed, for dressing, personal hygiene, and eating.
- Determine how much patient can safely do independently. Perhaps just opening containers or cutting meat is all that is needed to promote independence. Provide verbal cues to keep patient on track.
- Determine patient's food preferences and provide these foods if possible. Encourage the family to bring familiar foods from home if appropriate.
- Make sure that dentures are in place and that they fit correctly before serving a meal.
- Allow hot foods to cool to prevent burn injury.
- Simplify the meal routine. The patient may be able to cope with only one food or one utensil at a time. Provide finger foods if utensils are difficult to use.
- Reduce distraction during mealtimes. For instance, turn off the television or radio.
- Assess regularly for signs of dehydration. Offer fluids regularly.
- Make sure that patient can see his or her food and hear your instructions.
- Consider liquid supplements if eating solid food is too difficult.
- Assess for constipation.
- For patient with end-stage dementia, family may face decision on whether to pursue aggressive nutrition intervention if patient refuses to eat or is unable to swallow. Provide support for the family in attempting to weigh these difficult options. Consider offering ethics consultation or hospice assistance, if appropriate.

ALTERNATE NURSING DIAGNOSES

   Altered Family Processes
   Altered Thought Processes
   Ineffective Management of Therapeutic Regimen: Individuals
   Sensory/Perceptual Alterations
   Sleep Pattern Disturbance

Self-care Checklist

Ambulation:

Independent with steady gait _____
Uses cane _____ walker _____ wheelchair _____
Needs staff to accompany when walking _____ assist sitting/getting up _____
assist in/out of bed _____ assist up/down stairs _____

Effective techniques for assistance

Resists using necessary equipment/assistance: Yes _____ No _____
If yes, nursing approach: _____
_____

Feeding:

Independent _____   Adequate nutritional intake _____
Difficulty swallowing _____   Needs staff to locate dining area _____
Provide assistance prompts _____   Feed patient _____

Effective techniques for assistance

Requires special feeding routine: Yes _____   No _____
Requires special food/supplements: Yes_____ No _____
If yes, describe:_____
_____

Fluid intake:

Independent _____
Adequate amount _____
Needs staff to monitor daily amount of fluid intake _____
Provide prompts to drink _____ hold cup while drinking _____ drink with straw _____

Effective techniques for assistance _____
_____

Toileting:

Independent: Yes _____   No _____
If no, words/behaviors patient uses to express need to toilet: _____
Diarrhea _____ Constipation _____ Frequency _____
Uses bedpan _____ urinal _____ commode _____ adult diapers _____
Needs assessment of frequency/circumstances of urination _____ defecation _____
Needs staff to take to toilet at scheduled times (every hour _____ before going to bed _____)

Effective technique to encourage patient to use toilet _____
_____

Bathing/Hygiene:

Independent: _____
Areas of skin breakdown _____
Areas of paralysis _____
Needs staff to provide assistance and prompts _____
Wash certain body areas (list) _____
Full bath _____
Mouth care _____

Effective means for assistance _____
_____

Dressing/Grooming:

Independent _____
Hearing aid _____   Glasses _____
Needs staff to provide assistance and prompts _____
Change clothes _____
Provide grooming (for example, comb hair)
If yes, specify steps that require assistance or if total care is needed: _____

Effective techniques for assistance _____
_____

FIGURE 10–1. Self-Care Checklist

PATIENT AND FAMILY EDUCATION

- Provide simple instructions based on patient's current ability to comprehend.
- Teach the family techniques to control uncooperative and aggressive behavior.
- Give the family information about the disease so that they can better understand that the patient has no control over his or her behavior.
- Teach the family or caregivers about the need to avoid stress and fatigue for the patient because this can increase behavior problems.
- Encourage family to obtain material and newsletters from the Alzheimer's Disease and Related Disorders Association (ADRDA). Also encourage them to obtain a copy of *The 36-Hour Day* by Mace and Rabins.
- Alert family to signs of caregiver abuse.
- Teach the family or caregivers to build support systems to maintain a balance in their lives.
- Teach the family about the emotional strain created by caring for the confused patient. Educate them that, with Alzheimer's disease in particular, the family may go through a mourning process for the person that their loved one used to be. This process is complicated because the patient looks the same but no longer has the same personality. Adult children must be prepared to reverse roles and become caretakers.

CHARTING TIPS

- Document any changes in levels of confusion, memory, behavioral routines, or consciousness.
- Document which activities the patient cannot do.
- Document if patient is able to start an activity but requires a prompt to continue. Document words or physical directions that work as a prompt.
- Document stimulus that causes the patient to have catastrophic reactions, such as too much noise or too many demands at the same time.
- Document the patient's response to medications.
- Document any techniques that have been effective in calming patient.

WHEN TO CALL FOR HELP

- [ ] Sudden onset of confusion
- [ ] Episodes of patient's becoming physically combative
- [ ] Patient who becomes a danger to self or others because of poor judgment (driving, cooking, etc)
- [ ] Severe agitation unresponsive to medication or other interventions
- [ ] Delirium that does not remit or gets worse

COMMUNITY-BASED CARE

- Be sure that the family has the needed information on financial resources and legal information for power of attorney if patient is unable to care for himself or herself.
- Report all indications of abuse.
- Assist the family or caregivers to set a plan to provide them with needed rest and recreation. Encourage family and caregivers to seek out support of friends or clergy. Encourage attendance at local support groups.
- If the care demands become too much, families need to consider placing the patient in a nursing home, specialized Alzheimer's program, or day-care. Provide information on any specialized programs in the community and suggestions for what to look for in a facility. Provide families with support to make this difficult decision.
- Give specific information on this patient's management to home health agencies and skilled nursing facilities.
- Give information from local Alzheimer's Disease and Related Disorders Association on treatment programs, research, and facilities.
- Patients with end stage dementia may be appropriate for referral for hospice care when they are bedbound, experiencing repeated infections, and are having difficulty with eating and drinking.

Problems with Psychotic Thought Processes

THE PSYCHOTIC PATIENT

LEARNING OBJECTIVES

➢ Differentiate between schizophrenia and other psychoses.
➢ Describe effective interventions for the hallucinating and delusional patient.
➢ Describe possible nurses' reactions to the psychotic patient.
➢ Discuss specific interventions for the patient experiencing intensive care unit psychosis.

GLOSSARY

Delusional disorder—Persistent suspicions, persecutory ideation, and delusions or delusional jealousies with resentment, anger, and sometimes grandiosity without other signs of psychotic thoughts or mood disorders. Patients are usually able to maintain daily functioning.

Delusions—False, fixed beliefs that cannot be corrected by feedback and are not accepted as true by others in the same culture.

Good reality testing—The ability to accurately identify and evaluate events. Absence of delusions, hallucinations, and other distorted perceptions.

Hallucinations—Sensory experiences that are very real to the patient but that do not exist in external reality, occurring while the patient is awake and when no one else has a similar experience.

Poor reality testing—Defects in a person's ability to accurately assess external events and interactions with others.

Psychosis—Severe distortion of and withdrawal from reality accompanied by severe disorganization of the personality.

Schizoaffective disorder—Symptoms of major depressive disorder or the manic phase of bipolar disorder as well as some of the symptoms of schizophrenia.

Schizophrenia—A severe thought disturbance characterized by impaired reality testing, hallucinations, delusions, limited socialization; diagnosis requires the symptoms to last at least 6 months.

Caring for a patient who is hearing voices, believes that the staff is trying to kill him or her, or exhibits other bizarre behavior can be confusing, disorienting, frightening, and disarming for the nurse. Although nurses in the psychiatric setting may frequently see psychotic patients (over 50 percent of psychiatric beds are occupied by patients with schizophrenia [Berkow, 1992]), nurses in other settings may be unprepared for managing the psychotic patient (25% of all in-patient beds are occupied by patients with schizophrenia [Moller and Murphy, 2001]). These patients are often feared and shunned by healthcare workers.

Hallucinations and delusions can be frightening for both the patient to experience and the nurse to observe. Even hallucinations that begin as fairly innocuous experiences can become frightening or accusatory to the patient (Box 11–1). Subjects of delusions vary. Common delusions are described in Box 11–2.

Hallucinations, delusions, or other psychotic thought disorders occur in a primary psychiatric disorder such as schizophrenia, delusional disorder, brief psychotic disorder (caused by an episode of extreme stress), or severe depressive disorder. Physiologic changes or drug and alcohol use or withdrawal can also cause them. Whether or not the etiology of the symptoms is known, the basic interventions are similar.

Psychotic thought disorders lead to severe distortion of and withdrawal from reality, accompanied by major personality disorganization. This disorganization leads to hallucinations, delusions, and bizarre behavior such as catatonia (assuming inappropriate postures or becoming completely immobile), or echolalia (repetition of words heard).

Schizophrenia, a psychiatric diagnosis characterized by changes in cognitive, perceptual, affective, motor, and social domains, is one of the commonest forms of psychosis. Schizophrenics have psychotic episodes, but not all psychotic

---

BOX 11–1. Recognizing Hallucinations

Affected Sense	Example
Visual	"I watch gypsies bring different babies to my apartment each night."
Auditory (most common)	"The voices are calling me a prostitute."
Tactile	"When I touched my arm, I could tell my arm is made of stone."
Olfactory	"I don't want to stay in that room. I can smell the odors of the people who died there."
Gustatory	"I taste milk in my mouth all the time."
Kinesthetic (bodily or movement sense)	"It feels as if the rats in my head are eating up my brain."

---

episodes are caused by schizophrenia. The word *schizophrenia* refers to splits between different components of the personality, for example, what the patient says does not match the emotion shown. The onset of schizophrenia occurs between ages 17 and 25 for 75 percent of cases (Moller and Murphy, 2001). Schizophrenia is a chronic, disabling condition, although symptoms can be controlled with appropriate medication. All socioeconomic and cultural groups are affected, but schizophrenics tend to cluster in the lower socioeconomic levels because of their difficulty maintaining employment and functioning in society. Schizophrenic patients can also have features of depression, manic behaviors, or both (schizoaffective disorder).

BOX 11–2. Common Delusions

Delusion	Example
Grandeur (belief of exaggerated importance)	"I am Napoleon Bonaparte."
Paranoia (belief of deliberate harassment and persecution)	"The FBI is following me and wants to kill me."
Reference (belief that the thoughts and behavior of others is directed toward self)	"Those people on the TV show are talking to me."
Physical sensations (belief that parts of body are diseased, distorted, or missing)	"I have no blood in me."

Patients without a psychiatric illness who experience sensory deprivation or over stimulation can become psychotic. A common example is referred to as *intensive care unit* (ICU) *psychosis*. However, the patient does not need to be physically located in the intensive care unit to experience this problem. Psychological stress, sleep deprivation, sensory overload, and immobilization all contribute to the critically ill person's developing personality changes, hallucinations, and delusions. Physiologic changes such as hypoxia, renal failure, and response to medications also contribute.

ETIOLOGY

No single cause of schizophrenia has been identified. *Genetic* theories recognize possible hereditary tendencies because there is a higher incidence in families with one schizophrenic parent or sibling. *Biologic* theories have received increasing attention. Some causes may be brain dysfunction in the limbic system and prefrontal cortex or biochemical disruption in neurotransmitters such as dopamine. *Psychologic* theory focuses on deficits caused by severely inadequate parenting throughout development, with special recognition of the devastating impact of deprivation during the first years of life. The more research validates the genetic and biologic theories, the less psychological theories appear to be causal. Clearly, though, personality is affected by psychological development and in turn affects outcomes in patients with schizophrenia. *Cognitive* theories indicate that the patient with schizophrenia has problems with attention or information processing. The person is unable to filter stimuli, leading to disorganization of mental functioning. *Family* theory has examined communication patterns that present unrealistic and unworkable expectations for the susceptible individual.

Other types of psychotic disorders may develop in individuals with fragile egos who become flooded with anxiety under severe stress.

RELATED CLINICAL CONCERNS

Certain physical conditions and medications, drug and alcohol withdrawal, and sleep and sensory deprivation cause some type of brain dysfunction that may result in psychosis. Examples of physical conditions include brain tumors, head injuries, high fever, septicemia, AIDS, encephalitis, epilepsy, and hepatic encephalopathy. Box 11–3 lists the types of psychotic reactions caused by medications.

Disorders, medications, and environmental factors can alter cerebral perfusion and chemistry to create biologic states that mimic some psychiatric disorders, including exhibiting psychosis and thought disorders. The combination of medications, sensory and sleep deprivation, fear and anxiety, and illness make the patient in an intensive care unit at risk of experiencing psychotic episodes. If this occurs, a thorough assessment is essential to accurately determine the underlying cause.

A patient with a psychotic disorder may also misuse drugs or alcohol as a

---

BOX 11–3. Drugs Associated with Psychotic Reactions

- Amphetamines
- Antidepressants (particularly tricyclics)
- Anticholinergics (e.g., atropine)
- Anticonvulsants (e.g., carbamazepine, valproic acid)
- Antihistimines (e.g., diphenhydramine)
- Antiparkinsonians (e.g., L-dopa)
- Antituberculosis (e.g., isoniazid)
- Antivirals (e.g., acyclovir, amantadine)
- Antiarrythmics (e.g., lidocaine)
- Alcohol
- Beta blockers (e.g., propranalol)
- Corticosteroids
- H2-receptor blockers (e.g., cimetidine)
- Cyclosporine
- Digitalis
- Dilsulfiram (antabase)
- Anesthetics (e.g., ketamine)
- Antibiotics (e.g., cephalosporins, ciprofloxacin, sulfonamides)
- Opioids (e.g., morphine, hydromorphone)

Adapted from: Caine, ED, and Lyness, JM: Delirium, dementia, and amnestic and other cognitive disorders. In BJ Sadock and VA Sadock (eds.): Kaplan & Sadock's Comprehensive Textbook of Psychiatry, 7th ed., Philadelphia, Lippincott Williams & Wilkins, 2000; and Goff, DC, Henderson, DC, and Manschreck, TC. In NH Cassem (ed.): Massachusetts General Hospital Handbook of General Hospital Psychiatry, 4th ed., St. Louis, Mosby, 1997.

way to self-medicate for uncomfortable symptoms. These medications could intensify psychotic symptoms and confuse the diagnosis and treatment. Dual diagnosis is the term used to describe someone with a substance dependency and a major psychiatric disorder.

LIFE SPAN ISSUES

CHILDREN

Although schizophrenia is rare in children, it has been identified. Symptoms include inappropriate affect, hallucinations, and mutism. It is often confused with autism, which is the most severe developmental disability of childhood, but it is not the same disorder. Children with psychotic disorders can be treated with antipsychotic medications, but side effects such as sedation and weight gain are a concern.

Children of parents with schizophrenia are at high risk for developing the disorder. As children of the mentally ill, they are at risk for being victims of abuse because they may be inadequately protected as a result of parental illness. They are likely to take on more responsibility to care for the household and less likely to have developmentally appropriate social skills because of the poor skills of their parents. Because so many people with schizophrenia are homeless, their children may be living on the streets.

ADOLESCENTS

The diagnosis of schizophrenia is more common in adolescence. Teens may be more likely to experiment with drugs in an effort to self-medicate to deal with distressing symptoms of anxiety and hallucinations.

ELDERLY PEOPLE

Elderly schizophrenics often have fewer and less severe symptoms, especially hallucinations and delusions, although symptoms of emotional flattening and loss of motivation often continue. These patients often do not verbalize pain or discomfort, which leads to under-treatment of medical conditions. The first signs of physical illness in these patients may be changes in ability to perform activities of daily living. They are also more prone to the nonreversible drug side effect of tardive dyskinesia (constant involuntary movements). See Chapter 20 for further discussion. With elderly persons living longer and mentally ill people less likely to be institutionalized, it is believed that there will be an increase in the number of these patients in nursing homes and retirement settings.

A new onset of psychotic behavior in elderly people must be closely assessed to rule out physical illness or medication toxicity. Because elderly persons may already have some sensory deprivation, illness, and use a variety of medications, the simple fact of their being hospitalized can increase anxiety and can make them at risk for confusion and psychosis. Symptoms can easily be confused with those of dementia, which could lead to inappropriate treatment.

POSSIBLE NURSES' REACTIONS

- May avoid psychotic patients because the nurse feels that he or she lacks knowledge or experience with them.
- May feel strangely uncomfortable or detached because of patient's lack of emotional connectedness.
- May feel frustrated and angry and have unrealistic expectations regarding the patient's self care.
- May feel afraid because of patient's bizarre behavior. May fear violence and personal harm.
- May feel confused when patient responds unpredictably.
- May ignore patient's complaints because "he's crazy."
- May feel rejected if patient's extreme mistrust or fear of others is not understood.
- May feel that he or she has to control patient's bizarre behavior to be effective.
- May feel unable to intervene, leading to the nurse's giving up on the patient.

ASSESSMENT

Behavior and Appearance

- Strange or bizarre appearance, poor grooming, disheveled, eccentric clothing
- Unusual gestures, mannerisms, facial grimaces, posturing
- Neglect or difficulty performing activities of daily living
- Incoherent, repetitive speech; mumbling; talking to self
- May not answer questions or respond only partly; frequently asks that questions be repeated.
- May be watchful or withdrawn: head positioned, eyes moving, watching something that is not there.
- Socially unacceptable behavior and speech; may make up words
- Marginal functioning, such as being unable to maintain employment

Mood and Emotions

- Displays emotions inappropriate to situation such as crying when others are laughing
- Displays contradictory emotions at same time; unpredictable mood changes
- Flat affect
- Highly anxious, panic
- Difficulty controlling emotions: outbursts of rage, crying, laughing

Thoughts, Beliefs, and Perceptions

- Poor concentration
- Impaired ability for abstract and/or logical thinking
- Loose associations (ideas shift rapidly from one unrelated subject to another)
- Hallucinations; sensory distortions such as seeing objects or people change in size and shape
- Delusions
- Extreme sense of worthlessness; overwhelming, inappropriate guilt
- Decreased recognition of own body sensations, such as hunger, pain, and urge to urinate
- Depersonalization (sense of feeling separated from body)
- Suspicious; paranoid
- Extreme ambivalence; impaired decision-making ability; inability to problem solve
- Altered sense of self; uncertain where own body stops and external objects and people begin

Relationships and Interactions

- Dependent on others for basic needs
- Fear and distrust of others
- Unable to maintain close relationships
- Lack of social skills
- Interactions seem cold and detached
- Poor eye contact; withdrawn

Physical Responses

- Complaints of unusual or bizarre symptoms
- Blunting of pain

Pertinent History

- Psychiatric hospitalizations
- Ongoing or periodic outpatient psychotherapy
- Substance abuse
- Childhood behavior problems such as being isolated or described as "odd"
- Minor infractions of law
- History of suicide attempts

COLLABORATIVE MANAGEMENT

Pharmacologic

Although they are not cures, antipsychotic (or neuroleptic) medications can reduce and control many of the symptoms of psychosis. See Chapter 20 for a detailed discussion of these medications. Antipsychotics are especially effective in managing agitation, combativeness, and belligerence. Newer antipsychotics, often called atypical, such as risperidone and clozapine, are particularly effective in treating social withdrawal, flat affect, hallucinations, and delusions. These are now being used for patients with schizophrenia that is refractory to other antipsychotics. They have fewer extrapyramidal side effects than the older antipsychotics, but clozapine can cause agranulocytosis. Patients with schizophrenia may need to remain on these medications for the rest of their lives, and symptoms can recur if they stop taking them. Approximately 25 percent of patients with schizophrenia do not respond adequately to traditional antipsychotics (Moller and Murphy, 2001). For patients with chronic psychotic processes, finding the right antipsychotic with minimal side effect profiles can take months or even years of trial and error.

Antipsychotics can be given on an occasional basis to manage acute agitation, such as might be seen in ICU psychosis or drug reaction. They control the symptoms until the problem resolves or the cause can be treated.

NURSING MANAGEMENT

RISK FOR VIOLENCE EVIDENCED BY AGITATION, AGGRESSIVE BEHAVIOR RELATED TO DELUSIONS AND HALLUCINATIONS.

Patient Outcomes

- Able to maintain control of own behavior
- Demonstrates less anxiety
- Does not cause harm to self or others

Interventions

- Reassure patient that he or she is safe and that the staff will provide protection. Be aware that the psychotic patient is more timid and frightened than dangerous.
- Avoid putting patient on the defensive. Avoid ultimatums.
- Maintain nonstimulating environment. Use a calm voice with relaxed, nonthreatening body language.
- Ask if patient is hearing voices and if he or she can tell you what they are saying.
- Ask the patient if he or she is hearing "command" hallucinations, such as voices commanding him or her to act a certain way. If these commands are for dangerous behavior, monitor the patient closely.
- Reinforce the patient's ability to remain in control of his or her behavior.
- Be aware of signs that indicate tension level is increasing.
- Monitor patient's behavior closely. If having hallucinations or delusions that are very frightening, patient could inadvertently harm self or others (e.g., the patient has to protect himself or herself from a monster in the room or voices saying to kill himself or herself). Observe closely if this occurs and seek out additional assistance.
- The patient may interpret even the most innocent behavior as threatening (turning up the thermostat could be interpreted as turning on poison gas.)
- Administer ordered antipsychotic medications. Consider injectable ones for faster onset of action. Patient may need these medications administered frequently (rapid tranquilization) until behavior is controlled. Monitor closely for side effects including postural hypotension and extrapyramidal symptoms.
- Determine if use of touch calms patient or adds to his or her distress. Ask the patient's permission to be touched.
- Set limits on destructive behavior. Let the patient know what behavior is and is not allowed. Reinforce to staff members that everyone must support the same approach.
- If patient is out of control, use restraints only as last resort. See Chapter 8 on managing violent behavior and restraint application. For the psychotic patient, restraints can represent a relief from the tremendous anxiety and loss of control being experienced, or they can significantly increase anxiety and persecution delusions. Have adequate, trained staff available to manage potential violence.

> **ALTERED THOUGHT PROCESSES** EVIDENCED BY INABILITY TO EVALUATE REALITY; HALLUCINATIONS, DELUSIONS RELATED TO SCHIZOPHRENIA OR OTHER PSYCHOSES.

Patient Outcomes

- Demonstrates clear communication to others
- Maintains reality orientation (person, place, time, situation)
- Demonstrates improved ability to participate in treatment plan

Interventions

- Determine if patient's behavior is a chronic problem or if this is a new onset. If chronic, determine baseline behavior, medications taken, psychiatric care received, and provider. If new, determine possible causes.
- Make short, frequent contacts to help build trust by helping the patient feel secure.
- Focus on the present reality rather than future or past. Speak simply. Focus on concrete subjects. Keep directions simple. Give only one step at a time. Avoid theoretic or philosophical topics.
- Provide a quiet, nonstimulating environment.
- Use one form of communication at a time; avoid using a lot of hand motions while speaking.
- Although psychotic speech is unclear, listen for unconsciously symbolic communication.
- Avoid giving choices to severely disorganized patients to avoid provoking anxiety.
- If possible, problem-solve with the patient about ways to cope with anxiety.
- Provide frequent reality orientation: review location, date, and so on.
- Arrange for the same staff members to care for patient, if possible.
- Find ways to provide structure in patient's day; provide a written schedule to follow.
- Make sure patient is taking and swallowing prescribed antipsychotic medications. Recognize that hallucinations and especially delusions may take weeks to months to diminish fully once the medication is started.
- Patient can easily misinterpret what you are saying or doing. Obtain frequent feedback from patient.
- Monitor patient's decisions. Poor judgment may indicate an exacerbation.
- Ask the physician to arrange for a psychiatric consultation.
- For the patient who may be reacting psychotically to the stressful hospital environment:
  - Ensure that patient is able to get adequate rest and sleep.
  - Make sure patient is oriented to the time of day.
  - Explain equipment and noises and their significance to patient.
  - Call patient by name and personalize his or her care.
  - Encourage family to bring in personal belongings such as photographs.
  - Vary stimuli around the patient; for example, turn on music or TV at times.
- If the patient is hallucinating:
  - Ask patient directly about his or her hallucinations. For instance, you may say, "Are you hearing voices? What are they saying to you?" "Are they telling you to do anything or not to tell?"
  - Watch patient for cues that he or she is hallucinating: eyes darting to one side, muttering, or watching a vacant area of the room. Patient may deny hallucinations per imagined commands to do so.
  - Avoid reacting to hallucinations as if they are real. Do not argue back to the "voices."
  - Do not negate patient's experience, but offer your own perceptions. For

instance, you may say, "I don't see the devil standing over you, but I do understand how upsetting that must be for you."

- Focus on reality-based diversions and topics such as conversations or simple projects. Tell patient, "Try to not listen to the voices right now. I have to talk with you."
- Be alert to signs of anxiety in the patient, which may indicate that hallucinations are increasing.

• If the patient is having delusions:
  - Be open, honest, and reliable in interactions to reduce suspiciousness. Respond to suspicions in a matter-of-fact and calm manner.
    Ask patient to describe the delusions: for example, "Who is trying to hurt you?"
  - Avoid arguing about the content of the delusions, but interject doubt where appropriate: for example, "I don't think it would be possible for that petite girl to hurt you."
  - Focus on the feelings that the delusions generate, such as "It must feel frightening to think there is a conspiracy against you."
  - Once patient describes delusion, do not dwell on it. Rather, focus conversation on more reality-based topics. If patient obsesses on delusions, set firm limits on amount of time you will devote to talking about them.
  - Observe for events that trigger delusions. If possible, discuss these with patient.
  - Validate if part of the delusion is real, for instance, "Yes, there was a man at the nurse's station, but I did not hear him talk about you."

ALTERNATE NURSING DIAGNOSES

Ineffective Individual Coping
Risk for Injury
Risk for Self-Mutilation
Self-Care Deficit
Sleep Pattern Disturbance
Social Isolation

WHEN TO CALL FOR HELP

Self-mutilation
Suicide threats or attempts
Aggressive behavior escalating to violence
Hallucinations or delusions with increasingly violent, bizarre content
Patient's inability to care for self
Increasing staff anxiety and fear over patient's behavior

PATIENT AND FAMILY EDUCATION

- Teach patient signs of escalating symptoms.
- Teach patient effective interventions to control anxiety and fears, such as distraction.
- Review with patient ways to validate whether what is being experienced is real, such as asking others if they see or hear the same things.
- Make sure family or caregivers are aware of signs of escalating symptoms and provide suggestions for managing them. For chronic psychotic disorders, give the family written information on the diagnosis or suggest appropriate reading, such as *Surviving Schizophrenia: A Family Manual* by E. F. Torrey.
- Teach the importance of taking prescribed medications and ways to manage side effects.
- Teach the importance of informing the physician of new symptoms, delusions, physical symptoms, and pains.

CHARTING TIPS

- Document patient's behavior and content of delusions and hallucinations.
- Document the administration of medications, side effects, and patient's response to the medication.
- Document efforts and effectiveness in controlling patient's behavior.
- If restraints are needed, document the type used and appropriate monitoring provided.
- Document the family response to patient and the education and discharge plan.

COMMUNITY-BASED CARE

- Determine psychiatric care and provider. Reinforce the need to continue in treatment. Reinforce to the family or caregivers their responsibility for getting the patient to follow-up appointments. Give patient and family written referrals and specific appointments for psychiatric care.
- Emphasize to the family their need for emotional support. Refer to appropriate programs or support groups, such as local chapters of the National Alliance for the Mentally Ill.
- If the patient has a chronic psychiatric disorder, determine patient's functional ability. Referrals may be needed to programs to assist with employment skills and living arrangements.
- If patient has difficulty functioning in society, he or she may need to be transferred to a psychiatric hospital or more protected living arrangements, such as a halfway house, group living home, or day treatment program.
- Reinforce need to continue follow-up medical care. Give written specific appointments.

Problems Relating to Others

LEARNING OBJECTIVES

➢ Identify types of manipulative behaviors.
➢ Identify some possible nurses' reactions toward manipulative patients.
➢ Describe "staff splitting" and characteristic manifestations.
➢ Define confrontation and limit setting as therapeutic responses.
➢ List effective nursing interventions to deal with manipulative patients.

GLOSSARY

Adaptive manipulation—Skillful management or use of one's self to impact or change a situation to one's best advantage. It is goal oriented, used only when appropriate, considers others' needs and welfare, and is only one of several coping mechanisms used.

Antisocial personality disorder—A psychiatric disorder in which there is a pervasive pattern of disregard for and violation of the rights of others. Individuals with this disorder rarely feel motivated to change.

Borderline personality disorder—A psychiatric disorder in which there is a chronic state of instability with changes in relationships, self-image, and mood.

Maladaptive manipulation—Similar to an addiction and not goal directed, it is the predominant, continuous controlling of others whether or not it is appropriate, effective, or attains specific goals.

Personality disorder—A group of psychiatric disorders in which specific, pervasive patterns of inflexible, enduring maladaptive thinking about one's self and the environment cause difficulties in interpersonal relationships and the ability to do work.

Splitting—An unconscious defense mechanism found in certain manipulative people that causes them to experience others only in the extremes of love or hate, good or bad.

Staff splitting—An unfortunate staff response to a patient that leaves the staff members arguing and not coordinating with each other. The staff members whom the patient treats well think highly of the patient and the others do not.

The word *manipulation* usually conjures up negative images of pushy, untrustworthy individuals who are concerned only with getting what they want with no regard for other people's feelings, priorities, or needs. However, manipulation can be viewed more accurately as a tool that is not inherently bad and that can be used in either constructive or maladaptive ways. For instance, adaptive or constructive manipulation is an effective technique for a charge nurse making assignments to ensure the best use of nursing personnel to meet patients' needs while considering the nurses' preferences and learning needs. Some people use maladaptive manipulation strategies during periods of stress to avoid uncomfortable, anxiety-arousing feelings and to gain a sense of security. The patient may use manipulation to compensate for feeling overwhelmed, out of control, and frightened by illness, hospitalization, or personal or occupational concerns.

People who consistently use maladaptive manipulation regardless of the circumstances may have a personality disorder, most notably a *borderline* or *antisocial personality* disorder. They operate using ingrained behavior patterns that have been effective for them, and they may not be aware of their manipulative behavior, the cause-and-effect relationship between their actions and resulting consequences, or the possibility of alternative, effective approaches. This behavior can be very difficult to change because the person is repeatedly rewarded by achieving his or her goal when the manipulation is successful. People with borderline personality disorder manipulate to gain nurturance. They are so fearful of separation that they use manipulation to try to achieve a goal of maintaining closeness. They may exhibit both clinging and distancing behavior as they struggle with these issues (Townsend, 2000). People with antisocial personality disorder manipulate to gain power, possessions, or some other material gratification. Antisocial personality disorder is also associated with social irresponsibility and reckless or criminal behavior. Manipulative behavior from personality disorders can be either blatant or insidiously covert. The manipulative person may appear superficially pleasant. However, the person being manipulated often recognizes the impact or results even if he or she is unable to describe clearly how they occurred.

The first sign of a patient's use of maladaptive manipulative behavior may be the staff's growing frustration and anger. Manipulative patients may unconsciously project their own thoughts and feelings onto staff members and see one or some of them as a mirror image of themselves. As a result, the patient perceives the staff member(s) as manipulative, unreliable, and even verbally abusive. When the patient feels threatened, he or she tries to control the situation by manipulating, attacking, or avoiding the staff member(s).

Two effective techniques for working with manipulative patients are *confrontation* and *limit setting*. Both of these techniques need to be used consistently with concern for the patient. Although the word *confrontation* is usually associated with hostile, antagonistic battles, it is used effectively as an intervention to dispassionately point out to the patient a discrepancy among words, actions, or feelings. For instance, "You said you have not seen a doctor before coming to the ER, but you have a bottle of prescription drugs dated last week. Where did you get that?" *Setting limits* is teaching and maintaining boundaries of the nurses' and the patient's roles and acceptable behaviors. This may mean telling a patient what he or she may or may not do under certain conditions or in certain situations.

Despite protests, manipulative patients feel more secure and less out of control when their behavior is contained. Using these techniques, nurses can alleviate much of the patient's insecurity and help to create the appropriate boundaries of acceptable behavior. Before being successful at using these techniques, however, you need to feel comfortable being assertive and being in the role of an authority figure. The nurse's past experiences with authority figures and individual personalities influence his or her ability to master these techniques. It is important to realize that no one can completely control another person's behavior.

Manipulative patients who unconsciously block painful feeling by *splitting* their perceptions of people into the extremes of all good or all bad can have a very disruptive, divisive effect on the staff. *Staff splitting* is a possible response to splitting when the patient idealizes certain staff members, treating them as all worthy and good while viewing others as all bad and criticizing and devaluing them. The staff may respond similarly, each one either intensely liking or disliking the patient and eventually becoming alienated from each other (Box 12–1).

ETIOLOGY

According to *psychologic* theory, manipulative patients do not trust other people to like or accept them, to be responsive to them, or be responsible toward them. Consciously or unconsciously, they rely on manipulative behavior to demand that others supply what they need and want.

BOX 12–1. Warning Signs of Staff Splitting

A manipulative patient can have a devastating effect on the staff and functioning of the unit. Staff group behavior that can indicate that staff splitting has occurred includes:

- Diagnostic uncertainty with contradictory evaluation of patient.
- Groups of staff members feel emotionally isolated from one another. For instance, two or more staff members become suspicious of the motives and behaviors of other staff members toward the patient.
- Lunch hour and coffee break dominated by discussion of the specific patient.
- The nucleus of an in-group believe that only they can help the patient.
- Loss of morale and confusion in the out-group.
- Blurring of staff-client role boundaries (for instance, patient and staff discuss another staff member, staff share personal information with patient).
- Split in- and out-groups make accusations: "ins" accuse "outs" of being cold and insensitive; "outs" accuse "ins" of being too permissive and gullible and of spoiling patient.
- Splits between departments in a hospital agency structure.

Source: Adapted from Lego, S, Borderline personality disorders. In Varcarolis, E, Foundations of Psychiatric Mental Health Nursing. WB Saunders, Philadelphia, 1994. Reprinted with permission.

Manipulative behavior in healthcare settings may reflect the patient's ongoing, habitual mode of interaction, or it may be an escalation of milder, more common control mechanisms. In the hospital setting, the patient may regress and have unrealistic expectations that his or her every need will be instantly gratified. Disappointment results in fury and an increase in manipulative behavior.

Chronic manipulative behavior may result from childhood dilemmas if parents undermined attempts toward independence and autonomy. Manipulative individuals have come to suspect that any person or institution may try to control them, rendering them powerless and vulnerable to attack. Even being cooperative can be viewed as giving in or being weak, negatively affecting self-esteem. Authority figures are seen as being stronger and having too much control over the patient's life. The patient may seek ways to equalize the power by controlling staff, not complying with medical regimen, and making excess demands. Suicidal gestures may be a frantic attempt to regain control or block painful feelings of helplessness or dependence. Fear of rejection and abandonment or expectation of increased responsibility are also triggers for self-destructive acts.

The *learning* theory of manipulative behavior focuses on the concept that the behavior may have been learned in childhood based on adult role models, peers, and even the media. The *family* theory suggests that manipulative behavior may have been developed, especially in younger years, as the only way to cope with a severely dysfunctional family.

Antisocial personal disorder frequently arises from a chaotic home environment with early parental deprivation. There may be some genetic link

(Cadoret, 1994). Borderline disorder is associated with separation issues concerning parental figures. Personality disorders are generally associated with depression.

RELATED CLINICAL CONCERNS

This patient may rely on sedatives, analgesics, or other substances to reduce feelings of anxiety. These substances may trigger reduced inhibitions and increased aggressive responses.

LIFE SPAN ISSUES

CHILDREN AND ADOLESCENTS

Manipulative behavior begins in the earliest years, partly as a way to test the responses of parents and other caretakers. Toddlers have temper tantrums and quickly learn whether or not they can get their way. Children of all ages mimic the manipulative behavior of parents and siblings, such as making promises that are not kept. Or they may try getting permission from one parent after receiving a "no" from the other. They also learn from their peers. They may try to obtain privileges or possessions by saying that all their friends have these already.

Disturbed, maladaptive manipulative behaviors manifested in conduct disorders are seen in childhood and adolescence. Those who rely on deceitfulness can also display cruelty to animals or other children, destructiveness of property, and serious violations of rules. This can evolve into antisocial personality disorder in adulthood. These children may have experienced more severe deprivations such as multiple rejections, neglect, or abuse.

ADULTS

People who have successfully used manipulative behavior as children tend to become more proficient at this behavior as they grow older. They tend to flourish in systems where they are able to manipulate. People who are extremely manipulative and exploitative may violate laws and end up in the criminal justice system. Those who exhibit strong manipulative tendencies but are able to stay within legal confines may become successful in using people, personally and professionally, for their own goals.

ELDERLY PEOPLE

As people age and become more dependent on others for assistance in activities or socialization, they may resort more frequently or aggressively to manipulative behaviors to get their needs met. If guilt has been a favorite ploy, declarations such as "I don't want to be a burden" may be intended to stir guilt and get attention.

POSSIBLE NURSES' REACTIONS

- May feel angry, frustrated, or resentful for being tricked; may have lowered self-esteem if unable to stop the manipulation; or may feel embarrassed or humiliated.
- May feel helpless in relieving patient's apparent distress or when attempting to get patient to conform to nurse's expectations of reasonable conduct.
- May feel vulnerable and afraid of patient's attacks.
- May take manipulations personally and react defensively, especially when challenged in authority or position.
- May reject patient because the experience of coping with personal reactions is too draining and demoralizing.
- May avoid patient, spend minimal time needed to provide physical nursing care, or assign a different nurse to the patient each day.
- May compensate by becoming overcontrolling or engage in power struggles with patient.
- May experience desire for revenge, retaliation; may become punitive, want to counterattack by insulting, hurting, or embarrassing patient. May secretly hope things go wrong for patient.
- May experience guilt about negative feelings toward patient.
- May become overinvolved or overattached and wish to rescue patient.
- May feel total responsibility for patient's improvement or lack of improvement.
- May be punitive in setting limits or confronting the patient or may be inconsistent or hesitant in enforcing rules for fear of patient's reaction.

ASSESSMENT

Behavior and Appearance

- Frequent disregard of rules
- Argumentative
- Can be superficially charming and entertaining
- Demanding; the more staff try to cater to demands, the more they escalate
- Impulsive and unpredictable; lacks ability to tolerate frustration; can easily become out of control
- Uses threats to get demands met
- May use intimidation to control or feel superior
- Frustration causes more intense manipulative behavior
- Destructive toward self, others, property without taking responsibility
- Lies, cheats, steals
- Intense manipulation around medication; overuse of medication
- Noncompliant with health care treatment
- Undermines treatment of other patients, such as encouraging them to ignore doctor's recommendations or suggesting alternate treatments

Mood and Emotions

- Anger predominates. Behavior can be cutting, sarcastic, and vicious.
- Anxiety rises rapidly to panic, which precipitates impulsive actions. May not experience anxiety unless facing a threat to self-image or self-esteem.
- Views self as very vulnerable and frightened, even when being intimidating, or as totally invulnerable to harm or negative consequences, resulting in reckless behavior.
- Has labile moods and emotions. The more patient is in crisis, the more frequently moods and emotions may fluctuate over the course of a day. May appear resistant to depression or may have periodic depressive reactions.
- May have inflated or diminished self-esteem. If inflated, denies or distorts information that would lower self-esteem.

Thoughts, Beliefs, and Perceptions

- Thinking can contain gross distortions of some specific events or people and yet maintain accurate perception and good reality of others.
- Projects own thoughts and feelings onto others, resulting in feelings of fear and manipulation by others.

Relationships and Interactions

- May seek or avoid attention
- Exploitative with little real concern for others; limited capacity for empathy; demonstrates caring only to get own needs met
- Quick to recognize vulnerable areas in others
- Limited ability to see others for who they really are; distorted perceptions of how others experience self
- Needs to feel either in control or helpless and vulnerable (Life is seen as a seesaw competition. If someone else is up, then patient feels down)
- Does not feel a sense of obligation to reciprocate favors or helpful acts
- Devalues others to feel good about self
- Sees others as attacking or dangerous
- Feels and acts as if he or she were entitled to having needs met without comparable effort or cost
- Becomes a "special patient" to the staff
- Blames others for mistakes and problems without taking personal responsibility; confuses taking responsibility with being blamed, worthless, and vulnerable to attack
- Belief of being superior; cannot admit lack of knowledge and has great difficulty asking for assistance and information; obtains information by using indirect manipulation; unable to accept suggestions or criticism

Physical Responses

- Physical complaints that cannot be substantiated with testing
- Magnifies any subjective symptoms that cannot be measured
- With documented disability, usually requires more frequent medication and higher dosages; recovery takes longer than usual

Pertinent History

- Erratic, impulsive behavior with marked instability; frequent changes in jobs, relationships, and physicians
- Drug or alcohol abuse
- Long history of many physical complaints

COLLABORATIVE INTERVENTIONS

Multidisciplinary Team Communication

When staff members have extremely different experiences with the same patient, infighting among each other can occur when discussing care for the patient. These variations in experiences can occur between or among individuals in the nursing staff, different shifts, nurses and physicians, or all staff members and administrators. To overcome this staff splitting, the group needs to recognize the patient's dynamics and cooperatively share their different perceptions to gain a more complete picture of the patient. They need to identify whom the patient sees as "all good" or "all bad" and how this affects interactions.

Once the team has identified the problem behaviors, it is essential to formulate a united, consistent care plan. Each staff member should monitor the intensity of his or her individual reactions to the manipulative behavior. This will help to avoid becoming entrapped into feeling the need to be special or the only one who can help or avoid getting caught in power struggles. A supportive and coordinated multidisciplinary team approach helps neutralize the manipulative patient's ability to identify vulnerability in team members and discord in the health care organization.

Pharmacologic

If the patient is given tranquilizers to reduce anxiety, there is a risk for drug dependence and power struggles (e.g., patient may try to manipulate the nurse to get extra doses). Individuals with personality disorders may benefit from antidepressants to address depression and reduce impulsive behavior. The anticonvulsant carbamezepine has been used to improve mood stability. Herbal products may be used as a way to self-medicate uncomfortable symptoms.

NURSING MANAGEMENT

INEFFECTIVE INDIVIDUAL COPING EVIDENCED BY NONCOMPLIANCE WITH RULES AND TREATMENTS RELATED TO IMPULSIVE, MANIPULATIVE BEHAVIOR.

Patient Outcomes

- Decreased use of maladaptive, manipulative behaviors
- Complies with treatment regimen and hospital rules
- Uses effective coping patterns
- Demonstrates more adaptive methods of dealing with stress, such as using problem-solving skills

Interventions

- Carefully assess patient's mode of interaction and frequency over time before labeling behavior as "manipulative."
- Determine if the patient is using manipulation to indirectly express a need, anxiety, or distressful emotion. Active listening and empathetic responses to underlying issues can help diminish the patient's anxiety and need to control others.
- Approach patient in a calm and matter-of-fact manner, using a neutral tone of voice.
- Provide feedback to patient, who may not be aware that manipulative behaviors are being used. State specific observations about his or her style of interactions without arguing. If patient argues or denies, calmly repeat your observation without becoming defensive. Describe options and consequences. Follow through consistently with consequences.
- Don't state consequences that you do not have the authority to exercise.
- State which behaviors are not acceptable without personally rejecting the patient.
- Help patient identify when using manipulative behavior becomes an attempt to control anxiety. Encourage patient to identify triggers for anger and frustration.
- Encourage patient to verbalize feelings instead of acting them out. Ask the patient to identify what he or she is experiencing and what feelings and thoughts preceded the behavior.
- Evaluate whether patient's manipulative behavior increases or decreases when not reinforced by nurse's attention. Be aware that even when ignoring provocation is effective over time, there may be an initial escalation to test responses.
- Avoid power struggles and attempts to out-manipulate the patient. Point out that the patient is undermining his or her own care. State explicitly that the patient will not be forced to accept treatment and that each individual is responsible for the outcome of the treatment.
- Explain as early as possible rules and regulations and the reasons for them. If allowable limits are not stated, patient may push and test until they are clarified. If he or she attempts to break the rules, review firmly the stated expectations.
- Include the patient in decisions about limits and provide opportunities for personal decision making to enhance sense of control. When all rules are

rigid, the patient may feel a greater need to rebel. Be careful not to allow patient to dictate nursing decisions.

- Written contracts defining both staff and patient expectations can be most effective. Specifically define any consequences of patient's continued manipulation and lack of cooperation. Nurse and patient can sign contracts.
- Describe in detail on care plan the limits set and the consequences of breaking them. In periodic staff meetings and multidisciplinary case conferences, give current information and promote agreement about the patient, which will enable staff members to work more consistently and cohesively.
- Make sure all staff members are aware of limits and consequences. Confront colleagues who are observed not following the treatment plan.
- Consult with physician when patient seems to exaggerate complaints of pain or becomes preoccupied with timing of medications. The physician may decide to convert a PRN order to low doses of regularly administered medications to avoid power struggles.
- Assess for signs of substance abuse or withdrawal if patient has such a history or shows symptoms.

IMPAIRED SOCIAL INTERACTION EVIDENCED BY ATTEMPTS TO UNDERMINE, CONTROL AND INFLUENCE, AND CAUSE CONFLICT RELATED TO SPLITTING, DISTORTED PERCEPTIONS OF OTHERS, IMPULSIVITY, AND ANXIETY.

Patient Outcomes

- Uses acceptable methods to interact with others to communicate and obtain needs
- Positively responds to confrontation and limit setting
- Tolerates frustration and waiting
- Does not reject or denigrate the staff as "bad" when they are unable to respond in desired manner
- Develops a more trusting relationship with at least one staff member by sharing personal thoughts and feelings

Interventions

- Maintain assertive, centered, firm but fair, and even-toned stance when patient tries to manipulate or undermine you.
- Tell the patient that he or she may understand events and interactions differently than the staff does.
- Direct patient who complains about staff member to discuss the problem with implicated staff person. Do not allow yourself to be used as an intermediary; do not take sides.
- Use "I" statements indicating how patient made you feel. Avoid becoming defensive, which can escalate manipulative behavior.
- Confront the patient with your perception that he or she is trying to put you down. This can have an impact even if patient denies it.
- Take time to think about effective responses and to diminish the intensity

of your reactions if patient is trying to manipulate. Use stress reduction techniques.

- Role-play or discuss situation with other staff, if necessary.
- Return to original topic if patient tries to divert topic to a personal attack.
- Be aware of patient interactions that can increase staff divisiveness by blaming, accusations, or comparisons. Monitor your own responses.
- Provide praise and reinforcement when patient communicates directly and openly about needs and concerns.
- Use kind but firm approach. Clarify that setting limits is constructive and caring rather than punitive.
- Establish from the beginning that you take all of the limits very seriously. More flexibility can be introduced later as the patient takes more responsibility.
- Find neutral actions and topics for conversation. This will help to present you as a person interested in the patient and not just a rule keeper.
- Be aware that patient may need to test limits repeatedly to see whether there are repercussions and to be reassured that the staff will follow through on the consequences.
- Let patient know immediately that threats or verbal abuse are unacceptable, that you expect these will never be repeated, and state the consequences of repeated abuses.
- Confront patient when he or she attempts to undermine other patients' treatment.
- Do not allow patient to manipulate, flatter, seduce, bargain, or intimidate staff into granting him or her special status. Do not accept gifts or favors or share personal information, especially about any current difficulties.
- Never agree to keep a secret with a patient. Remind patient that the entire health team needs to be aware of patient's concerns in order to offer the best care.
- Assess interactions with family. If patient uses same approaches with them, family members may need information on changing their response.

ALTERNATE NURSING DIAGNOSES

Anxiety
Defensive Coping
Noncompliance
Powerlessness
Self-Esteem Disturbance

WHEN TO CALL FOR HELP

Threats or actions of physical harm to others or self, including suicidal threats or gestures

Undermining own or other's health care and unresponsive to nursing interventions

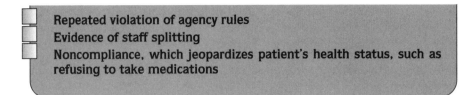

> Repeated violation of agency rules
> Evidence of staff splitting
> Noncompliance, which jeopardizes patient's health status, such as refusing to take medications

PATIENT AND FAMILY EDUCATION

- Teach patient to ask directly for what he or she wants and needs in words, not actions. Teach problem-solving skills.
- Help patient recognize that his or her desires may not require immediate action and that he or she may not always get desired responses.
- Explain the consequences of manipulative behavior.
- If a patient will not take responsibility for own actions, explain how his or her behavior contributed to the unwanted response or consequences and that taking responsibility is not the same as being blamed.
- Teach patient that understanding of one's own behavior and developing improved interactions are the avenues for developing stable support networks.
- Involve family in patient education. The same skills used in working with the patient may be helpful for the family.
- Provide information for family members of individuals with personality disorders. Psychiatric staff members may be helpful.
- Also Web site: www.mental-health-matters.com/borderline.html

CHARTING TIPS

- Describe specific manipulative behaviors objectively rather than just labeling the patient as manipulative.
- Develop a detailed treatment plan so that the team can respond consistently. Chart patient's responses to interventions.
- Document usage of PRN medication, reason for use, and patient's response.

COMMUNITY-BASED CARE

- Begin discharge planning as early as possible to decrease last-minute impulsive and inappropriate decisions the patient might make without consideration for consequences.
- Inform the family and patient together of patient's healthcare needs to reduce manipulative behavior with family.
- Inform referring agencies of patient's behavior and short-term treatment planning goals.
- If appropriate, make referrals for individual and group psychotherapy.

THE NONCOMPLIANT PATIENT

LEARNING OBJECTIVES

➤ Identify factors that contribute to a patient's noncompliance with treatment plans.
➤ List the principles of adult education that contribute to effective patient education.
➤ Identify nursing interventions to reduce noncompliance in the patient whose cultural beliefs impede compliance.
➤ List some nursing staff reactions to the noncompliant patient.

GLOSSARY

Compliance—Patient's accurately following a prescribed regimen of treatment.

Ineffective management of therapeutic regimen—A pattern of regulating and integrating into daily living a program for treatment of illness and the sequelae of illness that is unsatisfactory for meeting specific health goals.

Noncompliance—Patient's failure to follow therapeutic recommendations.

Compliance and *noncompliance* are terms that are used to describe patient behavior in response to information given about his or her health care. What makes a patient follow, change, or ignore health teaching is complex and may not always be related to the amount and quality of information provided. Nurses need to be aware that noncompliance is a symptom of an underlying problem and not the actual problem and that labeling behavior as "noncompliant"' can have negative connotations, such as blaming or criticizing a patient who is not following instructions. Once you have identified that the patient is noncompliant, you need to investigate what the illness and treatment mean to the patient as well as the other variables that influence the ability to comply. Because noncompliance can have a negative connotation, it can also be called ineffective management of therapeutic regimen.

The cost of noncompliance is greater than can actually be documented. Besides factors such as the cost of medications purchased but not taken or taken incorrectly, poor results of diagnostic tests caused by poor preparation, and more severe illness from not following recommended treatments, both patients and health care providers can experience a great deal of frustration. Although not the only reason for noncompliance, inadequate or inappropriate patient education is among the most common.

When teaching adults, the nurse needs to incorporate principles of adult learning (Box 12–2). Adults have different learning needs than children do. Adults are goal oriented. The goals need to be clearly identified and attainable, and they need to consistently be made aware of their progress toward their goal. Adults need to understand how the education will benefit them. Adults tend to learn better when they understand the rationale for what they are learning, apply what they learn immediately, and can compare what they are learning to knowledge from past experiences. Learning is inhibited when authoritarian teaching methods are used. Interpersonal relationships with teachers are important.

ETIOLOGY

There are many dynamics that contribute to noncompliance. For example, although the patient may fully understand the information and consequences of not following recommendations, he or she has the right to choose not to follow that advice. The patient's decision is in keeping with the principle of autonomy. In this situation, it is the health care provider's responsibility to ensure that the patient has all the information he or she needs to make that decision and then the responsibility of making the decision remains with the patient.

Other major factors contributing to noncompliance include:

- *Denial:* This may be a conscious or unconscious method of believing that he or she is not sick. By not checking blood sugars, the patient can block the diagnosis of diabetes from his or her mind.

BOX 12–2. Adult Learning Principles

- Adults need to participate in the learning process. Avoid directive approach. Give them some control.
- Adults need to understand the purpose behind any information they receive.
- Adults learn more effectively if past experiences are integrated into the teaching.
- Put new information to immediate use.
- Give specific feedback to learner of progress made in learning process.

- *Power struggles:* At times the patient who feels a lack of control over his or her body uses noncompliance as a way to maintain some control over a sense of destiny or over healthcare providers.
- *Counterdependence:* The patient could be concerned that following recommendations would increase dependency on others. Because dependency can enhance feelings of loss of identity, noncompliance becomes a statement of independence and individualism.
- *Loss of coping mechanisms:* Often health teaching involves asking the patient to give up habits that are part of the person's usual coping strategies. For example, smoking, diet changes, or exercise may need to be altered or avoided. If the patient has not yet developed alternative coping mechanisms, the anxiety created by the loss of these habits may be overwhelming.
- *Conflict with self-image:* Noncompliance may be a method of self-protection against the threat of an altered body image, particularly in individuals whose health and activity are a source of pride. Taking medication or imposing limitations on activity may represent a threat to the individual's self-image.
- *Fatalistic viewpoint:* A patient may believe there is no point to following instructions because of the belief that nothing will change the outcome.
- *Hidden benefits of illness:* Some people may consciously or unconsciously perceive benefits from the sick role, such as attention, avoidance of responsibility, controlling the destiny of another, or maintaining stability in a rocky relationship.
- *Self-destructive behavior:* A patient could be consciously or unconsciously participating in a wish to die or hurt himself or herself, possibly reflecting depression or suicidal tendencies. It could represent behaviors associated with a serious personality disorder.
- *Psychiatric disorder:* Psychiatric illness or altered thought processes may make consistent compliance with a health routine impossible.
- *Family influence:* Family members may discourage or undermine compliance because they are using denial, lack the understanding of the treatment, or unconsciously need to maintain the patient in the sick role.
- *Lack of economic resources:* If the patient has insufficient funds or no insurance, he or she may need to decide between eating or feeding the family and buying needed medications.
- *Lack of social resources:* Lack of funds, fear of being dependent on others, or lack of social contacts may cause the patient to miss appointments because there is no transportation.
- *Unsatisfactory relationship with health care team:* If the patient perceives the doctors or nurses as cold, uncaring, not knowledgeable, or authoritarian, he or she may resent or ignore instructions. This may stir up in the patient such issues as resentment of authority and feeling unrecognized as an individual. This patient may minimize or distort information given because of his or her emotional response. Long waits and uncomfortable waiting areas may also contribute to the poor relationship.
- *Lack of trust in information given:* Patient may not believe health information given because it has not proved useful in the past. Also, with the increase in media reporting of conflicting reports of studies, patients may think the information isn't trustworthy enough to warrant a change in lifestyle.

- *Cultural beliefs:* Cultural or religious beliefs may influence the way in which the patient views his or her illness and the treatments that are acceptable. For instance, women in some cultures may not allow a male health care provider to examine their breasts or a Jehovah's Witness may not accept a blood transfusion.
- *Inability to read or understand instructions:* Some patients may be too embarrassed to acknowledge that they cannot read English. This may apply to those who speak another language or even to those who do speak English. Literacy rates in the United States are dropping, so some patients who function well in society may not be able to read. Also, be aware that some patients will not admit that they do not understand language that is too technical or that contains too much jargon. To be understood by the majority, patient education materials should be written at the average reading level, which for most adults is the fifth to eighth grade level.
- *Uncomfortable side effects:* Patients may be noncompliant because of real or perceived side effects, especially with medications. The patient may be less likely to report them if they are embarrassing, such as impotence or incontinence. In addition, incorrect beliefs such as fear of becoming dependent on medications may cause some patients not to take medications. Noncompliance can become part of a negative cycle as the patient feels embarrassed or guilty for not following through and then begins canceling appointments to avoid health care providers.

RELATED CLINICAL CONCERNS

When patients are dealing with an acute crisis, most of their energy will be focused on just coping with the situation at hand. They will not be able to concentrate on learning until the crisis has subsided or they have made adaptations to deal with the situation. During this time, instruction should involve only what is absolutely necessary. You will need to be prepared to repeat much of the information provided as the patient may not remember what he or she was told.

Any physical or mental problem that impairs cognition will also interfere with learning.

LIFE SPAN ISSUES

CHILDREN

Following a particular treatment plan can be difficult for ill children and their family. Medications may affect behavior, alertness, or school performance. Incorporating a child's medical care into family life can create many stressors, contributing to noncompliance because the child may not be able to be responsible. It can be time consuming and difficult to administer. Working parents and single-parent families may not have the time to be able to supervise the child or take him or her for follow-up care. Because the child may not be able to communicate his or her needs, medical care can be difficult to monitor.

Parental noncompliance could have legal and ethical ramifications. Parents who refuse to give a child needed medical attention could be accused of negligence or even abuse. Parental autonomy to make decisions for their child may be overridden if it is determined the child is placed at some risk. In these extreme situations, legal intervention would be required.

ADOLESCENTS

Adolescents are particularly vulnerable to problems with compliance. Their attitude is often related to struggles with maintaining independence and rebelling against adult authority. In addition, any medical regimen that impacts body image puts additional demands on the teenager. Also, because the adolescent does not want to appear different from his or her peer group, complying with instructions may be particularly difficult. For example, a diabetic adolescent who is eating lunch with friends may be fearful to expose his or her dietary restrictions.

ELDERLY PEOPLE

Noncompliance is an extremely important issue for elderly people, who experience more chronic illness than the general population. Chronic illnesses often require multiple medications and are often combined with over-the-counter drugs and alternative therapies. Some elderly persons see more than one specialist and have a variety of prescriptions from the physicians they see or may be given contradictory treatment advice. They may become easily confused. Decreased muscle mass and increased fat stores may make individuals more prone to drug side effects. The elderly patient may need more assistance and time to explain instructions. If living alone, the elderly patient may have limited support for encouragement or reminding. Hearing and vision deficits as well as limited manual dexterity caused by arthritis can present other problems. In addition, cognitive impairments including poor short-term memory may inhibit the patient's compliance by causing him or her to forget instructions or how many pills have already been taken.

POSSIBLE NURSES' REACTIONS

- May become angry or frustrated because the time spent with patient seemed fruitless.
- May criticize or judge patient who does not follow instructions.
- May feel that situation is hopeless and makes less effort to communicate with patient.
- May judge self as inadequate or incompetent when patient does not follow instructions.
- May feel responsible for patient's noncompliance. Nurse may have difficulty recognizing that ultimately the responsibility for health care belongs to the patient.

ASSESSMENT

Behavior and Appearance

- Does not follow rules or instructions, demonstrated by:
  - Refusing to take or change medications
  - Continuing unhealthy habits
  - Missing medical appointments
  - Altering medical regimen
  - Challenging the necessity or helpfulness of treatments
  - Leaving facility against medical advice
  - Arguing without constructive resolution
  - Indicating understanding or agreement with treatment plan and then not following through
  - Hiding inability to read or comprehend educational material

Mood and Emotions

- Anger
- Depression
- Resentment
- Irritability
- Anxiety

Thoughts, Beliefs, and Perceptions

- Religious or cultural beliefs in contradiction with compliance actions
- Believes health care should be obtained only when symptoms are blatant or impairing needed activity
- Suspicions concerning motivations of health care professionals
- Lack of confidence in own abilities
- Denial of health care needs
- Psychotic thought process or suicidal thoughts

Relationships and Interactions

- May avoid sharing information with others about medical regimen
- Tendency to manipulate or control others
- Family not providing needed support
- Inconsistent relationship with health care team; at times may be very critical of them and other times more positive toward them
- Following instructions from only one particular nurse

Physical Responses

- Deterioration of health because of lack of compliance
- Blood or urine tests showing drug levels inconsistent with reported medication intake; discrepancies in other tests

Pertinent History

- Poor outcomes from previous medical treatment
- Poor relationships with past health care providers
- Noncompliance in earlier health care treatments

COLLABORATIVE MANAGEMENT

Multidisciplinary Team Communication

To ensure the best chance for patient compliance, a team approach is essential. All healthcare providers should be consulted to ensure a cohesive treatment plan and approach that the patient understands. This is a pivotal nursing responsibility because nurses coordinate most of the care provided, both in the hospital and in the home. Discrepancies in instructions from physicians, physical or occupational therapists, pharmacists, or other health care providers need to be discussed so that the patient is not left to choose whose advice to follow.

Pharmacologic

Noncompliance for medication regimen is a major health problem. Patients do not take medications for a variety of reasons including fear of side effects, lack of knowledge about the purpose of the drug, denial of the diagnosis, lack of money to pay for medications, and lack of support or reinforcement (Box 12–3).

NURSING MANAGEMENT

NONCOMPLIANCE EVIDENCED BY FAILURE TO ADHERE TO MEDICAL REGIMEN, FAILURE TO KEEP APPOINTMENTS RELATED TO HEALTH BELIEFS, CULTURAL INFLUENCES.

Patient Outcomes

- Verbalizes beliefs that influence noncompliance
- Demonstrates adherence to treatment plan
- Expected therapeutic goals realized

Interventions

- Develop a trusting relationship with patient. Communicate interest and openness to patient's needs and beliefs.
- Assess the degree of noncompliance and the underlying reason for it. One common area of noncompliance is in using medications. Many prescriptions are never filled or filled and never used. When seeing a patient in the

---

BOX 12–3. Factors that Influence Medication Compliance

Factors that Increase Compliance:

- Client's perception that illness is severe and medication is needed
- Client's knowledge of illness and treatment
- Moderate level of anxiety (useful worrying)
- Continuity and length of relationship with caregiver
- Return of unpleasant symptoms immediately on stopping medication
- Caregiver optimism regarding use of medication
- Written instructions
- Family support

Factors that Decrease Compliance:

- Numerous lifestyle changes required
- Uncomfortable side effects
- Lack of support for compliance
- Fear of independence and recovery
- Lack of immediate return of symptoms if medication is stopped
- Fear of drug dependence
- Long period when symptoms are controlled

Source: Adapted from Harris, B: Psychopharmacology. In Haber, J, Krainovich-Miller, B, McMahon, AL, and Price Hoskins, P. (1997): Comprehensive Psychiatric Nursing, 5th ed., St. Louis, Mosby, 1997, with permission.

hospital or in the home, always review the medications the patient has, how they are being taken, and the patient's understanding of why the drug is necessary. Check expiration dates, the name of the physician who ordered the drugs, and the instructions on the labels. Analyze whether the patient is taking more than one drug for the same reason, especially if they were ordered by different physicians.

- Encourage the patient to share beliefs or traditions that impact health care. Demonstrate to patient your interest in learning about these. Do not criticize or belittle these beliefs; rather, communicate your respect for them.
- Ask the patient to share rationale for avoiding the prescribed treatment. Resolve any misunderstanding the patient may have about the treatment, its side effects, or its potential outcome. Avoid insisting that the patient give up his or her beliefs. Never argue with the patient about the value of the beliefs. Instead, explain any negative outcomes that these beliefs may cause with his or her condition.
- In critical situations, the patient may need to be confronted more directly with life-threatening consequences of noncompliance (e.g., taking insulin).
- Enlist assistance of family, friends, caregivers, or, if beliefs are based in a particular culture, others with whom the patient may relate to, to explain the consequences of these actions on the patient's health status.

- Talk with family members about their beliefs about the patient's illness to determine their role in noncompliance.
- Obtain feedback from the patient to ensure that he or she understands the instructions given. Use an interpreter if needed.
- If appropriate, negotiate the best compromise with the patient. Have him or her commit to one or two areas in which he or she will comply rather than expecting the patient to give up all his or her beliefs completely.
- Identify one staff member who has the best relationship with patient to provide information.
- Recognize that it may be impossible to alter the patient's strong cultural or religious beliefs. Understand that in some cases illness, or even death, may be more acceptable and a higher priority than giving up one's beliefs.

INEFFECTIVE MANAGEMENT OF THERAPEUTIC REGIMEN (INDIVIDU-ALS) EVIDENCED BY ACCELERATION OF ILLNESS SYMPTOMS OR VER-BALIZED DIFFICULTY WITH REGULATING OR INTEGRATING PRE-SCRIBED REGIMENS RELATED TO COMPLEXITY OF THERAPEUTIC REGIMEN OR HEALTH CARE SYSTEM.

Patient Outcomes

- Identifies factors that contribute to noncompliance
- Demonstrates adherence to treatment plan
- Expected therapeutic goals realized

Interventions

- Encourage patient to share factors that contribute to noncompliance. Ask the patient to explain the rationale for actions taken or not taken.
- Avoid using medical jargon or abbreviations that may confuse or intimidate. Encourage open communication so that the patient will tell you when he or she does not understand something.
- Have patient perform a return demonstration or verbalize his or her routine to determine patient's understanding and determine areas of noncompliance.
- Assess whether other methods of teaching would be more appropriate, such as videos, role playing, pamphlets with more pictures, or pamphlets written at a lower reading level. Minimize any distractions during teaching sessions.
- Incorporate principles of adult learning in educating adult patients. For example, explain rationale, avoid lecturing or belittling the patient, involve patient in discussion, and allow patient to identify ways teaching can be incorporated into his or her lifestyle.
- Ensure that the patient is in the best physical and emotional state for learning to occur. Remember to repeat information that was previously given when the patient was dealing with the acute crisis. Avoid teaching if patient in pain or has other discomforts.
- Assess role of family in patient's health care regimen. Determine who provides care for patient at home, and determine the caregiver's role in the

noncompliance. Observe caregiver's technique if appropriate, and provide information as needed.

- Determine patient's understanding of using the health care system. Review ways to get appointments, arrange additional care such as home care, and how to contact health care providers. As needed, check with social service agencies to provide needed transportation, equipment, or other services.
- Help identify ways in which patient can individualize information. For example, if a patient works rotating shifts or travels extensively, you will need to focus your teaching on how to adapt the treatment plan to best fit into his or her lifestyle.
- Identify ways to reinforce patient's self-esteem and sense of competency. Provide positive reinforcement and recognition of patient improvement.
- Incorporate rewards as part of the teaching. For an adult, rewards may include those activities that increase self-esteem and a sense of control.

INEFFECTIVE INDIVIDUAL COPING EVIDENCED BY NOT DOING, PARTIALLY DOING, OR REVAMPING TREATMENT PLAN RELATED TO ANXIETY ABOUT ILLNESS, INADEQUATE COPING MECHANISMS.

Patient Outcomes

- Verbalizes anxieties and concerns
- Verbalizes acceptance and commitment to the treatment plan
- Demonstrates adherence to health care regimen
- Expected therapeutic goals realized

Interventions

- Encourage the patient to discuss worries and concerns regarding the illness. Determine patient's understanding of the illness, prognosis, and treatment plan. If patient's understanding is not accurate, review the appropriate information about the condition with him or her.
- Encourage the patient to express feelings verbally rather than act them out through noncompliance.
- Repeat and reinforce teaching. The patient's learning ability may be impaired by anxiety or physical status.
- Give patient some control in treatment regimen. Seek his or her ideas for adaptations that can be made. Identify other areas in patient's life where he or she can exert control. Consider negotiating a contract with the patient to reinforce compliance.
- For the patient who is impatient and perfectionistic, point out the need to develop realistic expectations of behavior changes. For example, he or she may not be able to lose weight and give up smoking at the same time.
- Approach the suspicious patient with the expectation of compliance. Keep directions clear and simple, and always be honest.
- Reinforce the idea that the patient is ultimately responsible for his or her own health.

- If major life changes must be made, break down expected changes into achievable steps that may be easier to accept and master. Develop a way patient can chart own progress.

ALTERNATE NURSING DIAGNOSES

Altered Thought Processes
Anxiety
Decisional Conflict
Ineffective Management of Therapeutic Regimen: Families
Knowledge Deficit
Powerlessness
Self-Care Deficit

WHEN TO CALL FOR HELP

☐ Patient refuses to comply with medical regimen, with life-threatening implications.

☐ Family or caregiver abuses patient or interferes with patient's compliance.

☐ Patient uses folk remedies or alternative health practices that complicate current medical condition.

☐ There is evidence of suicidal or psychotic thinking as reason for noncompliance.

☐ There is increased staff conflict over dealing with patient's noncompliance.

PATIENT AND FAMILY EDUCATION

- Determine appropriate materials available to assist in patient education including pamphlets, videos, closed-circuit health education channels in the hospital, or flip charts.
- Determine if appropriate educational materials are available from pharmaceutical and medical equipment companies. Many times they have excellent materials available at no charge.
- Identify appropriate times to provide education to patient and family. Realize that at times the patient may not be ready for teaching when the nurse is available. Other alternatives need to be identified.
- Identify other resources, such as diabetes educators, ostomy nurses, pharmacists, or dietitians, to assist in teaching. Be sure to coordinate teaching so that no conflicting information is given.
- Utilize appropriate adult learning principles for all education (Box 12–2).

CHARTING TIPS

- Document all identified factors that contribute to noncompliance.
- Use objective, nonjudgmental terms to describe behavior.
- Document the teaching plan and patient goals to ensure that all health care team members are providing the same information.
- Document all teaching given and patient and family response to the education.
- Document patient's verbalized reason for and effects of noncompliance.

COMMUNITY-BASED CARE

- Refer the patient for home health follow-up to evaluate home situation and its influence on compliance. Inform home health nurses of concerns regarding patient's compliance and any effective or ineffective strategies you have used.
- Identify practical issues that inhibit compliance such as lack of transportation, funds, or insurance. Then seek potential resources for assistance. Involve social worker, case manager, or community resources advisor for assistance.
- Refer to support groups, community education programs, or volunteer support programs, such as Reach for Recovery, or ostomy visitors. These people may provide needed reinforcement or role models for motivation and support.
- Ensure that the patient and caregivers have adequate information for follow-up appointments and future treatment and that they have needed phone numbers and resources to call for more assistance.
- Refer patient for follow-up counseling if persistent noncompliance is related to inadequate coping skills or psychiatric disorder.

THE DEMANDING, DEPENDENT PATIENT

LEARNING OBJECTIVES

➢ List the possible causes of underlying anxieties that could escalate a patient's demanding, dependent behavior.
➢ Select effective interventions for a patient who consistently needs to be the center of attention.
➢ Identify possible nurses' reactions toward demanding, dependent patients.

GLOSSARY

Dependent personality disorder—Behavior characterized by a pervasive and excessive need to be taken care of leading to submissive and clinging behaviors; fears of separations; a severe lack of self-confidence; difficulty making everyday decisions and difficulty expressing disagreement.

Entitlement—An unreasonable expectation that others will provide especially favorable treatment and automatic compliance.

(Healthy) narcissism—An adequate amount of self-love, acquired during early childhood, providing a healthy self-esteem without negating the needs of others.

Hidden dependency—Dependent behavior that is not obvious. Person may try to coerce others into behaving in ways that meet his or her needs.

Histrionic personality disorder—Behavior characterized by pervasive and excessive expression of emotion and attention-seeking behavior.

Interdependence—Having the capability for a normal balance between dependent and independent behaviors.

Narcissistic personality disorder—Behavior characterized by a pervasive pattern of an inflated sense of self-importance, need for admiration, and lack of empathy for others.

Regression—An individual's response to overwhelming anxiety by moving back to a much earlier, more comforting phase of childhood.

Both demanding and dependent patients can consume an enormous amount of nursing resources. When patients exhibit these behaviors, it is essential to identify the problems early so that efforts are not counterproductive and resources are not drained. Setting baseline behavior goals help the patient contain or deal with his or her needs to a tolerable degree for both the staff and the patient and prevent dysfunctional behavior from interfering with the planned healthcare regime.

The *demanding* patient consistently wants more than the nurse can or should give and asks for more than is reasonable. A request is usually expressed as an emergency, with absolute insistence that it is a legitimate, rightful claim. The *dependent* patient wants to be taken care of in more ways than is normal for an adult. Unable to function independently or with self-reliance, this individual has a sense of helplessness and powerlessness and either actively or passively expects others to take responsibility to meet his or her needs, make personal decisions, and provide support.

When a person is hospitalized, a dependent relationship occurs because basic rules of living, such as when to eat, are set by others. An adult with healthy coping mechanisms can usually adjust to this dependency role appropriately. However, the response is not so predictable in individuals who have consistently learned to use maladaptive coping mechanisms throughout their lives or in those whose situational stress have exhausted their normal coping abilities. When the patient deviates too much from commonly expected behaviors, misunderstandings and battles can be generated between the patient and staff. Maladaptive responses can include growing resentment at feeling so helpless, regression to a clinging neediness more characteristic of earlier years in life, fighting and refusing to follow rules, covert expressions of the need to be cared for with an overemphasis on physical symptoms, or relentless demands for affection.

Patients with certain types of personality disorders, particularly dependent, narcissistic, or histrionic types, normally exhibit a relentless demand for attention and need to be dependent on others. These individuals believe that their views are correct and that others must adapt to them. Because these behaviors are long-standing, they are very resistant to change. Additionally, the stress of illness and hospitalization can cause other individuals who normally function without the need to be demanding and dependent to exhibit these behaviors. This may occur when there is a growing resentment at being helpless or when normal coping mechanisms have been exhausted. This behavior can also be a normal temporary response in an individual faced with adjusting to a chronic condition, such as quadriplegia. An individual may express his or her intolerance for the dependent role by fighting, refusing to follow rules and meet expectations, or by overemphasizing physical symptoms.

ETIOLOGY

Psychologic theories examine early developmental experiences that inhibit successful independence contributing to demanding or dependent adult behavior and may even result in a personality disorder. For instance, a child may learn that to be heard and acknowledged, he or she must persist in making demands on parental attention. Both inadequately met needs and overindulgence during the first 18 months of life can discourage independence. If the child was not allowed to ask directly for what is needed, he or she may learn to get needs met by having physical symptoms, particularly if extra attention is received only during early bouts of illness, when physical care provided the only expressions of support and nurturing. If the child assumed the caretaker role for an ill parent, he or she may view illness as the main vehicle for obtaining care and assistance.

Patients who feel unloved and worthless or who are afraid to be alone may make frequent requests for the nurse to do things in an attempt to get attention. With attention given, the patient's anxiety decreases, and he or she becomes less demanding.

In hidden dependency, the patient can be very controlling, intimidating, dominating, or possibly even an overly caring caretaker. The patient does not seem obviously dependent but attempts to coerce others to behave in ways designed to meet his or her needs.

Patients with chronic personality disorders have a limited repertoire of coping skills and can respond to anxiety by becoming more dependent and demanding, regardless of whether such behavior is appropriate to the situation. These are also associated with low self-esteem and depression.

RELATED CLINICAL CONCERNS

Independent decision making and initiative taking can be adversely affected by dementia, depression, hearing and other sensory problems, and limited intellectual abilities. Dependent individuals may use drugs as a method of coping with intolerable feelings of anxiety and helplessness, which can lead to a pattern of substance dependency.

LIFE SPAN ISSUES

CHILDREN

Infants are expected to be totally dependent. Younger children are still expected to be dependent in the areas in which they have not yet matured to the point of being able to do things for themselves. As children grow older and physical, psychologic, cognitive, and social spheres develop, they are expected to do age-appropriate tasks, make decisions, interact, and exhibit independent behaviors. Children who must be more dependent because of illness or disabilities may have more struggles with these issues.

ADOLESCENTS

The struggle with dependence and independence is the hallmark of adolescence. At times teenagers are children and at other times they act like adults. They can have an inflated sense of self and self-importance with little empathy for others as a natural part of trying to form their own identities; however, this does not mean that they will develop a personality disorder. People in this age group may be influenced more by their peers, who are supports against the pressures of the adult world and its expectations. They often become dependent on peers for recognition and gratification. Parents can become confused by the frequent vacillation between responsible behavior and childlike dependency, especially in earlier adolescent years.

ADULTS

Dependency can be manifested in fears of leaving the home of origin, difficulties maintaining jobs, and remaining financially dependent on parents. Brief periods of dependency during times of stress can be normal.

ELDERLY PEOPLE

As individuals age, they may experience an accompanying increased dependence based on losses in agility, speed, or strength. Some elderly people face illnesses along with the loss of previous support systems. Old friends and relatives may die or become preoccupied with their own growing limitations. Elderly persons who are treated as children incapable of making independent decisions and behavior may eventually respond with dependent and demanding behaviors.

For an elderly individual with a narcissistic personality disorder, adjusting to physical and occupational limitations can be particularly difficult, often straining family relationships.

POSSIBLE NURSES' REACTIONS

- Nurses have different tolerance levels for demanding, dependent behaviors. Patient may be considered difficult by one nurse but not by another. The extremes of these behaviors are usually considered difficult by all.
- May experience frustration and anger with the constant demands.
- May expect thanks or reward for meeting patient's needs.
- May feel guilty about not meeting all the patient's stated needs and question own competence. May try to avoid the patient.
- May not recognize that giving too much to patients who can do things for themselves is detrimental to the patients' emotional and physical health.
- May confuse appropriate limit setting with being overly harsh and withholding.
- May be punitive or hesitate to be firm with patients because of anger and fear about being punitive. It may also seem easier just to give in to the patient's demands.
- Nurses with strong dependency needs or who are inexperienced may ini-

tially overidentify with patients and try to meet all of their demands. May resent giving so much and not being appreciated.

ASSESSMENT

Behavior and Appearance

- Intrudes into personal space and time of others
- Unkempt appearance, either actual inability to provide self-care or an unconscious attempt to get others to provide care
- Demanding assistance although able to do things for self
- Manipulative behavior, such as:
  ∘ Arguing or begging
  ∘ Crying, clinging
  ∘ Calling nurse "mean," "hardhearted," "a bad person," "incompetent"
  ∘ Dwelling on health problems and medical history
  ∘ Complaining of feeling used and victimized by others
  ∘ Constantly seeking attention, suggestions from others
- Disregard of facility rules
- Regression; wanting to be totally taken care of, fed, repeatedly reassured, or comforted
- Frequent use of call lights
- Repeated visits to nurses' station
- Demands to have physician called several times each day
- Use of family visits to demonstrate helplessness; getting relatives to make demands on staff
- Sense of entitlement

Mood and Emotions

- Frequently angry; may be expressed in passive-aggressive behavior
- Fears being alone or abandoned
- Anxiety

Thoughts, Beliefs, and Perceptions

- Believes that each request is an actual problem requiring instant attention
- Low self-esteem with chronic feeling of helplessness and inadequacy
- Resistant to interpretations that point out reason for behavior (may experience this as an attack)

Relationships and Interactions

- Self-absorbed, with little interest in others' concerns or problems
- Frequently clings to others
- Sometimes nagging
- Fights or reverses roles and becomes a helper to others if unable to tolerate or acknowledge own dependency needs

- Dependent relationships with significant others (SOs), in which other person makes all decisions, answers for patient
- Others dislike caring for or being with patient for long periods

Physical Responses

- Overconcern about health and preoccupied with symptoms
- Frequent requests for and preoccupied with medications, especially for pain or anxiety
- Adverse drug interactions if prescriptions taken from several different doctors who are not aware of each other's involvement

Pertinent History'

- Long history of medical problems, some of which linger atypically for an unusually long time or do not quite match patterns of usually diagnosed diseases; does not respond to usual treatments
- Goes from one doctor to another in search for diagnosis and treatment for complaints that show no physical basis
- Multiple hospitalizations
- Unnecessary surgery

COLLABORATIVE INTERVENTIONS

Pharmacologic

Multiple medications, perhaps from different prescribing doctors, can generate a host of problematic adverse effects. Psychiatric medicines may also be used. A tendency for dependency may lead to increase risk for dependency on medications. Confusion and lethargy in elderly patients, which can lead to more dependent behavior, can be caused by overmedicating or too many types of medications. A pharmacologic review can be helpful in these instances. Antidepressants can be used for depressive symptoms.

NURSING MANAGEMENT

POWERLESSNESS EVIDENCED BY DEMANDING, DEPENDENT BEHAVIORS RELATED TO ANXIETIES GENERATED BY ILLNESS, DISABILITY, AND/OR HOSPITALIZATION.

Patient Outcomes

- Displays less demanding, dependent behavior and conveys needs more directly and appropriately
- Provides increased amount of self-care as physical condition permits
- No longer exaggerates physical complaints to gain attention, support, and concern

Interventions

- Assess baseline:
  - Consult with family or SO to determine if behaviors are normal for the person.
  - Evaluate if the patient is demanding in all situations or only in specific ones and if he or she exhibits this behavior only with certain people.
  - Identify the specific behaviors the patient uses to express dependency.
  - Determine whether the patient's helplessness is consistent with his or her medical problem or if patient is more independent when not in view of others.
- State limits and rules in advance. Discourage unnecessary or excessive time spent at the nurses' station. Discourage asking for nurses' assistance when the patient is aware that the nurse is on break, at lunch, or leaving at the end of the shift.
- Assess the required amount of assistance the patient needs and provide help when it is needed. Diplomatically point out unreasonable demands: "We're concerned about your overall well-being. In our experience, patients feel more effective and better about themselves when they do as much as they can. Let's discuss what you're realistically able to do right now and what the nurses need to provide."
- Make an extra effort to communicate concern:
  - Demonstrate active listening. Sit down rather than stand up during the talk. Repeat statements or reflect feeling being expressed, as necessary.
  - Be consistent. If you have told patient that you will speak with him or her at a specific time and are unable to do so, explain reasons and reschedule.
  - Give feedback to demonstrate that you understand what patient is asking for, feels, or needs. Encourage patient to describe his or her fears and anger over the loss of control.
- Explain that identifying each situation as an emergency makes it difficult to determine what is an actual emergency.
- Determine if the patient has had previous bad experiences with healthcare providers or institutions. He or she may need reassurance that proper treatment is being given.
- Give support and reassurance to allay fears when first attempting behaviors that will lead to more independence. Assure the patient that you will be available if needed.
- Help patient to distinguish between feeling helpless and being helpless. Provide a progress list of at least one new activity per day, however small, that he or she can do independently.
- Encourage the patient to identify and verbalize real sources of anger. Ask how he or she usually handles anger. Suggest ways to redirect anger into positive activities.
- Encourage patient to make independent choices. Accept different preferences and opinions.
- Do not take an overly directive approach because it can reinforce dependency.
- Identify and point out patient's strengths; provide praise whenever used.

- Determine whether some of the patient's expressed needs are better met by other professionals.

> **INEFFECTIVE INDIVIDUAL COPING** EVIDENCED BY DEMANDING, DEPENDENT BEHAVIOR RELATED TO CONTINUOUS AND ONGOING PERSONALITY DISTURBANCE THAT HINDERS ABILITY TO DO HEALTHCARE TASKS EFFECTIVELY AND COMMUNICATE CONCERNS APPROPRIATELY.

Patient Outcomes

- Uses less dependent behavior with fewer unnecessary demands for nurses' attention
- Uses appropriate methods to gain attention and support
- Verbalizes appropriate degree of health concerns
- Makes informed choices
- Initiates and carries through tasks

Interventions

- Obtain history from patient and SOs to determine patient's baseline style of interaction before illness or hospitalization. Those who have displayed demanding and dependent behaviors as a lifelong pattern may present more complexities.
- Be aware that patients who have long-standing, ingrained, demanding, dependent patterns will be resistant to change. Be patient and explain limit setting as often as needed.
- Determine realistic expectations for behavioral changes and expect that any changes will occur in small gradual steps.
- If the patient becomes upset because you are not presently able to spend time with him or her, determine a convenient time and provide assurances that patient will have your undivided attention.
- Assess whether the patient is inappropriately using the volunteers or other healthcare workers or is interacting inappropriately with visitors or other patients.
- Do not personalize remarks made by patients who need to feel superior. If the patient wants to speak only with the charge nurse or doctor, let those individuals explain the limits of their availability.
- Be aware when patients are using seductive behaviors to gain attention, control, or unnecessary assistance. Mild behaviors can be ignored to discourage future use. Persistent behaviors need firm confrontation.
- Assess for the use of manipulative behaviors to gain attention or dependence. Encourage methods to increase self-esteem that can decrease the patient's need for approval from others.
- Analyze behaviors to determine what needs the patient may be expressing when he or she asks the staff to perform tasks that could easily be done independently.
- Point out to the patient ways in which he or she has control of some situations.
- Assess the cause of a problem with independent decision making. If it is

caused by a lack of information, provide all the information you can. If the patient always has difficulty making decisions, teach effective problem-solving skills.

- Recognize your own tolerance for demanding, dependent behavior. Ask for assistance or temporary reprieve if necessary. For extremely dependent patients, strive for a balance between rotating staff to help decrease dependency on one nurse and providing consistent nursing care.
- Be especially diplomatic in correcting patient's behavior. Narcissistic patients may react to criticism or defeat with rage, disdain, or counterattack. If this occurs, help the patient regain a perspective on feedback and response.
- Maintain your own perspective when receiving praise from dependent or histrionic patients as well as the devaluing or ignoring of your efforts and contributions by more narcissistic patients, who tend to take all the credit.
- Praise independent and interdependent functioning. Reassure the patient that he or she will not be forgotten nor abandoned by the staff when more independent. Reward less demanding behavior by spending more time with the patient.

ALTERNATE NURSING DIAGNOSES

Anxiety
Decisional Conflict
Impaired Social Interaction
Self-Care Deficit
Self-Esteem Disturbance

WHEN TO CALL FOR HELP

When the patient is "burning out" staff with insatiable, unreasonable requests

When the patient's demands or needs for assistance become so unrealistically prolonged that it impairs staff's ability to adequately care for other patients

When the patient is not getting good medical care because of staff anger

If the patient seems resistant to all interventions attempted

PATIENT AND FAMILY EDUCATION

- Teach decision-making skills, such as problem identification, listing possible solutions, considering possible outcomes of each, and evaluating each outcome. Teach the patient to draw upon past experience and intuition when making decisions. Point out potential stumbling blocks such as choices that lower self-esteem or violate values or goals. Caution the pa-

tient that there may not be a perfect solution. Teach the concept of collaborative decision making.
- Teach the patient to recognize personal strengths.
- Explain to the patient that in delegating personal decision making to another, one still must retain personal responsibility for one's own life. He or she will have to live with the consequences of the decision.
- Teach the patient to distinguish situations that require immediate attention from those that do not. Explain that identifying each situation as an emergency makes it difficult to determine what is an actual emergency.
- Teach the patient to identify which problems require assistance. Teach the patient to use frustration as an opportunity for problem solving.
- Teach relaxation techniques.
- Teach the family members to identify when they are promoting dependent behaviors and to examine alternatives. Teach approaches that the staff members have found effective.
- Teach the patient the difference between providing good nursing care and catering to excessive demands.

CHARTING TIPS

- Document specifics of demands and their frequency. Note if they occur at similar times or in relation to similar events.
- Document actual patient responses to specific interventions listed in the treatment plan. Avoid subjective opinions about the behaviors.
- Document frequency of requests for PRN medications.
- Document details of unusual physical complaints.

COMMUNITY-BASED CARE

- Anticipate increased dependency and demanding behavior as discharge from one level of care becomes imminent; reduce anxiety by discussing concerns as early as possible.
- Involve patient in discharge arrangements.
- Anticipate that discharge will probably be a difficult time if the patient will be going to a facility with different caretakers and less staff.
- If patient is going home, assess what services patient will need at home and discuss arrangements with patient and family.
- Ensure that patient has specific plans for follow-up appointment with physician.
- Remind patient who is about to be transferred to a skilled nursing care facility to continue to use the methods learned for expressing needs.
- Discuss with the next caregivers the interventions that have been effective.
- If the patient's behavioral patterns continue to significantly impair health care and the patient is distressed about this, discuss the possibility of seeking psychotherapy.
- Communicate patient concerns and behaviors to referring agencies.

Problems with Substance Abuse

THE PATIENT ABUSING ALCOHOL

LEARNING OBJECTIVES

➢ Identify factors that contribute to the etiology of alcoholism.
➢ Formulate appropriate nursing interventions for patients experiencing problems with alcohol abuse.
➢ Describe common nurse's reactions to the patient abusing alcohol.
➢ Describe the characteristics of codependency.

GLOSSARY

Alcohol intoxication—Excessive alcohol use that leads to maladaptive behavior and at least one of the following: slurred speech, incoordination, unsteady gait, nystagmus, impairment in attention or memory, and stupor.

Alcoholism—A complex progressive disease characterized by signifi-

Binge drinking—Pattern of periodic intervals of heavy use of alcohol with intervals of no or little use.

Blackouts—Lapses of memory resulting from persistent heavy drinking. During blackouts the person may appear to function normally while drinking but cannot recall events afterwards.

Codependency—Maladaptive coping behaviors that prevent individuals from taking care of their own needs because they are preoccupied with the thoughts and feelings of another. Also known as "enabling behavior."

Detoxification—The process of withdrawal of alcohol from the body through supervised medical interventions to prevent complications.

Dual diagnosis—Diagnosis of both a substance dependency and a major psychiatric disorder.

Korsakoff's syndrome—Severe memory impairment related to thiamine deficiency from long-term alcohol use. Characterized by confabulation and inappropriate cheerfulness.

Tolerance—the need for increasing amounts of a substance to achieve desired effect.

Alcohol remains the most used and misused drug in America. Alcohol use is socially accepted throughout our culture, is included as part of celebrations, religious rituals, and social occasions, and is often used as a relaxant. Nearly 90 percent of all American adults have used alcohol at some time in their life (DSM-IV-TR, 2000).

The move from social use of alcohol to alcoholism can occur very quickly in some people and over many years in others. In the past, alcoholism was viewed as a defective character trait, a weakness, or a moral flaw. Since the 1950s, it has been realized that alcoholism is a complex disease that responds to proper treatment.

Studies indicate that about 7 percent of Americans are dependent on alcohol at any one time, and 14 percent report alcohol dependence at some time in their life (DSM-IV, 1994). This includes daily or binge drinking that negatively affects the way one lives. Three times as many men as women are reported to have a drinking problem; however, it is suggested that women are more secretive in their drinking behavior, and, therefore, drinking by women may be underreported. Alcohol is often used along with other substances, especially in younger individuals, often to alleviate or enhance the effects of other drugs (e.g., to relax after using a stimulant).

Alcohol is a central nervous system depressant that produces mind-altering and mood-altering effects. Twenty percent of alcohol consumed is absorbed directly into the bloodstream through the stomach. The remainder moves through the digestive system and is absorbed more slowly. Drinking rapidly on an empty stomach or consuming drinks with higher alcohol content will lead to a more rapid rise in blood alcohol level. One ounce of distilled liquor, 5 ounces of wine, and 12 ounces of beer have equivalent amounts of alcohol. It is known that, given the same amount of alcohol, women have higher blood alcohol concentrations than men, even when size is taken into consideration. This is because of differences in fat and body water content, making women more prone to long-term effects of alcohol.

Alcoholism has a tremendous impact on the individual, the family, and society. Spouses and especially children are particularly vulnerable to become victims of alcohol-related abuse. They may experience violence or emotional and physical neglect, and they may blame themselves for the alcoholic's abusive state. Amazingly, 43 percent of U.S. adults have been exposed to alcoholism through a spouse or blood relative. Alcoholism is truly a family crisis. (National Council of Alcohol and Drug Dependence, 2001).

The impact of alcohol abuse on society includes crime, traffic accidents and fatalities, suicide, industrial accidents, fires, and decreased workplace productivity. People with major psychiatric disorders may also have an abuse problem if they use alcohol to self-medicate for the psychiatric symptoms.

ETIOLOGY

Because alcoholism runs in families, there is currently support for the *genetic* and *biologic* theories as the cause of alcoholism. Studies show that children of alcoholic parents are four times more likely to develop alcoholism with sons being at greater risk (DSM-IV, 1994). The risk remains even if the children are not raised in the same home as the alcoholic parent. One current theory suggests that there is an inherited deficiency in some neurotransmitters that leads to a greater tendency to develop dysphoria or feelings of discomfort. Alcohol then becomes learned as a way to relieve these uncomfortable feelings. Also, because it is known that cross-tolerance develops when an individual moves from alcohol to barbiturates or benzodiazepines, it is believed that a specific neurotransmitter is involved. Individual biological differences in response to alcohol may contribute to susceptibility to more problems.

A number of *psychologic* factors are recognized as contributing to alcohol abuse. One of the most important looks at the link between depression and alcoholism. Alcoholics may have a higher incidence of depression and low self-esteem. Alcohol becomes a way to relieve those feelings. Each time a drink makes the person feel better, it reinforces this behavior. Difficulty managing anxiety and low self-esteem has led to identification of common coping styles (Table 13–1). Denial is the major defense mechanism used when the person is unable to acknowledge the role that alcohol plays in his or her life.

Alcohol use can severely affect the dynamics of the family relationship. Family members use protective behaviors, sometimes called "codependent" or "enabling behaviors," to control or hide the alcoholic's behavior so that a sense of normalcy can be maintained. Affected family members care for and attempt to control the behavior of the alcoholic at the expense of their own needs. The family does not realize that this type of behavior reinforces the

TABLE 13–1. COMMON COPING STYLES OF ALCOHOLICS

Coping Style	Definition	Behaviors
Denial	Person minimizes or does not acknowledge the problem or the results of the problem even when strong evidence is presented.	• "I only have 2 drinks a day, I could stop any time." • Refuses to admit drinking problems that are obvious to others. • Family may participate in denial by covering up the problems created by the drinker.
Projection	Blames others for their drinking and behavior.	• Avoids taking responsibility for own unacceptable behavior. • "My brother is the one with the problem. He drinks more than I do." • "I'd stop if everyone would leave me alone."
Rationalization	Justifies intolerable behavior by giving plausible excuses.	• Excuses reinforce denial. • "My kids are always in trouble. They make me drink." • "I only drink beer."
Minimizing	Avoids conflict by reducing the impact of the behavior.	• Places less value on the behavior and the impact of the problem. • "You worry too much." • "I'm not hurting anyone."
Manipulation	Plays one person against another in order to get one's way or cover up or avoid a problem.	• Convinces one or two people that he or she will improve if they will help. • If he or she fails it is the fault of the helper.
Grandiosity	Maintains a sense of superiority and irresponsibility particularly evident when intoxicated.	• Lacks concern for others feelings.

drinking patterns and dysfunctional behavior. Examples of these behaviors include minimizing the drinking, finding excuses for the drinker's alcohol use, attempting to control the drinking by diluting bottles or pouring out liquor, covering up for the drinker's unacceptable behavior, and self-blame for the drinking. Family members and friends of the person abusing alcohol are also at an increased risk of emotional or physical abuse.

Social and cultural factors may also contribute to the development of alcoholism. Certain cultural groups have higher incidences of drinking problems, which may represent an increased acceptance of heavy alcohol use. It may be part of socially expected behavior. One's social circle may play a role in how alcohol is used as one observes its use by friends or family to avoid problems, become a risk taker, and so on.

RELATED CLINICAL CONCERNS

Alcohol abuse plays a major role in a variety of health problems including gastritis, liver failure, and pancreatitis. Heavy drinkers are at higher risk for oral cancers. Twenty-five percent of admissions to general hospitals are related to an alcohol problem, including being treated for consequences of drinking (National Institute of Alcohol Abuse and Alcoholism, 2001).

Alcohol is toxic to many major organs, especially the heart and liver. The patient with heart disease who abuses alcohol is at increased risk of complications, including hypertension. Liver metabolism may be compromised, and therefore drugs metabolized by the liver may need dosage adjustments.

Hingson (1993) noted that alcohol is a contributing factor in the following: 50 percent of trauma fatalities, 40 to 50 percent of falls, 30 percent of motor vehicle accidents.

LIFE SPAN ISSUES

NEONATES

Fetal alcohol syndrome is now recognized as being caused by alcohol abuse during pregnancy, when rapidly growing fetal brain cells are exposed to alcohol. The end result can be an infant born with mild to moderate developmental disabilities, hyperactivity, and growth deficiencies.

CHILDREN AND ADOLESCENTS

Alcohol use by children and adolescents has shown an alarming increase in recent years. Access to alcohol from the home or from friends can make it readily available. Sixty-two percent of high school seniors have been drunk (National Institute of Alcohol Abuse and Alcoholism, 2001). Teens who start drinking at age 15 are 4 times more likely to develop alcoholism than those who start at age 21. (National Council of Alcoholism and Drug Dependence, 2001).

As with adults, children learn from parents, peers, or television and movie images suggesting that alcohol can be a defense against feelings of depression, low self-esteem, or anxiety. It may also represent an acting out against parental authority or enhance a sense of closeness with peers. Children who grow up in a home where one or both parents have an alcohol abuse problem may have an increased risk of abusing alcohol. However, even those children who intensely dislike their parents' drinking behavior may use alcohol as a coping mechanism because they have not learned more appropriate ones. Children and adolescents who become intoxicated are at increased risk of injury related to motor vehicle and bicycle accidents because they usually do not drink in the home. They are also at increased risk of alterations in growth and development because of nutritional deficiencies and because they often do not learn to deal effectively with normal anxiety and other uncomfortable emotions. Adolescents and young adults are more prone to binge drinking, which has been associated with life threatening effects from alcohol intoxication.

ELDERLY PEOPLE

Alcohol abuse is often unrecognized and undertreated in the over-65 age group. Our society generally does not view the older population as an at-risk group. Because alcohol abuse is often a lifelong pattern, elderly people may continue their earlier struggles with alcohol. Because of changes in metabolism with age, it may take less alcohol to begin to cause intoxication or other problems. Others may start drinking in later life as they face increasing problems, such as isolation, loss of spouse, and changes in health status. Alcohol may produce significant health problems in elderly persons, particularly if they have impaired liver function. Mental changes from alcohol use may be confused with dementia. It is a major factor in falls, burns, and suicide attempts. The brain in elderly people is more susceptible to the depressant effect of alcohol, and therefore depression may mask the signs of alcoholism. Other signs might be unexplained falls, poor nutrition, and self-neglect. Use of multiple medications with alcohol can exacerbate alcohol's effects. Withdrawal programs for this age group may require specialized care because of the increased health risks.

POSSIBLE NURSES' REACTIONS

- May view alcohol abuse as a personality defect or weakness rather than a health problem.
- May avoid, criticize, or reject the patient. This may trigger guilt feelings, and the nurse may try to make up for these feelings by being overly sympathetic.
- May have feelings of disgust for the patient.
- May have unresolved feelings related to a past family or personal history of substance abuse.
- May feel helpless to facilitate change, especially in a patient with a long history of alcohol problems.

ASSESSMENT

Behavior and Appearance

- Signs of intoxication include odor of alcohol, slurred speech, loud talking, loss of inhibition, loss of coordination, and poor judgment
- Sudden onset of signs of withdrawal
- Frequently talks or brags about alcohol use
- Exhibits extremes of behavior from euphoria to irritability
- Justifies drinking or the need to drink
- Refuses to discuss drinking or lies about drinking
- Drinks large quantities of alcohol
- Needs to drink increasingly more to get same effect
- Unable to stop drinking once he or she starts
- Overreacts when questioned about drinking pattern

- Reports drinking a much smaller amount than is accurate
- Two or more affirmative responses to the CAGE questionnaire (Box 13–1) suggests dependence, further assessment required

Mood and Emotions

- Depression
- Remorse after a binge
- Low frustration tolerance
- Anxiety
- Low self-esteem

Thoughts, Beliefs, and Perceptions

- Evidence of defense mechanisms of denial, rationalization, projection, and minimizing
- Thinking about alcohol supply and plans to obtain it
- Blackouts
- Hallucinations

Relationships and Interactions

- Dependent
- Resentful of authority
- Manipulates others to avoid confrontation, conflict
- Blames others for drinking
- Argues with family about drinking

BOX 13–1. CAGE Questionnaire

To determine the patient's perception of his or her drinking problem, you may ask the following questions. Two or more affirmative answers strongly suggest dependence on alcohol.

1. Have you ever felt you should cut down your drinking?
2. Have people annoyed you by criticizing your drinking?
3. Have you ever felt bad or guilty about your drinking?
4. Have you ever had a drink first thing in the morning to steady your nerves or get rid of a hangover?

Source: Mayfield, D, McLeod, G, and Hall, P: The CAGE Questionnaire: Validation of a new alcoholism screening instrument. Am J Pyschiatr 131:1121, 1974, with permission.

Physical Responses

- Blood alcohol level (0.08 to 0.10 is legal limit to define intoxication in most states) or positive polydrug panel (may be negative, depending on time since last consumption). Blood level is less useful in elderly people because of altered metabolism. Urine testing can be a less invasive approach.
- Amylase may be elevated if liver damage is present. Blood sugar may indicate hyper- or hypoglycemia. Serum magnesium may be low from alcohol damage to the nervous system. Hemoglobin may be low if bleeding is present
- History of falls, burns
- May have signs of gastrointestinal bleeding, ascites, or jaundice
- May be underweight and show signs of malnutrition and dehydration
- Korsakoff's syndrome from prolonged thiamine deficiency creates a secondary dementia marked by ataxia, confabulation, and peripheral neuropathy
- Withdrawal symptoms may occur 8 to 24 hours after last alcohol use. Analgesics and recovery from anesthesia can precipitate an acute withdrawal reaction. This emphasizes the importance of quick diagnosis to institute detoxification
- Alcohol-related delirium (also known as delirium tremens) is a medical emergency with a 20 percent mortality rate if left untreated. Complications include pneumonia, dehydration, electrolyte imbalance, respiratory failure, and status epilepticus (Box 13–2).

Pertinent History

- Previous history of alcohol or polydrug use
- Psychotic, depressed, or manic behavior
- Blackouts, seizures, or delirium
- Alcohol-related police record, possibly including motor vehicle violations or accidents, physical violence, or child or spouse abuse
- May have history of being abused as a child
- Erratic work record because of alcohol abuse
- One or both parents with history of alcohol problems

COLLABORATIVE MANAGEMENT

Pharmacologic

Symptoms from alcohol withdrawal generally start within 4 to 12 hours of cessation of heavy drinking. Symptoms are the most intense on the second day. Protocols for detoxification from alcohol include pharmacologic treatment to prevent or reduce the development of alcohol-related delirium. Sedation with longer-acting central nervous system depressants is substituted for shorter-acting alcohol. Benzodiazepines such as diazepam (Valium) and chlordiazepoxide (Librium) are the drugs of choice because they have anticonvulsant actions and are relatively safe. The drugs are usually adminis-

---

BOX 13–2. DSM-IV Criteria for Diagnosis of Alcohol-Related Syndrome

Alcohol abuse—Maladaptive pattern of alcohol use that is manifested by one or more of the following within the same 12 months:

1. Inability to fulfill major role obligations at work, school, and home
2. Recurrent legal or interpersonal problems
3. Reduction or absence of important social, occupational, and recreational activities
4. Participation in physically hazardous situations while impaired, for example, driving a car, exacerbation of a symptom

Alcohol dependence—Maladaptive pattern of alcohol use leading to impairment by 3 or more of the following occurring at any time during the same 12 months:

1. All criteria for alcohol abuse
2. Presence of tolerance to drug
3. Presence of alcohol withdrawal syndrome
4. Ingestion of alcohol to relieve or prevent withdrawal
5. Taking more alcohol over longer period of time than intended
6. Unsuccessful or persistent desire to cut down or control use
7. Great deal of time spent in getting, taking, and recovering from alcohol

Alcohol withdrawal—Cessation of alcohol use which has been heavy and prolonged and has at least 2 of the following within several hours to a few days:

1. Autonomic hyperactivity (high blood pressure, tachycardia, fever)
2. Hand tremor
3. Insomnia
4. Nausea and or vomiting
5. Anxiety
6. Transient visual, tactile, or auditory hallucinations or illusions
7. Grand mal seizures

Alcohol-induced delirium—An organic mental disorder with symptoms in excess of the usual withdrawal (formerly called "delirium tremens") or intoxication symptoms that occurs after cessation or reduction of long-term heavy drinking or during intoxication. In someone with a history of substance use, symptoms include:

1. Impaired consciousness
2. Changes in cognition including memory, language, disorientation, hallucinations (especially tactile such as feeling bugs crawling on one's body)
3. Develops over short period of time (hours to days) and fluctuates over a day.

Source: Adapted from DSM-IV, 1994, and DSM-IV-TR, 2001.

---

tered on a routine basis and then tapered down by 20 to 25 percent per day until withdrawal is complete. Shorter-acting tranquilizers such as oxazepam (Serax) and lorazepam (Ativan) may be used if patient has liver disease. Anticonvulsants may also be needed. Detoxification may be done in an alcohol treatment unit or hospital or at home, if adequate supervision is available.

The inpatient setting needs to be used if the patient is at risk for alcohol related delirium, has multiple comorbidities, or is elderly.

Disulfiram (Antabuse) has been used for chronic alcohol abuse. This drug inhibits impulsive drinking because it produces an extremely uncomfortable physical reaction when alcohol is ingested. The drug is taken daily and stays in the system for 5 days after the last dose. If the patient is exposed to alcohol while the drug remains active, he or she may experience headache, tachycardia, nausea, vomiting, flushing, sweating, and changes in blood pressure, as well as potentially serious reactions including shock and cardiac arrhythmias. Because of the risks involved with using this drug, the patient must have the ability to understand the reaction if alcohol is ingested and give informed consent. The patient must be instructed to avoid inhaling substances that could contain alcohol, such as paint or wood stains, and refrain from using any substances with alcohol, including those with hidden sources such as some mouthwashes, elixirs, skin preparations, or colognes. The drug metronidazole (Flagyl) may cause a disulfiram-like reaction when alcohol is also ingested. Antabuse is best used for the motivated patient who is less subject to impulsive behavior and does not have a psychiatric history.

Naltrexone has also been used to prevent the euphoria associated with alcohol intake. Other commonly used medications include beta blockers, clonidine, and haloperidol (for hallucinations).

Dual-diagnosis patients present a challenge as they usually need to continue to take their psychiatric medications during the detoxification process. These medications need to be closely monitored. Alcohol may have been a way to self-medicate the disturbing psychiatric symptoms such as anxiety and low self-esteem for these patients.

Alternative approaches may include herbs and plants such as chamomile for insomnia, valerian for anxiety (should not be taken with sedatives), kava kava for anxiety (should not be used with sedatives or alcohol). Multivitamins, thiamine, and magnesium therapy is indicated in chronic alcoholics to prevent neurologic complications. Patients must also maintain hydration.

Twelve-Step Program

The Twelve-Step Program of Alcoholics Anonymous (AA) is generally accepted as part of every alcoholic's treatment program. AA's philosophy mandates that the individual become sober and never drink or use mood-altering substances again. The person acknowledges that he or she is powerless over alcohol, is always considered recovering, and is never cured. One drink could cause a downward spiral to heavy drinking. The best outcomes occur when the AA group members are of similar age and cultural background.

AA uses sponsors who have been sober for longer periods to support new members. The alcoholic needs to attend regular, even daily group support meetings and work on the Twelve-Step Program. AA chapters are found in virtually every community in the United States. The only requirement for membership is the desire to stop drinking. Alcoholics Anonymous has been the model for other self-help groups, including Gamblers Anonymous and Cocaine Anonymous. Family members of alcoholics can participate in self-help groups following the same model, including Al-Anon for spouses and friends, Al-a-Teen for adolescents, and Adult Children of Alcoholics (ACoA). Additional approaches may include behavioral, group, and marital therapies.

NURSING MANAGEMENT

INEFFECTIVE DENIAL EVIDENCED BY LACK OF ACKNOWLEDGMENT OF ALCOHOL ABUSE RELATED TO IMPAIRED ABILITY TO ACCEPT CONSEQUENCES OF OWN BEHAVIOR.

Patient Outcomes

- Acknowledges own drinking problem
- Expresses feelings while under nurse's care
- Demonstrates problem-solving skills
- Abstains from alcohol and drug use or significantly reduces intake
- Asks for assistance with drinking problem

Interventions

- Help patient identify disturbing feelings by listening to concerns and helping him or her put labels on possible emotions. Patient may have used alcohol to deny feelings and needs assistance to identify them.
- Foster problem solving. Explore with the patient, the coping mechanisms that are more appropriate than alcohol to deal with the specific causes of stress and anxiety.
- Talk with patient about the normal range of personal emotions.
- Discuss behavioral inconsistencies.
- Maintain a positive attitude. Communicate the idea that patient can overcome his or her problems.
- Work with patient to set realistic small goals for abstaining from alcohol and managing his or her problems. This may require structured planning for how to get through the next day without a drink. Encourage use of readings and meditations.
- Reinforce the Alcoholics Anonymous philosophy of "one day at a time." This means setting a goal of not drinking today rather than thinking about not drinking for the next year.
- Develop a trusting relationship. When the patient feels safe with a staff member, encourage examination of the negative consequences of his or her behavior. Recognize that this relationship could become too threatening to the patient and he or she may try to sabotage it or reject the nurse. This is all part of the struggle to face one's problems.
- If patient states, "I could stop drinking any time," have him or her identify what could be done right now to stop. Look for windows in denial that might indicate the slightest insight and focus.
- Set limits on manipulative behavior. Some patients may have learned to be very charming. The goal of these behaviors is to avoid dealing with the real problems.

> **RISK FOR INJURY** EVIDENCED BY DISORIENTATION, LACK OF COOR-
> DINATION, OR AGGRESSIVE OR DISRUPTIVE BEHAVIOR RELATED
> TO ACUTE ALCOHOL INTOXICATION, WITHDRAWAL, AND/OR DELIRIUM.

Patient Outcomes

- Remains free from injury while under care of the nurse.
- Sleeps at least 6 hours at night.
- Has reduced incidence of medical complications.
- Exhibits appropriate behavior.

Interventions

- Monitor vital signs, seizures, and changes in mental status closely for 5 days after withdrawal from alcohol.
- Monitor closely for signs of withdrawal and report to physician to begin early treatment. With appropriate management, severe complications can be prevented. Recognize that the patient may be using several drugs, so the signs of alcohol withdrawal may be masked or delayed.
- Follow agency policy or protocol for detoxification for high-risk patients.
- Maintain a quiet, calm environment. Use a soft voice and calm, supportive approach to reassure patient.
- Keep a night light on. Institute fall precautions. Encourage staff or family to stay with patient to ensure safety.
- Avoid restraints if at all possible by adequate use of medication.
- If the patient has pain from another medical condition, such as trauma or surgery, be sure to treat the pain. Do not withhold analgesia for fear that it will reinforce addictive tendencies.
- Promote use of relaxation techniques and herbal teas to reduce tension and help with possible insomnia.
- Monitor for complications, including cardiac arrhythmias or diabetes.
- Monitor food intake. Encourage fluids and a high-carbohydrate diet. Discourage use of dehydrating foods and fluids such as coffee, tea, and chocolate. Administer vitamins as ordered.

> **INEFFECTIVE FAMILY COPING: COMPROMISED** EVIDENCED BY OVER-
> RESPONSIBLE BEHAVIOR TO CONTROL THE ALCOHOLISM RELATED TO
> ANXIETY IN THE FAMILY SYSTEM.

Patient Family Outcomes

- Demonstrates assertive response when faced with abusive behavior
- Expresses feelings about the impact of alcohol on the family
- Demonstrates reduced number of behaviors that take responsibility for patient's drinking
- Attends support group meetings

Interventions

- Recognize that alcoholism is a health problem that affects all family members. Monitor response of all family members to patient's behavior.
- Give feedback to individuals about overresponsible behavior. Encourage them to recognize the signs and feelings associated with it. Explain how efforts to contain the patient's drinking merely delay the needed confrontation.
- Assist family members to set limits on the urge to "rescue" the patient. Give suggestions on coping mechanisms to reduce the stress. They need support to accept the idea that they are not responsible for patient's drinking or behavior.
- Educate family members about availability and purpose of group support programs. Talk to them about meeting with a chemical dependency specialist for assistance. Participate in a planned intervention technique under the supervision of the specialist when the patient is confronted by family and friends about his or her drinking problem.
- Give person permission to take care of own needs first.
- Teach the family assertive responses to abuse or criticism from others, especially the patient.
- Encourage them to express emotions, both positive and negative.
- Reinforce the idea that ultimately the individual with the drinking problem is the only one who can control his or her own behavior.
- Recognize the fact that family members may unconsciously sabotage patient's recovery in order to maintain the security of the status quo. Remain as objective as possible and avoid becoming involved in family conflicts.
- Prepare patient for changes in relationships with family and friends that may occur once he or she has stopped drinking. There may be some individuals who no longer like the patient when he or she is sober. Patient needs to reexamine these relationships.

ALTERNATE NURSING DIAGNOSES

Altered Nutrition: Less Than Body Requirements
Altered Thought Processes
Noncompliance
Risk for Violence to Self
Sleep Pattern Disturbance

WHEN TO CALL FOR HELP

Escalation of aggressive, belligerent behavior to violence
Need to apply restraints
Intoxication

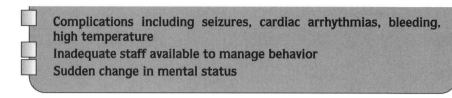

- Complications including seizures, cardiac arrhythmias, bleeding, high temperature
- Inadequate staff available to manage behavior
- Sudden change in mental status

PATIENT AND FAMILY EDUCATION

- Reinforce strategies to avoid exposure to alcohol. For example, caution patient to avoid contact with drinking friends. Teach patient to avoid his or her old habits that included drinking, and remove all alcohol from the home. Teach patient and family to read labels of products purchased. Avoid products with alcohol in them such as mouthwashes and cough syrup. Avoid any mood-altering substance that could be used as a substitute for alcohol.
- Provide information about the addictive process and how it affects all aspects of one's life. Review "one-day-at-a-time" philosophy.
- Provide information on nutrition and how to address possible vitamin and mineral deficiencies.
- Provide information to patient and family on managing potential seizures.
- Provide health teaching on the potential of gastrointestinal bleeding and liver disease. Encourage patient to avoid using products containing aspirin.
- Educate patient and family on the hazards of drinking in pregnancy and the effects of alcohol on driving and working.
- Teach strategies to replace alcohol with more healthy activities such as sports, hobbies, and journal keeping.
- Reinforce relaxation measures.
- Prepare patient for need to develop social contacts who do not dri nk.
- Reinforce education to family on avoiding overresponsible responses.
- Prepare the patient for the fact that intense emotions may be more painful without alcohol. He or she may need extra help at these times.
- Remind patient to tell every physician seen about his or her history to ensure that doctor will prescribe medications appropriately.
- Useful Web sites include ncadd.org (National Council on Alcoholism and Drug Dependence).

CHARTING TIPS

- Document vital signs and any evidence of symptoms of withdrawal and delirium.
- Describe in detail the patient's level of consciousness and mental status.
- Document the patient's response to the medications being used for withdrawal.
- Document the family's response to patient's behavior.
- Document any observations of continued alcohol use.
- Document any actions taken to prevent violent behavior.

- If restraints are necessary, document the type, the time the patient was in restraints, the reason why they were applied, the patient's response to treatment, when limbs were released, and the care given to the patient while in restraints.

COMMUNITY-BASED CARE

- Provide information to patient and family on location and phone numbers for local chapters of AA, Al-Anon, Al-a-Teen, as needed.
- Encourage the patient and family to begin or continue counseling or provide referral to alcohol counseling programs.
- Encourage the patient to follow up with medical appointments
- Arrange for follow-up home health visits for patients being discharged from detox treatment to home.
- Provide information to referring agencies, such as home health agencies or nursing homes, on patient's drinking patterns and the treatment program.

THE PATIENT ABUSING OTHER SUBSTANCES

LEARNING OBJECTIVES

➤ Differentiate between substance abuse and dependence.
➤ Identify common reactions of the nurse to the substance abuser.
➤ Describe important nursing considerations of abusing amphetamines, cocaine, hallucinogens, nicotine, opioids, and sedatives.
➤ Identify nursing diagnoses and interventions in caring for the substance abuser.

GLOSSARY

Binge—Pattern of periodic intervals of heavy use of substances with intervals of no or little usage.

Cross-tolerance—State in which the effect of a substance is reduced because the individual has become tolerant to a similar drug.

Detoxification—Process of withdrawal of a drug from the body through supervised medical intervention to prevent complications.

Drug tolerance—Need for higher and higher doses to achieve same desired effect.

Dual diagnosis—Individual with a mental disorder who is also a substance abuser. The substance is often used to self-medicate to relieve psychiatric symptoms.

Flashback—Transient recurrence of a disturbance in perceptions associated with hallucinogens that are reminiscent of those experienced when taking the drug. Sometimes referred to as a "hallucinogen persisting perceptual disorder."

Polypharmacy—Taking more than one substance at any given time.

Substance abuse—The maladaptive and consistent use of a drug accompanied by recurrent and significant adverse consequences often related to physical hazards, multiple legal problems, and recurrent social and interpersonal problems.

Substance dependence—Cluster of cognitive, behavioral, and physiologic symptoms indicating that the individual continues use of the substance despite significant substance-related problems.

Withdrawal—Negative physiologic and psychologic reactions that occur when the drug is reduced or no longer taken.

Using mind- and mood-altering substances is probably as old as the human race. Today many people use medications or other substances to relax, sleep, and increase energy. Prescription and over-the-counter psychoactive substances such as caffeine, tobacco, alcohol, painkillers, tranquilizers, and common cold treatments are both socially acceptable and commonly used. It is interesting that we accept these substances to help us feel better but loathe people who are dependent on or abuse drugs. People who eventually become substance abusers also take drugs to feel better, possibly as a way to avoid some problems and stressors. Eventually, though, the need to obtain and use the drug negatively affects all aspects of the person's life, including family, job, friends, and other responsibilities. Many people who use drugs retreat to the company of others who share their lifestyle, beliefs, and drugs. Polydrug use is particularly common, as individuals use one drug to counteract or enhance the effects of the first drug.

There is a significant difference between substance dependence and substance abuse. According to the DSM-IV-TR, *substance dependence* is characterized by a pattern of repeated self-administration of a drug that usually results in tolerance, withdrawal, and compulsive drug-taking behavior. *Substance abuse* is characterized by compulsive use in which the individual continues to use the drug even in the face of problems, including inability to fulfill major role obligations at work, school, or home; recurrent use in situations in which it is physically hazardous; recurrent legal problems related to the substance use; and recurrent social or interpersonal problems related to drug use.

Substance abuse is a major health problem for individuals in all ages and socioeconomic groups; however, abuse rates are highest in the 18- to 24-year-old group (DSM-IV-TR, 2001). Patterns of use vary in relation to cost and availability. It is difficult to say which substance is the most abused because often more than one drug at a time is used to control side effects. The National Household Survey on Drug Abuse n 1996 reported that 36 percent of the US population have used illicit drugs in their lives and 12 percent have used prescription drugs for nonmedical purposes. The economic impact of drug abuse is tremendous, including crime, medical costs, accidents, and loss of workdays in addition to the resulting family dysfunction.

The American Nurses Association (1997) estimates that 10 to 20 percent of nurses have substance abuse problems, with 6 to 8 percent being impaired as a result of alcohol and drug use. Stressful jobs, a tendency to perfectionism coupled with a feeling of inadequacy, and knowledge about and access to drugs increase the risk of substance abuse in this population. Because they do not fit the image of an addict, nurses often minimize or deny their problem.

Many states have now developed Diversion Programs to provide treatment and rehabilitation confidentially.

ETIOLOGY

The causes of drug abuse are similar to those of alcohol abuse; however, because of the wide range of drugs abused, there are some differences.

Biologic theories look at the role of specific neurotransmitters. Various drugs activate slightly different areas of the brain or brain circuits. Cocaine has been studied in more depth than some of the other drugs, and it is believed that there may be a deficiency of dopamine and norepinephrine that creates more of a craving for that drug. With opioids, it is theorized that there may be some abnormality in opioid receptors and endorphins.

Psychologic theories view drug dependence as an attempt to adapt to severe emotional distress. Low self-esteem and anxiety become masked under the influence of the drug. Drugs relieve feelings of depression and dependency and may be used to suppress anxiety, particularly after a traumatic event such as rape or violent crime. Individuals with tendencies toward antisocial behavior and difficulties with impulse control and frustration tolerance may use substances as a way to control anxiety that contributes to antisocial behavior. In addition, the role of the family and tendency to codependent relationships (see the preceding subsection on alcoholism for complete discussion) also exist with substance abuse. Drug abusers use many of the same coping mechanisms that alcoholics do, including denial, projection, and manipulation (see Table 13–1). Substance abuse can also be a way to cope with overwhelming traumas such as physical and mental abuse.

Sociocultural views recognize that certain drugs may be more likely to be used, depending on peer group, income, or culture. Acceptable behavior within a group, access to specific drugs, and status related to specific drugs may all be influencing factors. For example, crack cocaine has spread quickly within the low-income groups because of its easy availability and low cost.

RELATED CLINICAL CONCERNS

There is no evidence to suggest that an individual will become dependent on drugs by taking analgesics for pain. In fact, McCaffery and Ferrell (1994) report that less than 1 percent of individuals who take analgesics for a painful condition become addicted to that substance. Individuals who have developed drug tolerance require larger amounts of medications to relieve pain. This should not be confused with addiction.

Individuals with a substance abuse problem may experience withdrawal symptoms when hospital admission prevents them from taking the addictive substance. This is an important consideration when analyzing assessment findings. For instance, when a patient who has been hospitalized and NPO for 2 days experiences headaches and irritability, it may be related to caffeine withdrawal. In certain instances, withdrawal symptoms for more potent substances can increase the risk of complications. For example, the confusion resulting from amphetamine withdrawal may cause a postoperative patient to attempt to get out of bed, tear out tubes and intravenous lines, and possibly fall.

A new category of substance referred to as "club drugs" have been used increasingly by young people. These include ecstasy, ketamine, and rohypnal. Rohypnal has been associated with "date rape." When this short-acting benzodiazepine is slipped into an alcoholic drink, the victim becomes incapacitated and unable to resist a sexual assault. Ecstasy (also called MDMA) is a stimulant/hallucinogenic that can destroy neurons in the brain leading to brain damage.

The effects of high-risk behaviors that contribute to HIV, hepatitis, and bacterial endocarditis from infections and shared drug paraphernalia cause additional clinical concerns. Individuals may be more prone to high-risk behavior when under influence of drugs because inhibitions are suppressed.

LIFE SPAN ISSUES

NEONATES

Cocaine use during pregnancy presents severe problems for the exposed neonate. Complications include lower birth weight, decreased head circumference, preterm delivery, and placental abruption. Long-term problems can include conduct disorders. There is often a lack of prenatal care associated with the pregnancy as well because the mother may be fearful of seeking medical care.

CHILDREN AND ADOLESCENTS

Children and adolescents today are at high risk for exposure to substance use and abuse because of the easy availability of drugs in the schools and community. Peer pressure, experimentation, curiosity, and rebellion, as well as trying to find ways to cope or escape from problems, may be part of the etiology. Alcohol, tobacco, and marijuana are most frequently used. Drug use often begins while experimenting with peers. When the child experiences a sense of well-being and power, drug use continues. The child may then become drawn into the drug culture and possibly into a gang, which provides a support system for continued use. Children and adolescents are more likely to have abuse problems than dependence disorders. Adolescents who are victims of abuse and gay teens are particularly vulnerable to drugs as a way to cope with painful feelings (Tweed, 1998).

Children as young as 7 years have been identified as using inhalants, which are an easily available substance to children and younger teens when household items such as hair spray and aerosol whipped cream can be used.

Signs of substance abuse in this group may be indicated by change in functioning at school, loss of interest in sports, change in sleep patterns, increased isolation or change in social network.

ELDERLY PEOPLE

Substance use and abuse in elderly people are complicated because they routinely take a greater number of prescribed and over-the-counter drugs and have diminished tolerance to many medications. The individual, family, and health professionals often deny this problem in elderly persons. This may be because family members and health care professionals are reluctant to accuse an older person of drug abuse. The signs of abuse may also be masked or mistakenly attributed to the use of another drug the person is taking. The older adult is more likely to abuse prescribed tranquilizers, sedatives (especially benzodiazepines), and some analgesics. Falls, unexplained accidents, increased lethargy, loss of memory and attention span, and unexplained confusion may be signs of a drug abuse problem. Use of illicit drugs is relatively uncommon in elderly people, but it may increase in the future as young and middle-age addicts grow older.

POSSIBLE NURSES' REACTIONS

- May have strong negative feelings, viewing the patient as weak, immoral, or responsible for his or her own problems.
- May fear the patient's manipulative, provocative behavior and potential for criminal or violent behavior.
- May tend to minimize patient's concerns or discomforts because of resentment or fear of being manipulated.
- May distance self from patient because of own discomfort.
- May have a rescue fantasy of being the one to help this patient. The nurse may then become repeatedly disappointed when the patient returns to drug use.
- May view patient's cure as hopeless.
- May allow personal or family experience with substance abuse to influence response to the patient.

ASSESSMENT (TABLE 13–2)

Behavior and Appearance

- May talk frequently or brag about using drugs
- May have an in-depth knowledge of drugs and how they work
- Dramatic behavior changes, for instance, may be suddenly euphoric, drowsy, more outgoing
- Wears sunglasses indoors because of photophobia or to hide dilated or pinpoint pupils
- Unpredictable behavior
- Grandiosity, overconfidence
- Disheveled appearance
- In children and adolescents, loss of interest in school, drop in grades

TABLE 13–2. COMPARING COMMONLY ABUSED SUBSTANCES

Drug	Intoxication	Overdose	Withdrawal	Nursing Considerations
Amphetamines, including dexedrine and methamphetamines	*Signs:* Euphoria, high energy, impaired judgment, anxiety, aggressive behavior, paranoia, and delusions (often seen with long-term use)	*Signs:* Ataxia, high temperature, seizures, respiratory distress, cardiovascular collapse, coma, death *Treatment:* Supportive	*Signs:* Depression, agitation, insomnia, confusion, vivid dreams followed by extreme lethargy *Treatment:* Antidepressants, counseling, suicide precautions	• Used in weight reduction programs and to treat benzodiazepine abuse. • May cause a paradoxical reaction in children. • Remains in urine for up to 3 days.
Cannabis, including marijuana and hashish	*Signs:* Euphoria; intensified perceptions; impaired judgment and motor ability; increased appetite; weight gain, sinusitis, and bronchitis with chronic use; anxiety, paranoia; red conjunctiva	*Signs:* Extreme paranoia, psychosis *Treatment:* Antipsychotics	*Signs:* None	• Most widely used illicit drug. • Remains in urine for up to 7 days. • May exacerbate psychiatric symptoms in mentally ill patients. • May negatively affect fertility. • May therapeutically reduce nausea and vomiting, intraocular pressure, and stimulate appetite.
Cocaine, including crack	*Signs:* Euphoria, grandiosity, sexual excitement, impaired judgment, insomnia, anorexia; nasal perforation associated with inhaled route; psychosis associated with long-term abuse	*Signs:* High temperature, seizures, transient venospasms possibly causing MI or CVA, coma, death *Treatment:* Supportive	*Signs:* Fatigue, depression, anxiety, suicidal behavior *Treatment:* Support counseling, antidepressants	• Crack is smoked or injected IV; has a rapid onset and high dependency rate. • Cocaine is inhaled, snorted or injected IV. • High risk of acquiring HIV, hepatitis, bacterial

(Continued)

219

TABLE 13–2. COMPARING COMMONLY ABUSED SUBSTANCES (*Continued*)

Drug	Intoxication	Overdose	Withdrawal	Nursing Considerations
				endocarditis, and osteomyelitis from shared IV needles or promiscuous sexual relations. • May be used to control appetite. • Flashbacks can occur for up to 5 years. • Could precipitate a psychiatric disorder in susceptible persons.
Hallucinogens, including LSD and mescaline	*Signs:* Dilated pupils, diaphoresis, palpitations, tremors, enhanced perceptions of colors, sounds, depersonalization, grandiosity	*Signs:* Panic, psychosis with hallucinations, cerebral tissue damage, death *Treatment:* Diazepam or chloral hydrate; quiet environment antipsychotics	*Signs:* None	
Inhalants, including glue, gasoline, and paint thinner	*Signs:* Euphoria, impaired judgment, blurred vision, unsteady gait	*Signs:* Psychosis with hallucinations, cardiac arrhythmias, CNS depression, coma, cerebral tissue damage, death *Treatment:* Supportive	*Signs:* None	• Most available substance for younger children. • May be difficult to detect specific substance used. • Particularly irritating and/or flammable substances can cause trauma and burns in nose, mouth, and airways.
Nicotine, including cigarettes, chewing tobacco, and nicotine gum or patch	*Signs:* Produces a sense of anxiety reduction, relief from depression, and satisfaction	*Signs:* None	*Signs:* Insomnia, depression, irritability, anxiety, poor concentration, increased appetite *Treatment:* Transdermal	• Since most medical facilities do not allow smoking, inpatients may experience withdrawal symptoms.

Drug	Signs of Use/Intoxication	Withdrawal	Overdose	Nursing Implications
		nicotine patches in decreasing doses, nicotine gum and clonidine for severe anxiety, behavioral modification		• Less than 25% of individuals are successful with first attempt to quit. • Monitor for weight gain. • Monitor for hypotension with clonidine.
Opioids, including heroin, morphine, meperidine, and codeine	*Signs:* Euphoria, drowsiness, impaired judgment, constricted pupils	*Signs:* Yawning, insomnia, anorexia, irritability, rhinorhea, muscle cramps, chills, nausea, and vomiting, feelings of doom and panic *Treatment:* Detoxification, possibly with clonidine for severe anxiety and methadone, naloxone, or burenorphine to block euphoria	*Signs:* Dilated pupils, respiratory depression, seizures, cardiopulmonary arrest, coma, death *Treatment:* Naloxone, supportive	• High risk of acquiring HIV, hepatitis, bacterial endocarditis, and osteomyelitis from shared IV needles. • Monitor for hypotension with clonidine.
Phencyclidine (PCP, angel dust)	*Signs:* Impulsive behavior, impaired judgment, belligerent, assaultive behavior, ataxia, muscle rigidity, nystagmus, hypertension, numbness or diminished response to pain	*Signs:* None	*Signs:* Hallucinations, psychosis, seizures, respiratory arrest, stroke *Treatment:* Gastric lavage; cranberry juice or ammonium chloride to acidify urine (if awake); quiet environment; haloperidol or diazepam; fluids	• Have adequate staff available since behavior is unpredictable and patient may become violent. • May consider using four-point restraints. • Drugs remain in urine for several weeks. • Avoid using phenothi-

(Continued)

TABLE 13–2. COMPARING COMMONLY ABUSED SUBSTANCES (*Continued*)

Drug	Intoxication	Overdose	Withdrawal	Nursing Considerations
				azines because they can potentiate the effects of PCP.
Sedatives, hypnotics, and anxiolytics including barbiturates and benzodiazepines	*Signs:* Slurred speech, labile mood, inappropriate sexual behavior, loss of inhibitions, drowsiness, impaired memory	*Signs:* Hypotension, nystagmus, stupor, cardiorespiratory depression, coma, death *Treatment:* Benzodiazepine antagonist (flumazenil); induce vomiting, if awake; activated charcoal; cardiorespiratory support	*Signs:* Insomnia, hand tremor, agitation, nausea and vomiting, anxiety, tinnitus (with benzodiazepines), seizures, and cardiac arrest *Treatment:* Detoxification using gradually reduced dosages of a similar drug, anticonvulsants, and support and counseling	• Abrupt barbiturate withdrawal can be life-threatening. • Alcohol will potentiate drug effects. • Cross-tolerance may develop between alcohol and other CNS depressants. • Detectable in blood and urine. • Shorter-acting benzodiazepines have a greater risk of producing addiction and more severe rebound anxiety than longer-acting ones.
Club Drugs including Ecstasy (MDMA)	*Signs:* Euphoria, muscle relaxation	*Signs:* Confusion, hallucinations, severe anxiety, hypertension, seizures, high temp *Treatment:* Supportive	*Signs:* Not physiologically addictive, but psychologic dependence can cause depression, flashbacks	• Can cause memory loss and brain damage. • Physical response may be exacerbated by dehydration.

Mood and Emotions

- Mood swings
- Low frustration tolerance, angers easily
- Angry outbursts
- Anxiety, especially associated with discussion of drug use
- Emotional reactions related to change in medication regimen, particularly changes in analgesics
- Depressed; verbalizes self-deprecating thoughts

Thoughts, Beliefs, and Perceptions

- Denies impact of drug use
- Rationalizes that he or she can stop using any time
- Persistent belief that drug is for medical use only
- Obsessive thoughts about drug use and access to drug supply
- Suicidal ideations

Relationships and Interactions

- Change in circle of friends and isolation from family
- Blames others for need to use substances and other problems
- May become more isolated as fears of exposing habit to others increases
- Charming, charismatic, or manipulative with others

Physical Responses

- Needle tracks (raised marks from repeated IV injections) may be seen in antecubital space, wrist, feet, behind knees, or in tattoos.
- Recent injection sites may be red and swollen.
- Abscesses and ulcerations may be present.
- There is evidence of drug(s) in urine testing. Each drug varies as to how long it remains in the body. Check with the laboratory for specifics.
- Pupil response varies from constricted to nonreactive with different drugs.

Pertinent History

- History of withdrawal symptoms, overdosage, complications from past drug use
- Psychiatric disorders
- Family history of drug or alcohol abuse
- Criminal record and other legal problems
- Daily or binge drug abuse or dependence
- History of eating disorders

COLLABORATIVE MANAGEMENT

Treatment for substance abuse frequently requires a multidimensional approach including pharmacologic for detoxification, individual and group counseling, Twelve-Step Program, and education. Most treatment can be done on an outpatient basis except for high-risk detoxification.

Pharmacologic

Medications are used in detoxification programs for many drugs, including opioids, barbiturates, sedatives, and tranquilizers. They are used to control withdrawal symptoms and discourage continued use of the abused substance. Most are used for only short periods until withdrawal is complete; however, in some cases they may be used for longer periods to control cravings for the drug. Methadone, a synthetic narcotic that resembles morphine and heroin but does not produce the euphoric effects, is used daily on a long-term basis to treat heroin addiction. Both physical and psychologic dependence are maintained on methadone, but the euphoric effects of heroin are blocked. Patients usually make daily trips to a methadone clinic to obtain the drug. Buprenorphine, an opioid with agonist and antagonist action, has been used as an alternative to methadone. Naltrexone also reduces the euphoric sensation from narcotics, and clonidine decreases discomfort during narcotic withdrawal.

Bromocriptine and amantadine, dopamine agonists, are used to decrease craving during cocaine withdrawal.

Benzodiazepines and sedative withdrawal is more risky because of the risk for seizures and delirium. Tapering the dose of the identified or similar drug, along with anticonvulsants and antidepressants, is usually used.

Dual-diagnosis patients may require medications for treatment of their psychiatric diagnosis, but efforts are made to avoid sedatives and tranquilizers. Patients with anxiety or psychotic disorders may be using illicit drugs as a way of controlling hallucinations or anxiety.

Complementary approaches to treatment of substance abuse might include acupuncture, biofeedback, and massage. Herb and plant products to treat distressing symptoms may be helpful and include chamomile, valerian, kava kava, and St. John's wort. The last is contraindicated if the patient is taking antidepressants, narcotics, or amphetamines.

Twelve-Step Program

The Twelve-Step Program has been used to treat substance abuse and includes groups such as Narcotics Anonymous, Cocaine Anonymous, and Pills Anonymous. The philosophy mandates that the individual remains free from the substance and acknowledges that he or she is powerless over the chemical. Individuals need to attend group meetings routinely. Sponsors who have been drug free for longer periods provide support for new members. Family members can also participate in self-help groups following the same model.

Counseling

Drug rehabilitation also includes counseling to restore physical and emotional stability, identify the person's usual coping mechanism and work to adopt more effective ones, and develop a sense of self-worth and self-esteem.

NURSING MANAGEMENT

INEFFECTIVE DENIAL EVIDENCED BY LACK OF ACKNOWLEDGMENT OF SUBSTANCE ABUSE PROBLEM RELATED TO IMPAIRED ABILITY TO ACCEPT CONSEQUENCES OF OWN BEHAVIOR

Patient Outcomes

* Acknowledges substance abuse problem
* Abstains from substance use
* Participates in treatment plan

Interventions

* Convey acceptance of patient. Avoid criticizing, preaching to, or attacking the patient to get his or her attention.
* Promote trust by listening to concerns and treating patient as an individual.
* Give patient specific feedback on any behavior that appears drug related. Identify defense mechanisms such as blaming others or rationalizing behavior. Encourage personal responsibility for own behavior.
* Provide information on treatment approaches, such as Cocaine Anonymous (CA) or Narcotics Anonymous (NA).
* Help patient identify and share the possible emotions he or she is feeling.
* Help patient see link between substance use and personal and medical problems. Give the patient the opportunity to identify these, if possible.
* Assist patient to identify ways in which drug use affects daily life. Encourage being specific and honest.
* Set limits on manipulative behavior and realistic consequences for this behavior. Recognize that patient may exhibit charming, charismatic behavior, making limit setting more difficult. Never cover up for the patient or act entertained by drug use.
* Recognize that the drug effects may overwhelm the patient's motivation to stop. However, do not ignore signs of patient intoxication. Become familiar with your institution's policies for suspected drug use such as conducting a room search or confiscating drugs.
* If patient indicates that he or she wants to participate in a treatment program, immediately contact appropriate resources, such as a social worker, to facilitate admittance to a program.

INEFFECTIVE INDIVIDUAL COPING EVIDENCED BY ANXIETY, WITHDRAWAL SYMPTOMS, INABILITY TO FUNCTION WITHOUT DRUGS IN

RECOVERY RELATED TO INADEQUATE COPING SKILLS TO MANAGE STRESSORS WITHOUT DRUGS

Patient Outcomes

- Participates in treatment plan
- Demonstrates alternate coping mechanisms to deal with stress that do not involve drugs
- Verbalizes need to continue in treatment
- Abstains from substance use

Interventions

- Help patient to focus on getting through each day without drugs rather than the overwhelming thought of never using them again.
- Give reinforcement for ability to delay gratification and tolerate frustration. Provide information on possible coping mechanisms to reduce stress and tolerate discomfort. Review alternative ways to cope with anger. Role-play dealing with stressful situations.
- Explain the long-term physical effects of drug use, such as short attention span, that affect daily life.
- Prepare patient for the possibility that family and friends may have difficulty relating to him or her when he or she is not using drugs. For instance, friends may seem to abandon the patient who no longer wants to participate in their drug-related activities. The patient will need to prepare to accept this and work on changing these relationships or developing new ones.
- Help the patient discuss realistic future plans and life changes to make when no longer using drugs. Help to identify steps to achieve these goals.
- Encourage participation in support groups or visits or phone contacts with sponsors.
- Monitor to see if visitors are bringing in drugs.

RISK FOR INJURY EVIDENCED BY DISORIENTATION, LACK OF COORDINATION, OR AGGRESSIVE OR DISRUPTIVE BEHAVIOR RELATED TO SUBSTANCE INTOXICATION, OVERDOSE, OR WITHDRAWAL

Patient Outcomes

- Remains free from injury
- Reduced incidence of medical complications related to substance abuse
- Sleeps at least 6 hours a night

Interventions

- Recognize that many people who abuse drugs can function in society fairly well. Early signs of withdrawal may occur during hospitalization with no access to drug supply. Suspicious symptoms should be assessed carefully so that treatment can be instituted as early as possible.
- Determine which substances the patient has been using. Take a careful his-

tory from patient or family and friends (if applicable). Obtain ordered urine and blood for drug screening, and carefully monitor the patient's clinical condition and behavior. Recognize that many patients are using more than one substance, including alcohol.

- Institute fall and seizure precautions, as appropriate.
- Recognize that many substance abusers have poor nutritional habits because of anorexia, emotional changes, or inadequate intake. Monitor food and fluid intake. Encourage adequate fluids and nutrition.
- Administer ordered medications to ease symptoms and monitor for adverse and therapeutic effects. Monitor for signs of aggressive, agitated behavior. Avoid restraints if at all possible.
- Promote rest and sleep by maintaining a quiet environment and encouraging use of relaxation techniques and herbal teas.
- Patients with painful medical conditions need to have analgesics. The substance-abusing patient may need higher doses of analgesics and benefit from a regular dosing with a long-acting analgesic rather than p.r.n. administration. This avoids the euphoria effect from the analgesic.

ALTERNATE NURSING DIAGNOSES

Altered Thought Processes
Impaired Social Interaction
Knowledge Deficit
Risk for Infection
Self-Care Deficit
Self-Concept Disturbance

WHEN TO CALL FOR HELP

Escalation or onset of aggressive, belligerent behavior or violence

Change in level of consciousness unrelated to underlying medical condition

Need to apply restraints

Inadequate staff available to manage behavior

Suspected criminal activity related to drug use, selling drugs

---

PATIENT AND FAMILY EDUCATION

- Encourage patient to inform health care providers about drug use because this information will influence drug and dosage selections for needed medical treatments.
- Use caution when using over-the-counter drugs, diet pills, sedatives, and herbal products.

- Teach family members about need to adjust some aspects of their relationship with patient. Help them to identify possible behaviors that could be reinforcing substance use. Give them specific feedback if you observe any of these behaviors.
- Encourage patient to establish new routines and activities that do not involve drug use. This may include avoiding old circle of friends and developing hobbies or new interests.
- Provide information on risks of exposure to HIV, hepatitis, and other infections. Encourage patient who is at risk to obtain blood tests to determine exposure, and teach health practices to reduce risk to self and others.
- Help patient recognize potential fears and changes that may occur when he or she changes his or her life to live without drugs.
- Provide information on the health impact of specific substances patient is abusing.
- Provide information on treatment of substance abuse to patient and family.
- Educate patient and family on effects of drugs on pregnancy, on the job, or operating mechanical equipment.

CHARTING TIPS

- Document behavior associated with intoxication, overdose, or withdrawal.
- Document any indications of inappropriate drug use.
- Describe patient behavior after visits from family or friends.
- Describe response to treatments.
- Describe pain or anxiety behaviors and need for analgesics or tranquilizers.

COMMUNITY-BASED CARE

- Provide referral information on clinics, hotlines, halfway houses, drug treatment programs, and counseling that assist drug abusers.
- Inform referring agencies of patient's history.
- Arrange for follow-up psychiatric home health visit to reinforce drug treatment program as needed.
- Encourage follow-up medical appointments.

Problems with Sexual Dysfunction

LEARNING OBJECTIVES

➢ Define sexuality and sexual health for adults.
➢ Differentiate the major sexual dysfunctions found in men and women.
➢ Identify therapeutic interventions for common sexual dysfunction
➢ Describe common nurses' reactions to patients with issues about sexual functioning.

GLOSSARY

Dyspareunia—Persistent genital pain in either a man or woman before, during, or after sex.

Female sexual dysfunction—Includes inhibited desire, orgasmic dysfunction, and vaginismus.

Impotence—Erectile dysfunction or inability to attain or maintain an erection sufficient to complete intercourse.

Male sexual dysfunction—Includes inhibited desire, erective incapacity, premature ejaculation, ejaculatory incompetence, and ejaculatory pain.

Premature ejaculation—Persistent and recurrent ejaculation with minimal sexual stimulation and before the person wishes it.

Sexual dysfunction—A change in sexual health or function, which the individual views as unrewarding or inadequate. Sexual dysfunction is usually related to one or more of the following: lack of knowledge or incorrect information; biologic or physiologic causes, such as diabetes, drug or alcohol use, hormonal disorders; change in or loss of body part; ineffective coping or poor relationships; or organic problems (impotence, premature ejaculation, vaginismus, and orgasmic dysfunction).

Sexual response cycle—Includes excitement, plateau, orgasm, and resolution. Gender, age, culture, experience, and expectation affect each of these stages.

Sexually transmitted disease—Any disease that can be contracted by sexual contact; also called venereal disease. Symptoms range from merely annoying to life threatening.

Vaginismus—Involuntary spastic constriction of the lower vaginal muscles.

Human sexuality is a complex phenomenon encompassing biologic, psychologic, and sociocultural aspects. Biologic aspects include the anatomy and physiology of sexual development and sexual activities; psychologic aspects include gender identity, sexual self-concept, and valuing one's self as male or female; and sociocultural aspects include sexual orientation learned from the value systems of family, peers, and community. All these aspects are interrelated, influencing the individual to experience and value the self as masculine or feminine, seeking and giving affection and striving to meet basic needs for love and belonging (King, 1999).

A sexually healthy person has the following characteristics:

- Behavior agreeing with gender identity (persistent feeling of one's self as male or female)
- Ability to participate in loving and committed relationships
- Physical ability to find erotic stimulation pleasurable
- Ability to make decisions about sexual behavior that are compatible with values and beliefs, cultural norms, and social mores
- Ability to make adjustments in sexual functioning appropriate to limitations and changes resulting from illness, injury, or other events such as unavailability of a partner.

Human sexuality can be healthy, satisfying, and enriching, as defined by the preceding characteristics; or it can be the source of physical and mental distress (LeMone & Jones, 1997; Fergusson, 1998). Sexuality encompasses a person's feelings about himself or herself and how to interact with others. Sexuality and sexual behaviors are influenced by age, knowledge, marital status;

230

resources; values; social, spiritual, and cultural norms; and emotional and physical health (Poorman, 2001).

Society today allows people to experience various types of adult relationships. Once believed to be the legal and moral right of only married people, sexual activity is now considered by many individuals to be acceptable for any consenting adult. More people are involved in relationships that were not considered acceptable just a decade or two ago, such as premarital sex, open marriages, remarried or blended families, unions of never-married adults, single-parent families, and homosexual relationships. Sexual preferences are considered a matter of personal choice, and homosexuality is no longer considered a mental illness (King, 1999; Levine, 1999; Torkelson & Dobal, 1999).

All aspects of human sexuality may be affected by acute and, especially, chronic illness. Ill health is one of the greatest detriments to sexual expression, not only because it focuses energies toward recuperation but also because it often lowers an individual's sense of personal worth and attractiveness, and indirectly, sexual desire. The most common dysfunctions in women are arousal and orgasmic dysfunction. Common dysfunctions in men are impotence and premature ejaculation.

A diagnosis of sexual dysfunction is made when an individual identifies a problem with sexuality (not when the caregiver is uncomfortable with the patient's sexual preference) or when antisocial sexual behavior results in harm to others. Individuals have the right to make choices regarding their sexual options and should be offered education about them, such as information on appliances and strengthening exercises for cord-injured patients. However, they do not have the right to inflict discomfort or harm on others (Taylor, 1999). Changing social norms for sexual behavior have recently made deviations from "traditional" sexuality more acceptable. Some individuals who adopt alternative modes of sexuality (e.g., homosexuality) experience little or no conflict internally or externally and thus may not be subject to problems of sexual dysfunction. However, some members of society continue to experience extreme discomfort with less traditional sexual expression (Townsend, 2000).

Competence and success in handling problems with sexual dysfunction depend on the nurse's knowledge, experience, and comfort with his or her own sexuality. It can be difficult for some nurses to assess a patient's sexual problems or intervene for inappropriate sexual behavior. It may be useful in these situations to confer with a nurse colleague, especially a nurse specialist or a mental health practitioner with training in sexual counseling (Poorman, 2001).

Nurses should not feel that they need to be sex therapists. They can, however, help resolve some sexual problems created by the patient's illness and the limitations it creates. To be prepared to deal with this aspect of patient care, the nurse should:

- Be knowledgeable about sexuality and sexual norms.
- Use this knowledge to understand others' behavior and reactions to sexuality in health and illness.
- Be aware of differences in cultural and individual attitudes and perspectives regarding sexuality.

- Assist patients' adaptation to an optimal level of health regarding their sexuality.
- Make appropriate referrals for patients with more complex sexual dysfunction.

ETIOLOGY

The human sexual response cycle stages (excitement, plateau, orgasm, and resolution) describe the type of responses people have during sexual activity. Sexual dysfunction can occur at any of these stages. There is seldom any single cause of unsatisfying or inadequate sexual experiences.

It is estimated that 15 to 25 percent of patients seen in family practice have concerns about sexual function. One of the most common causes of sexual dysfunction, in particular erectile dysfunction (impotence) in men and decreased desire in women, is the wide range of medications prescribed for common medical and psychiatric illnesses. Virtually all antipsychotic and antidepressant medications and a variety of other psychotropic medications can cause disruptions in sexual function. Antihypertensives are also implicated in disorders of sexual desire, arousal, and orgasm (Table 14–1). Illicit drugs and alcohol should not be overlooked in evaluating sexual disorders. Many patients believe that alcohol and other drugs decrease sexual inhibitions, whereas in reality they decrease sexuality and ability to perform sexually. Major tranquilizers, cocaine, and even tobacco have been implicated in sexual disorders (Finger et al., 1997).

TABLE 14–1. DRUG CATEGORIES THAT ALTER SEXUAL BEHAVIOR

Drug Type	Probable Effects
Antihypertensives	Produce vasodilation and decreased cardiac output, depress CNS; cause impotence in men and decrease vaginal lubrication in women
Antidepressants	Peripheral blockage of nervous innervation of sex glands; may have positive effect because they decrease depression
Antihistamines	Block parasympathetic nervous innervation of sex glands
Antispasmodics/anticholinergics	Inhibit parasympathetic innervation of sex glands
Sedatives and tranquilizers	Block autonomic innervation of sex glands; may have positive effect as they produce tranquilization and relaxation, may have negative effect influencing libido
Oral contraceptives	Remove fear of pregnancy
Alcohol	In small amounts, may increase libido, in large amounts, impairs neural reflexes involved in erection and ejaculation, chronic use may cause impotence
Opioids	Central sedation causes impotence in chronic users
Cancer chemotherapy agents	May produce temporary sterility or neurotoxicity in men, causing impotence
Estrogen	Suppresses sexual function in men
Diuretics	Chronic use may cause impotence

Adapted from Finger, WW, Lund, M, and Slagle, MA: Medications that may contribute to sexual disorders. Journal of Family Practice 44:33–43, 1997.

Physiologic causes include disruption of neural pathways as seen in spinal cord injury or prostate surgery; impaired circulation as seen in diabetes or peripheral vascular disease; and hormonal changes as in testicular or ovarian dysfunction. Physiological factors are likely to be consistent across time and situations, whereas disorders with psychogenic causes are likely to be situation or mood specific. *Psychologic* causes include unresolved internal conflicts, low self-esteem, discordant relationships with current or past partners, feelings of dependency or abandonment, and depression. *Sociocultural* factors include cultural or religious myths or beliefs that inhibit sexual activity.

Sexual disorders are categorized by DSM-IV-TR (1999) into six major categories:

1. Sexual desire disorders, including hypoactive sexual desire in men or women, and extreme aversion to genital sexual contact
2. Sexual arousal disorders, including female sexual arousal disorder and male erectile disorder
3. Orgasmic disorders in both men and women, also known as delayed or premature ejaculation in men
4. Sexual pain disorders, including dyspareunia in men or women, vaginismus in women
5. Sexual dysfunction caused by General Medical Condition and Substance-Induced Sexual Dysfunction
6. Paraphilias: repetitive sexual fantasies or behaviors involving use of a nonhuman object (fetishism), nonconsenting partners (voyeurism, and exhibitionism), or activity that causes humiliation or harm (masochism, sadism, and pedophilia)

RELATED CLINICAL CONCERNS

In nonpsychiatric settings, most nurses see sexual dysfunction related to medical problems, traumatic injuries, or surgical procedures. Sexual dysfunction may be a temporary concomitant of an illness or treatment, or it may be a permanent consequence of chronic illness or injury. Sexual problems associated with illness or injury can be classified into four groups:

1. Lack of interest in or desire for sexual activity
2. Physical incapacity for or discomfort during sexual activity
3. Fear of precipitating or aggravating a physical illness through sexual activity
4. Use of illness as an excuse to avoid feared or undesired sexual activity

Surgical procedures resulting in changes in sexual functioning include urologic procedures for prostatic hypertrophy; intestinal surgery for colitis, ileitis, or Crohn's disease; and most other fecal or urinary diversion surgeries for neoplasms. Loss of external or internal body parts or functions; relocation of orifices, such as hysterectomy, mastectomy, colectomy, and cystectomy; and amputations can all lead to changes in both physical and mental components of sexual functioning. How a surgical procedure influences postoperative sexual functioning depends on the:

- Reason for surgery, diagnosis, and prognosis related to sexual functioning
- Significance of loss of childbearing and fertility functions
- Knowledge of anatomy and physiology of sexual structures and functions
- Meaning, assumptions, and values related to sexual identity
- Type and rationale for premorbid sexual activity

The main difference between a health disruption resulting from chronic illness and surgical or accidental trauma is the irreversible effect on nerves, blood vessels, and hormonal supply usually associated with surgery and trauma.

Most of the drugs reported to affect sexual functioning directly (see Table 14–1) act on specific neurotransmitters. There is evidence that the primary neurohormone in mobilizing sexual behavior is dopamine, whereas serotonin is the major inhibitor. Therefore medications that block dopamine receptor sites and drugs that deplete dopamine interfere with central control of sexual function, whereas drugs that depress serotonin concentrations in the brain are expected to stimulate sexual function.

Many sexual responses are mediated through the parasympathetic nervous system; therefore, parasympatholytic or cholinergic blocking drugs may cause impotence in men and problems with vaginal lubrication in women. Orgasm and ejaculation are primarily functions of the sympathetic, adrenergic, and nervous system, and therefore drugs such as anticholinergics may interfere with potency and orgasm.

Ganglionic blocking drugs, such as antispasmodics, impair both sympathetic and parasympathetic nervous system function. Drugs that stimulate or depress the central nervous system can affect sexuality, particularly antianxiety agents and narcotics and many of the substances used socially such as caffeine, alcohol, cocaine, marijuana, and amphetamines. Many therapeutically useful drugs have some adverse effect on sexual function.

LIFE SPAN ISSUES

CHILDREN

Masculinity and femininity are defined culturally. Although chromosomes determine sexual identity before birth and by physical appearance of the genitals at birth, postnatal factors greatly influence the way children perceive themselves and others sexually.

Gender identity is usually firmly established by the age of 18 months. In rare cases in which gender was misassigned at birth because of physical abnormality or accidental damage was suffered, it is considered almost impossible to reassign a child to the opposite sex after age 2 years.

Research on infantile sexuality indicates that both male and female infants are capable of sexual arousal and orgasm. By age 3 children are very aware of how they are alike or different from their parents. Research supports early masturbation experiences in 15 to 20 percent of 5- to 8-year-olds. By age 10 to 12, children are preoccupied with pubertal changes and beginnings of romantic interest in the opposite sex.

ADOLESCENTS

American culture has very ambivalent feelings about adolescent sexuality. Although teachers and parents realize the importance of psychosocial development, most want to avoid anything that will encourage teenage sex. Trends in teen sex for the past 2 decades include more teens engaging in premarital intercourse, and the average age of first intercourse is decreasing. Recently the previously increasing trend in incidence of teen pregnancy has decreased in most areas of the U. S. A major concern at this time is sex education regarding sexually transmitted diseases, birth control, and the development of satisfying, long-term relationships with same-sex and opposite-sex friends.

ADULTS

During this period of the life cycle, from about age 20 to 65, every adult must deal with numerous issues that may lead to temporary or long-term sexual dysfunction. Developing sexual relationships, choosing a marital partner, attitudes about premarital or extramarital sex, infidelity, divorce, remaining single, and raising children are just a few of the issues. After age 45 to 50, a decrease in hormonal activity, menopause, and other physical changes in both men and women may decrease biological drives. In general, healthcare providers should feel comfortable encouraging both sexes to continue healthy sexual activity during adulthood (Townsend, 2000).

ELDERLY PEOPLE

There are many myths and stereotypes about sexuality and elderly people. The most important factor in sexual activity in older adults is the availability of a healthy relationship between two healthy partners. The most significant health issues affecting sexuality for older people are fear of heart attack, post-stroke dependency, fatigue related to chronic obstructive pulmonary disease, erectile dysfunction related to diabetes and impotence related to treatment for prostate cancer in men, inadequate lubrication in women, and arthritis causing movement limitations. Surgical procedures that are more common in the elderly persons, such as prostatectomy, mastectomy, hysterectomy, and ostomies, also affect the older adult's sexuality. Institutionalization is a particular problem for elderly people because the staff at such facilities may not understand or be sensitive to the sexual needs of their residents.

POSSIBLE NURSES' REACTIONS

- May be shy or insecure about the sexual aspects of their professional role, even though they are sanctioned to touch others in an intimate and personal manner and to ask personal questions, including questions about sexual matters, related to their patients' health.
- May experience anxiety, even revulsion, when dealing with sexual questions or behaviors while caring for their patients.

- May deny their own or their patients' sexuality by avoiding any verbal or behavioral interaction regarding sexual function, for instance, avoiding subject of sex, responding to sexually oriented questions in a vague manner, or using euphemistic expressions like "private parts" or "down below" when referring to genitalia.
- May use hospital rules to sidestep patients' sexual concerns. For example, they may assign male staff members to male patients when sexual behaviors or concerns develop.
- May not recognize or may actually encourage patients' becoming emotionally involved with them.
- May experience pity for patients who are unable to perform some sexual acts after injury such as spinal cord injury. May feel insulted, denigrated, or angered by patient behaviors such as flirting, pinching, and exposing body parts.
- May feel uncomfortable dealing with sexual dysfunction in patients.
- May have a mistaken belief that the seriously ill do not have sexual needs or desires and may show a lack of tolerance and empathy for a patient's sexual concerns during illness.

ASSESSMENT

See Box 14–1 for guidelines for an interview with a patient with a sexual problem.

BOX 14–1. Guidelines for an Interview with a Patient Having a Sexual Problem

These questions serve as a guideline. Adjustments in the focus and depth of the assessment depend on the nature of the patient's problem and the nurse's level of comfort in discussing sexual concerns.

1. Does patient's current physical condition affect level of sexual function?
2. Does patient have concerns about body image or self-esteem related to illness, injury, or surgery?
3. What does patient know about potential or expected changes in sexual function related to the illness, injury, or surgery?
4. What significance does the physical change or limitations have on the patient's perceptions and understanding of sexual function?
5. What are patient's previous sexual patterns?
6. What does patient's spouse or significant other (SO) understand and believe about the patient's sexual function and the impact of the illness, injury, or surgery?
7. What is patient's outlook and prognosis regarding sexual function?
8. What is patient's level of comfort and willingness to discuss sexual function with health professional, spouse, others?
9. Would patient and SO benefit from more education, counseling, or therapy?

Behavior and Appearance

- Reluctance to answer questions related to sexual functioning
- Concern over changes in sexual performance, body image
- Withdrawn, isolated, embarrassed
- Inappropriate sexual acting out, such as pinching or teasing the nurse, exposing genitalia, or wearing seductive clothing
- May verbalize changes in functioning caused by illness, injury, or surgery

Mood and Emotions

- Fear about future limitations of sexual performance or attractiveness
- Fear, anxiety, or guilt about sexual abilities or loss of function resulting from illness, injury, or surgery
- Presence of stressors affecting sexual functioning, such as job problems, financial worries, religious conflict, value conflict with family or partner, separated or divorced partner
- Discomfort over lack of privacy, frequent physical exams, or invasive procedures
- Depression over lack of sexual satisfaction or loss of relationships

Thoughts, Beliefs, and Perceptions

- Lack of knowledge or incorrect information about sexual functioning
- Change in self-concept or body image caused by illness, injury, or surgery
- Denial or misinterpretation of partner's reactions to sexual functioning
- Denies any concerns about sexual functioning but acts in a sexually inappropriate manner with staff or others

Relationships and Interactions

- Sexual dissatisfaction or decreased sexual desire
- Altered relationship with significant other
- Partner unavailable, unwilling, or abusive
- Poor past sexual relationships, absent or negative sexual teaching

Physical Responses

- Painful intercourse
- Inability to complete intercourse, early ejaculation, impotence in men
- Menopausal changes in women because of age, surgery, or medications (such as chemotherapy) causing vaginal dryness and lack of interest

Pertinent History

- Physical diseases or injuries affecting sexual functioning
- History of depression
- History of sexual abuse or rape
- Alcohol or other substance abuse

- Previous sexual dysfunction, such as impotence, painful intercourse, premature ejaculation, or lack of lubrication in women

COLLABORATIVE MANAGEMENT

Pharmacologic

Any patient experiencing sexual dysfunction needs a thorough assessment of all medications being taken. Then alternative drug choices as well as changes in doses and timing can be tried. There is a limited role for medications to enhance sexual functioning. Hormonal therapy may be appropriate treatment in some cases. For example, postmenopausal women may benefit from estrogen replacement therapy to reduce discomfort during intercourse. Antidepressants can contribute to sexual dysfunction in some, but in others they have been known to increase desire and reduce depression. Any medications that would increase patient comfort such as analgesics may also be helpful to reduce pain during sexual contact. Sildenafil (Viagra) is the first oral medication to treat impotence. A variety of herbal products are used by individuals of different cultures to enhance sexual functioning (e. g., ginseng, saw palmetto).

Sex Therapy

A patient may need to seek out individual, couple, or group therapy to treat sexual dysfunction. Many mental health professionals have specific training for sexual dysfunction. In addition, the patient may wish to seek out a professional who has obtained certification as a sex therapist from a national organization.

NURSING MANAGEMENT

SEXUAL DYSFUNCTION EVIDENCED BY IMPOTENCE, PREMATURE EJACULATION, VAGINISMUS, DYSPAREUNIA, OR OTHER CHANGES IN SEXUAL BEHAVIOR RELATED TO ILLNESS

Patient Outcomes

- Relates valid, accurate information regarding sexual anatomy and function
- Able to verbalize correct information about previously believed myths and misinformation about sexual matters
- Identifies alternate sexual expressions that are pleasurable
- Discusses sexual functioning using correct information

Patient and Partner Outcomes

- Participate in treatment or practices that mediate problem or facilitate and enhance current sexual functioning

Interventions

- Create an atmosphere of understanding, openness, and acceptance between patient and nurse.
- Eliminate or reduce causes for patient to feel embarrassed while discussing sexual functioning.
- Provide privacy and be nonjudgmental and supportive.
- Begin with other subjects, such as physical or family questions, then move on to questions on biologic aspects of sexuality, such as age at menarche and onset of sexual development, before discussing sexual behaviors or fears. Focus on general knowledge and expectations before moving on to specific individual concerns.
- Determine patient's knowledge and attitudes about sexuality and sexual function.
- Focus on patient's knowledge of anatomy and functioning of body parts that may be affected by disease, injury, or surgery.
- Pay attention to attitudes and words used by patient.
- Identify any misinformation, myths, or beliefs that may affect patient's adjustment to changes in sexual functioning. Validate correct information and correct erroneous information.
- Accept person's feelings and concerns; explore cultural, social, religious, and parental influences on current beliefs.
- Provide new information appropriate to patient's maturational or educational level; include spouse or partner as appropriate.
- Discuss with patient and partner the various etiologies for specific diagnoses; explain cause of problem, if known; provide information about its treatment and prognosis.
- Encourage couple to talk over the effect of dysfunction on their relationship.
- Discuss alternate methods of sexual gratification with patient or partner.
- Refer to a urologist or other specialist for further evaluation regarding surgical procedures for penile implants, or vaginal reconstruction when appropriate.
- Refer for further evaluation, counseling, or therapy, if indicated.

> **SEXUAL DYSFUNCTION** EVIDENCED BY IMPOTENCE, PREMATURE EJACULATION, LACK OF SEXUAL DESIRE OR AROUSAL OR OTHER DISSATISFYING CHANGES IN SEXUAL BEHAVIOR RELATED TO INABILITY TO ADAPT TO LIFE STRESSORS, E.G., DIVORCE, DEATH, LOSS OF JOB, DEPRESSION.

Patient Outcomes

- Identifies stressors affecting sexual function
- Identifies constructive coping patterns and sexual practices
- Resumes previous sexual activity

Interventions

- Assess for factors causing patient's ineffective coping and their influence on sexual function.
- Help the patient to understand and discuss the relationship between life stressors and poor sexual functioning.
- Help patient to determine which stressors can be changed and which he or she has no control over.
- Discuss the modifications of or changes in ways of dealing with stressors. Assist in problem solving for alternatives.
- Help the patient identify alternative methods to reduce sexual energy when partner is unavailable or unwilling, such as the role of regular physical exercise, alternative sexual practices (self-stimulation, increased social activities if spouse or partner is absent or deceased). Provide educational materials, as needed.
- Refer patient or partner for further counseling or therapy, as indicated, such as consider referrals to marriage counselor, sex therapist, social services as indicated by patient's specific problems.

> **ALTERED SEXUALITY PATTERNS** EVIDENCED BY ACTUAL OR ANTICIPATED NEGATIVE CHANGES IN SEXUAL ACTIVITY AND/OR IDENTITY RELATED TO CHANGES IN OR LOSS OF BODY PART OR PHYSIOLOGIC LIMITATIONS.

Patient Outcomes

- Shows increased acceptance of change in or loss of body part
- Identifies practices that assist in restoration of sexual function despite change in or loss of body part
- Identifies practices that conserve energy and oxygen requirements for sexual activity
- Discusses change in or loss of body part and its influence on sexual functioning

Patient and Partner Outcomes

- Identifies mutual concerns
- Shows increased acceptance of change or loss
- Identifies and uses practices that assist in satisfying sexual functioning

Interventions

- Determine the level of acceptance or adaptation of the patient or partner to the changed or lost body part or function. Note patient's reactions, such as anger, depression, or denial. Explain normal feelings about loss, grief, and change.
- Convey an attitude of acceptance. Be sensitive to the patient's cues that a

concern exists, and encourage any attempts to discuss the problem or fear.

- Respect the patient's need for privacy.
- Facilitate the partner's and family's understanding of patient's condition and concerns.
- Encourage need to share by listening and answering questions.
- Include spouse or partner in counseling and teaching if he or she express readiness. Also include spouse or partner in discussions about fear of future losses, fear of rejection by loved ones, and fear of physically hurting partner.
- Help the patient realize that body changes and losses are acceptable to others by spending time with the patient, appropriate touching, and teaching about care during regular nursing care.
- Ask about strengths of relationship with partner and encourage discussion of alternative sexual activities.
- Do not assume that patient knows about how the illness or injury affects sexuality. Many patients do not ask questions or give any indication at all about their concerns.
- Check to see whether the patient understands medical terminology by asking for feedback on what he or she comprehends. Use pictures and verbal explanations when providing information or giving instructions.
- Provide information over short, repeated visits so that patient has time to think over what you have discussed and to formulate questions for later clarification.
- Check which medications the patient is taking, and inform the patient about any adverse effects on sexual function.
- Encourage the patient to resume sexual activity as close to previous pattern as physically possible. Teach specific information applicable to individual physical condition:
  - For the patient with an ostomy, provide information on ways to control drainage odor.
  - Refer to enterostomal nurse specialist for assistance with appliances. Refer to other specialists as needed.
  - For the patient with cardiac or respiratory disease, teach techniques for conserving oxygen and reducing cardiac workload.
  - Identify the symptoms that indicate sexual activity should be terminated.
  - Provide information on specific techniques if patient is unable to move legs because of arthritis or spinal cord injury.
  - Teach patient to take pain medication before sexual activity for pain caused by arthritis, cancer, and so on.
- Promote the use of alternative methods of sensory and perceptual stimulation, such as body massage.
- Refer the patient and partner to further educational material, self-help support organizations, and therapy as needed. Many self-help groups offer support related to sexual concerns; these include the United Ostomy Association, Arthritis Foundation, American Cancer Society, organizations for the disabled, and Reach for Recovery.

ALTERATION IN SEXUAL BEHAVIOR PATTERNS EVIDENCED BY INAPPROPRIATE SEXUAL BEHAVIOR IN THE MEDICAL SETTING RELATED TO INEFFECTIVE COPING.

Patient Outcomes

- Decreases or eliminates sexual acting-out behavior
- Shows willingness to discuss meaning of behavior and its impact on others
- Uses other behaviors for maintaining sexual identity
- Finds more appropriate ways to meet sexual needs in medical setting

Interventions

- Assess meaning of sexual behavior as release of sexual needs or anxiety, aggression, fear of loss of identity, reaction to change in or loss of body part, or need for closeness.
- When inappropriate behaviors occur, identify what happened before acting out.
- Discuss behaviors with patient and attempt to understand meaning of behavior to patient.
- Give patient feedback about staff reactions to behaviors. Help patient to understand their impact on other patients and staff. Point out which behaviors are most disturbing.
- Set clear limits with patient about what specific behavior is inappropriate.
- Discuss more appropriate ways for patient to meet sexual needs, such as exercise, reading, or spending private time with partner.
- Ensure that the patient knows that sexual acting out is not needed to maintain nurse's interest or concern as a person.
- Provide time to talk with or give physical care to patient when sexual behaviors are not occurring.
- Provide opportunity for the patient to express feelings about sexual identity and the impact of illness, injury, or surgery on body image and self-concept.
- Discuss and negotiate ways to provide privacy during long-term hospitalization.
- Provide structured activity or active games. If appropriate, ask volunteers to arrange for activities outside the current environment.
- Conduct care plan conference to discuss problem and appropriate interventions. When embarrassed or frustrated by sexually acting-out patient, get backup from other staff members, consultants, or administrator who can assist in setting limits and determining care plan goals.

ALTERNATE NURSING DIAGNOSES

Self-Concept Disturbance
Impaired Social Interaction
Ineffective Individual Coping
Knowledge Deficit
Social Isolation

WHEN TO CALL FOR HELP

☐ Onset of sexually "acting-out" behaviors inappropriate to medical setting

☐ Increased staff complaints or conflict over management of patient behavior

☐ Increased staff anxiety over dealing with sexually inappropriate behavior

☐ Increased sexually inappropriate behavior in other patients

☐ Patient's sexual behavior interfering with treatment

☐ Staff inability to provide needed information or counseling to patient

PATIENT AND FAMILY EDUCATION

- Review with the patient and sexual partner, if requested, any effects of medications that may affect sexual function. Reinforce need to report these to physician so that alternatives can be found.
- Teach probable causes and treatment for sexual dysfunction if patient and partner request this information.
- Provide information on birth control and prevention of sexually transmitted diseases, as appropriate.
- Provide information on the impact of surgery, illness, and medication on sexual functioning.
- Ensure patient has needed information about use of special devices and drugs, e.g., penile implants, Viagra.

CHARTING TIPS

- Use objective, nonjudgmental terms to describe the patient's sexual behavior.
- Document the patient's sexual concerns even if you do not feel comfortable providing information or education.
- Document the selected interventions for dealing with inappropriate sexual behavior on the patient care plan for consistency.
- Document the patient's understanding of cause and treatment of sexual dysfunction. Include responses of family members if they are involved in patient education and treatment.

COMMUNITY-BASED CARE

- Consult with physician and inform patient and partner about appropriate resources related to sexual dysfunction.
- Provide referrals to appropriate support groups.
- Inform other healthcare professionals of patient's inappropriate sexual behavior if patient is being transferred to another facility.
- Inform patient and partner about expected changes in sexual behavior or dysfunction as disease progresses or patient is rehabilitated.
- Provide referral information for further sexual counseling or therapy if needed.

Problems with Pain

LEARNING OBJECTIVES

➢ Differentiate between acute, recurrent, and chronic nonmalignant and malignant pain.
➢ Examine the reasons for underassessment and undertreatment of pain.
➢ Describe important factors to be considered in the assessment of pain.
➢ Describe the role and routes of opioid and nonopioid analgesics in pain management.
➢ Discuss the importance of alternative (nonpharmacologic) methods of pain relief.

GLOSSARY

Acute pain—Pain that lasts from seconds to usually less than 6 months after the noxious stimulus. Usually subsides as healing takes place.

Addiction—A psychological process, in contrast to drug tolerance, that involves the repeated use of a drug or drugs for psychological, not medical, reasons. Patients who are psychologically dependent on a drug (addicted) will continue to desire the drug even though the pain is resolved.

Cancer pain—Usually placed in a category of its own. Even if it lasts over 6 months, it is often treated like acute pain because of its progressive nature. Sometimes referred to as malignant pain.

Chronic pain—Lasts for 3 to 6 months or longer after the noxious stimulus. Types of chronic pain include recurrent acute pain with potential for recurrence over a prolonged period, with pain-free intervals between episodes; chronic acute pain, which may last months or years, but has a high probability of ending; and chronic, benign pain, which occurs almost daily and has existed for 6 or more months.

Drug tolerance—A physiologic response of the body, not under the person's control, in which the drug loses its effectiveness after repeated use. Occurs in almost all patients using opioids longer than 7 to 10 days. Needs to be taken into consideration when determining correct dosage of analgesic because the patient may require increased doses to achieve the same effect.

Pain—An unpleasant sensory and emotional experience arising from actual or potential tissue damage caused by a noxious stimulus.

Pain tolerance—Duration and intensity of pain that an individual is willing to tolerate at any one time. Pain tolerance changes within an individual from one pain experience to another.

Placebo—Any medical or nursing measure that works because of its implicit or explicit therapeutic intent rather than its chemical or physical properties.

Referred pain—Pain felt at a site other than the injured or diseased organ or body part. The pain of coronary artery insufficiency, for example, is often referred to the left shoulder, arm, or jaw, and pancreatic pain may be referred to the middle back.

> *Pain is what the person experiencing it says it is, exists when and where he or she says it does. The patient is the authority about his own pain.*
> (McCaffery, 1968)

Pain is a universal experience occurring in all age groups and is the most frequent reason why people seek health care. Much progress has been made over the last decade in understanding pain mechanisms and the epidemiology of pain. The subject is important for all clinicians because the frequency and perhaps the severity of pain may increase now that progress in medical science has increased survival through old age and chronic illness, now affecting more people than ever before.

Studies continue to show that pain is underassessed and undertreated by healthcare professionals. The classic study by Marks and Sachar (1973) reported that 73 percent of hospitalized medical patients experienced moderate to severe pain despite receiving parenteral opioid analgesics. Recent research indicates that nurses and physicians continue to undertreat pain in patients because they do not understand pain management principles, they fear causing the patients' dependence on opioids, and they have poor knowledge of opioids, adjuvant therapies, and the components of pain assessment (McCaffery and Ferrell, 1997a, 1997b). Despite the establishment of federal guidelines on pain management (Agency for Healthcare Policy and Research, 1992 and 1994), many patients of all ages still suffer unnecessary pain in all healthcare settings and at home. [Twycross, 1999 and Weiner et al., 1999) In 2001, the Joint Commission on Accreditation of Healthcare Organizations implemented pain management standards that mandate frequent assessment and appropriate interventions.

Pain is a multidimensional and complex phenomenon, requiring effective assessment and management. Many disciplines are involved in pain management in a variety of clinical settings. Optimal pain management depends on cooperation among the different members of the healthcare team throughout the patient's course of treatment (Stratton, 1999).

The nurse usually has the most significant influence on management of the patient's pain because of having the most frequent contact with the patient. Consequently, the nurse is in a unique position to identify the patient who has pain; to appropriately assess the pain and its impact on the patient and family; to initiate action to alleviate pain using available resources, and to evaluate the effectiveness of those actions.

Patients vary greatly in their responses to pain and its interventions, as well as in their personal preferences and expectations regarding pain relief. Therefore rigid prescriptions for the management of pain are inappropriate. An effective pain management program will incorporate the following requirements and principles:

1. Pain intensity and relief must be assessed and reassessed at regular intervals in a consistent manner (Fig. 15–1).
2. Patient preferences must be respected when selecting methods of pain management.
3. Each institution must develop an organized program to evaluate the effectiveness of pain assessment and management.
4. Establishing positive relationships between patients and healthcare professionals is an important part of successful pain control. Patients should be informed that information about options to control pain is available and they are welcome to discuss their concerns and preferences with the healthcare team.
5. Unrelieved pain has severe negative physical and psychologic consequences. Aggressive pain prevention and control can yield both short-term and long-term benefits. Although complete elimination of some pain may not be practical or even desirable, techniques are now available to make pain reduction a realistic goal.
6. Prevention is better than treatment. Pain that is established is more difficult to control. The goal should be reduced pain at all times, with "round-the-clock" medications if needed.

INITIAL PAIN ASSESSMENT TOOL

Patient's Name _____ Age _____ Date _____

Diagnosis _____ Physician _____

Room _____

Nurse _____

I. LOCATION: Patient or nurse mark drawing.

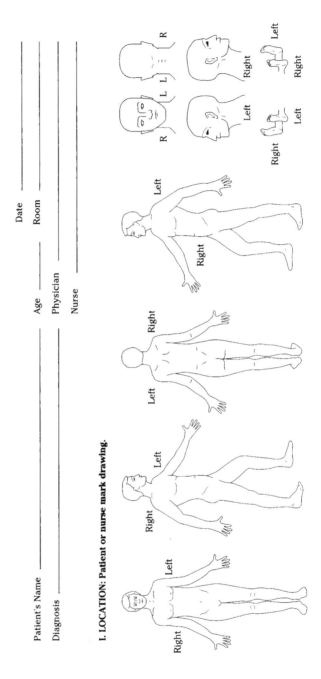

II. INTENSITY: Patient rates the pain. Scale used _____

Present: _____

Worst pain gets: _____

Best pain gets: _____

Acceptable level of pain: _____

III. QUALITY: (Use patient's own words, e.g., prick, ache, burn, throb, pull, sharp) _____

IV. ONSET, DURATION VARIATIONS, RHYTHMS: _____

V. MANNER OF EXPRESSING PAIN: _____

VI. WHAT RELIEVES THE PAIN? _____

VII. WHAT CAUSES OR INCREASES THE PAIN? _____

VIII. EFFECTS OF PAIN: (Note decreased function, decreased quality of life.)

Accompanying symptoms (e.g., nausea) _____

Sleep _____

Appetite _____

Physical activity _____

Relationship with others (e.g., irritability) _____

Emotions (e.g. anger, suicidal, crying) _____

Concentration _____

Other _____

IX. OTHER COMMENTS: _____

X. PLAN: _____

FIGURE 15–1. Initial Pain Assessment Tool (From McCaffery, M, and Pasero, C: Pain: Clinical Manual, 2nd ed., St. Louis, Mosby, 1999, with permission.)

ETIOLOGY

The exact mechanism of transmission and perception of pain are not completely understood; however, neurophysiologic, psychologic, and sociologic research has contributed to the formation of pain theories.

The gate control theory, originally proposed in 1965 by Melzack and Wall, suggests that pain occurs when smaller-diameter type A nerve fibers and very small diameter type C fibers are stimulated. These afferent, or sensory, fibers penetrate the dorsal horn of the spinal cord and end in the substantia gelatinosa. When the sensory stimulation reaches a certain critical point, the "gate" opens and allows nearby transmission cells to project the pain message to the brain. In contrast, the large-diameter type A sensory fibers inhibit pain transmission. When these fibers are stimulated, fast-conducting afferent fibers oppose the smaller fibers' input and activate the substantia gelatinosa "gate" to close, thus blocking nerve transmission.

This theory explains why external methods of pain control work. For example, stimulating the large-diameter type A fibers by massage, applying heat or cold, acupuncture, or transcutaneous electric nerve stimulation (TENS) can override sensory input in the smaller-diameter type A fibers and block pain transmission at the gate. Cognitive techniques, such as distraction, biofeedback, relaxation, and guided imagery, operate through the efferent fibers, closing the gate.

In the 1970s, the body's own internally secreted opioid-like substances, called endorphins, were identified. Research found that the brain triggers the release of endorphins, which lock into the narcotic receptors at nerve endings in the brain and spinal cord to block the transmission of pain signals, preventing the impulse from reaching consciousness. This research has helped to explain why pain perception and the need for analgesia can vary greatly from one person to another. Endorphins are depleted with prolonged pain, recurrent stress, and the prolonged use of morphine or alcohol. Endorphin levels are increased during brief pain episodes, brief stress, physical exercise and sexual activity, massive trauma, some types of acupuncture, and some types of transcutaneous nerve stimulation; and possibly with placebos. Much of the recent research in this area supports patient-controlled interventions for pain (Ellis, Blouin & Lockett, 1999).

The multiple opioid receptor theory is one of the newest theories. It recognizes that not all opioids work the same way and some cannot be switched back and forth without adverse consequences. There are at least three types of opioid receptor sites in the spinal column. Each type binds somewhat differently with different types of opioids. For example, opioids like Stadol or Nubain (agonist-antagonist drugs) antagonize the effects of other narcotics like morphine and can contribute to withdrawal rather than pain relief. Knowledge of this theory enhances appropriate selection of analgesics (Ripamonti, Zecca, & Bruera, 1997).

Gender and social and cultural factors also affect the pain response by influencing how the individual interprets pain and how he or she responds emotionally. Through family, social, and cultural values and attitudes, the patient learns which types of pain responses are appropriate within his or her group.

Of course, family and social influences change as a child matures. By the time adulthood is reached, the individual may have modified or even rejected many family values or taken on the values of another subgroup. If the patient's values conflict with those of his or her family, additional stress and anxiety may be felt. This may explain why certain patients act differently when family members are present (Fillingim, 2000; Wessman & McDonald, 1999).

Other factors influencing pain behaviors may include the body part involved, the patient's socioeconomic status and religious beliefs, and experience with folk medicine or alternative therapies. A patient's language and vocabulary affect the way in which pain is described. Do not be too quick to assume that you understand what the patient is trying to say, especially if his or her native language and ethnic background are different from yours.

RELATED CLINICAL CONCERNS

Chronic pain is a significant health problem. For example, 10 to 15 percent of adults in the U.S. are estimated to have some form of disability from back pain (Borsook, et al., 1996). In addition to disrupting employment, chronic pain can contribute to family problems and social isolation. Acute pain is associated with anxiety; chronic pain is more associated with depression. Chronic pain patients are also at higher risk for dependence and abuse of medication because their pain is often not relieved and they begin taking larger doses in hopes of obtaining relief. Healthcare professionals may become frustrated and eventually deny the patient the pain medications, leading the patient to seek alternative ways to obtain relief. The chronic pain patient usually requires a multidisciplinary pain team.

The physiologic and psychological risks associated with untreated pain are greatest in frail patients with other illnesses, such as heart or lung disease, those undergoing major surgical procedures, and very young or very old patients. Untreated pain can contribute to complications because the patient is unable to cough or deep-breathe or get adequate rest or nutrition. Uncontrolled pain in dying patients contributes to the wish to hasten death. In patients with psychiatric diagnoses such as depression, schizophrenia, dementia, malingering, and hypochondriasis, pain may be the chief presenting complaint. Treating the underlying psychiatric disorder should lead to reduction in pain. Patients with alcohol or drug withdrawal syndromes need special consideration in their pain management, especially if they also have other medical problems.

Each individual experiences and expresses pain in a unique manner, depending on age, gender, culture, and previous pain experience (Box 15–1). All pain is real to the person experiencing it, regardless of its physical or psychological etiology. Each person's ability to tolerate pain is also unique. Depending on the situation, pain tolerance can vary even in the same individual. Anxiety or depression can decrease pain tolerance. Most people with severe or prolonged pain also have emotional changes related to their pain.

About one third of all patients with a diagnosed physical cause for their pain respond to placebos. Nurses should be aware that a positive response,

> **BOX 15–1. Factors Influencing Pain Tolerance**
>
> **Factors that may increase or decrease tolerance:**
>
> - Past experiences with painful stimuli (e.g., surgery, trauma, illness)
> - Knowledge about cause of pain, its treatment, and probable outcome
> - Personal meaning of pain (e.g., recurrence of cancer, day off from school or work)
> - Knowledge and experience in coping with pain, willingness to try new techniques
> - Stress, fatigue, energy levels
> - How others treat person when he or she has pain (e.g., secondary gains)
> - Available resources (e.g., money for treatment)
> - Interactions with healthcare providers (e.g., preventive approach: pain is treated early or patient has to prove that pain is "real" before anything is done to help relieve it)
> - Cultural background: some cultures encourage the expression of even mild discomfort, whereas others expect stoic, quiet tolerance of even very severe pain
>
> **Factors that usually decrease pain tolerance:**
>
> - Disbelief on the part of others
> - Lack of knowledge about pain, pain-relief measures
> - Fears about addiction, loss of control over pain
> - Poor experiences with past pain-relief efforts
> - Disability, increasing or long-term
> - Fatigue and monotony

meaning that the patient gets relief after taking the placebo, cannot be used to prove that the pain is psychologically induced. Sometimes just listening to the patient, acknowledging the pain, and the act of giving a medication can enhance pain relief.

The benefits of adequate and consistent pain management are significant: earlier and easier mobilization, shorter hospital stays, increased productive rehabilitation, and earlier return to previous work or lifestyle; or if the patient is terminal, increased comfort and peace of mind. These outcomes should be expected and worked toward with every patient experiencing pain (McCaffery & Ferrell, 1997b; de Rond et al., 2000; and Raines, 2000).

LIFE SPAN ISSUES

CHILDREN

Research indicates that younger children, including neonates, may experience some pain more intensely than older children. For children who cannot communicate verbally about their pain, one needs to assess pain by observing physiologic changes, nonverbal behavior, and vocalizations, such as crying or groaning. Consult parents or guardians about how the child expresses pain at home. Knowledge of the child's age and developmental level gives insight into how pain may be expressed (McGrath & Finley, 1999; Twycross, 1998).

If painful procedures are needed, be sure they are performed outside the child's room or playroom so that his or her bed, room, and playroom continue to be safe places. If the child is verbal, try to use his or her words for pain when asking about the discomfort. The Faces Pain Rating Scale is particularly geared to children as well as adults with dementia (Fig. 15–2).

Most dosage recommendations for opioid analgesics in children are not supported by double-blind studies, and underdosing is especially common. Initial recommended doses must be viewed as educated guesses and should be adjusted either up or down according to the individual child's response. Toddlers and older children may obtain pain relief from cutaneous stimula-

FIGURE 15–2. Pain Rating Scales (*Sources:* (A) Agency for Health Care Policy and Research. Management of Cancer Pain, 1994. (B) Wong-Baker FACES Pain Rating Scale from Wong, DL, et al. Whaley and Wong's Nursing Care of Infants and Children, ed. 6, St. Louis, Mosby, 1999. Copyrighted by Mosby-Year Book, Inc. Reprinted with permission.)

tion like massage and TENS and distraction, similar to adults. Adolescents may report more pain than younger children, especially if the pain is chronic.

ELDERLY PEOPLE

Pain is not an inevitable part of aging; however, elderly people are at greater risk for many disorders that may result in pain, such as arthritis, cardiovascular disease, osteoporosis, falls, hip fractures, and cancer. Elderly patients may deny pain more frequently than other age groups because they fear the consequences of admitting pain, such as longer hospitalization or more tests, or they have the mistaken belief that pain is normal for their age. Special efforts must be taken to adequately assess pain, especially in confused elderly people (McGuire & Graffam, 1995; Wynne, Ling, & Remsburg, 2000). Dementia patients are particularly vulnerable to undertreatment of pain because of their inability to express themselves.

Polypharmacy is of special concern in elderly persons. Because of the physiologic changes that occur with aging, drug half-life and clearance times are increased in elderly people, and this can lead to increased and unexpected side effects and toxicity, making pain control more difficult in this group. Unrelieved pain may also contribute to confusion and dementia. Adjuvant analgesics must be used with caution in elderly patients because sedation, confusion, and the sedative and anticholinergic effects of many of these drugs may compound constipation. Low starting doses are recommended. Long-acting analgesics may be more likely to cause side effects.

POSSIBLE NURSES' REACTIONS

- May rely more on physiologic changes or signs such as vital signs, body movement, facial gestures, and other nonverbal behavior than on patients' own verbal reports to assess patient's pain.
- May become immune to patient's expressions of pain.
- May have difficulty accurately assessing the patient's pain. Varying opinions among staff members over interpretation of behaviors suggesting pain and selected pain control modalities can lead to very divisive conflicts among staff members.
- May feel extremely frustrated over what can be done to help the patient.
- May fear causing a patient's addiction if the patient requires narcotics for an extended period of time.
- May think that the need for greater pain control is more acceptable for certain types of pain, such as cancer pain.
- May believe that patients will always accurately report pain when they have it.
- May become frustrated over what to do when a patient denies having pain to the physician but continues to request pain medication from nursing staff.
- May feel manipulated by patients who staff members believe are faking pain for the purpose of obtaining more medication.

ASSESSMENT

ACUTE PAIN

Behavior and Appearance

- Verbalizes pain rating and describes location and character of pain
- Guarded positioning
- Tense or grimacing facial expression
- Rubbing, pulling at, splinting, or protecting painful area
- Fatigued, lethargic
- Crying or moaning
- Restless

Mood and Emotions

- Fearful, anticipating more pain
- Angry, irritable, frustrated
- Depressed, hopeless, withdrawn
- Feeling out of control or helpless about pain if relief is inadequate

Thoughts, Beliefs, and Perceptions

- Wide variations in beliefs about pain, its causes, and methods for relief
- May be confused and unable to concentrate
- Lack of information or misinformation about pain control methods
- Decreased motivation to participate in activities of daily living
- Unwillingness to try alternative pain-relief methods
- Lack of trust in caregivers if pain not relieved

Relationships and Interactions

- Patient may withdraw socially or have angry outbursts related to pain.
- Secondary gains may influence pain behaviors. For instance, family members may cater to patient's needs more attentively if he or she is in pain.
- Caregivers may avoid the patient because of previous experiences when he or she was in pain, may have feelings of helplessness.

Physical Responses

- Increased blood pressure, pulse, respirations
- Diaphoresis
- Tremors
- Redness and swelling around painful area

Pertinent History

- Previous pain experiences
- Effect of pain on work, sleep, eating, elimination, and sexual patterns
- Previous and current use of narcotics or other analgesics
- Drug or alcohol dependency
- Litigation pending after injury or an accident
- Medical problems, surgical procedures, and injuries

CHRONIC PAIN

Behavior and Appearance

- Verbalizes pain rating or describes pain
- Presence of pain for more than 6 months
- Difficulty maintaining job or other activities
- Frustration, fatigue
- Changes in skin color over painful area
- Changes in muscle tone and reflexes

Mood and Emotions

- Depression
- Hopelessness
- Suicidal ideations
- Anger and bitterness
- Preoccupied with pain
- Fear that caregiver will give up on patient and pain problem

Thoughts, Beliefs, and Perceptions

- Fear that pain is intractable and will always affect family, work, social life, finances, and mood
- Perceives others as not believing that he or she is in pain
- Fears losing control over the pain and that the medication will lose effectiveness or be withdrawn before pain resolves
- Has misinformation about effectiveness or alternative pain-relief methods
- Lacks trust in caregivers who do not acknowledge or treat his or her pain

Relationships and Interactions

- Social isolation and withdrawal
- Family or work relationships may have changed since pain became chronic
- Patient's dependency increases with pain
- Patient withdraws from usual activities and friends
- Patient experiences decreased social activities and reduced satisfaction with relationships and diminished sexual interest
- Family experiences fear and frustration about the patient's using pain for secondary gains

Physical Responses

- Anorexia or weight gain
- Impaired mobility
- Insomnia
- Intermittent pain relief with rest; pain recurring with increased stress or certain activities

Pertinent History

- Pain of more than 6 months' duration
- Changes in mood, sleep, appetite, and activity patterns
- Constipation related to prolonged use of narcotics
- Litigation pending after injury
- Prolonged use of medication without effective pain relief
- Physical dependency on pain medications, other drugs, or alcohol since pain became chronic
- Financial problems caused by cost of medical care
- Possible multiple medical complaints, little satisfaction with treatment
- Seeking out numerous doctors for treatment

COLLABORATIVE MANAGEMENT

Pharmacologic

Several types of drugs are available to treat pain. Selection is based on the cause of the pain, its intensity and duration, and the patient's response. Mild intermittent pain may be treated with salicylate analgesics or nonsteroidal anti-inflammatory agents. More severe, acute pain may need opioid analgesics. Determining the most effective medication requires careful assessment of the cause of the patient's pain and his or her perception of the pain and underlying condition.

Factors that influence the effectiveness of medication to relieve pain include:

- Route of administration
- Amount and frequency of dosage
- Anticipated onset and duration of action
- Method of drug's action (central versus peripheral)
- Previous experience with medication

The patient experiencing pain needs to be constantly reevaluated to ensure that he or she receives maximal relief with the least potent drug. For instance, a surgical patient may require parenteral opioid analgesics immediately after surgery. As healing occurs, the drug can be titrated to a less invasive method and a lower dose while still maintaining adequate pain control. An equianalgesic list (Table 15–1) gives the dose and route of administration of one drug that produces approximately the same degree of analgesia as the dose and

TABLE 15–1. OPIOID ANALGESICS COMMONLY USED FOR SEVERE PAIN

| Name | Equianalgesic Dose (mg) | | Starting Oral Dose | | Comments | Precautions and Contraindications |
	Oral	Parenteral	Adults (mg)	Children (mg/kg)		
Morphine-like agonists						
Morphine	30	10	15.30	0.30	Standard of comparison for opioid analgesia. Sustained-release preparation (MS Contin, OramorphSR) release drug over 8–12 hours.	For all opioids, caution in patients with impaired ventilation, bronchial asthma, increased intracranial pressure, liver failure
Hydromorphone (Dilaudid)	7.5	1.5	4–8	0.06	Slightly shorter duration than morphine	
Oxycodone	20	—	15–30	0.30		
Methadone (Dolophine)	20 acute 2–4 chronic	10 acute 2–4 chronic	5–10	0.20	Good oral potency, long plasma half-life (24–36 hours)	Accumulates with repeated dosing, requiring decreases in dose size and frequency, especially on days 2–5
Levorphanol (Levo-Dromoman)	4 acute 1 chronic	2 acute 1 chronic	2–4	0.04	Long plasma half-life (12–16 hours)	Accumulates on days 2–3
Fentanyl	—	0.1	—	—	Transdermal fentanyl (Duragesic) 25 µg/hour, roughly equivalent to sustained-release morphine, 45mg/day. Oral transmucosal fentanyl citrate now available for treatment of	Because of skin reservoir of drug, 12-hour delay in onset and offset of transdermal patch; fever increases dose rate

...breakthrough pain in chronic cancer pain patients already taking around-the clock opioids.

Drug	Parenteral	Oral		Comments
Oxymorphone (Numorphan)	—	1		5 mg rectal suppository = 5 mg morphine IM	Like IM morphine
Meperidine (Demerol)	300	75	Not recommended	Slightly shorter acting than morphine	Normeperidine (toxic metabolite) accumulates with repetitive dosing, causing CNS excitation; avoid in children with impaired renal function or who are receiving monoamine oxidase inhibitors
Mixed agonist–antagonist					
Nalbuphine (Nubain)	—	10		Not available orally, not scheduled under Controlled Substances Act	Incidence of psychotomimetic effects lower than with pentazocine; may precipitate withdrawal in narcotic-dependent patients
Butorphanol (Stadol)	—	2		Like nalbuphine	Like nalbuphine

Source: Adapted from American Pain Society: Principles of Analgesic Use in Treatment of Acute Pain and Cancer Pain (ed 4), Skokie, IL, American Pain Society, 1999.

route of administration of another drug. There are many differences among individual patients, so these lists serve only as guidelines to the relative equivalences of various analgesics. Dose and time intervals must be titrated for each patient (Agency for Health Care Policy and Research, 1992, 1994). Chronic pain patients may need opioids, and the long-acting preparations are particularly useful because they avoid the fluctuating blood levels of analgesics.

Patients on one or more other medications need to be evaluated for possible drug interactions. Drug pharmacokinetics may change because of alterations in cardiac, renal, and liver function; respiratory rate; and gastrointestinal absorption. Fever, sepsis, burns, and shock also affect drug effectiveness. Patients with psychiatric conditions who take antianxiety agents or psychoactive drugs must also be evaluated for possible drug interactions, in particular, the added sedative effects of opioids and many of the psychotropic drugs. Clinicians should be aware that patients in these categories might not respond as expected to pain medication (Borsook et al., 1996).

A variety of herbal products are being used to treat pain, including capsicum ointments, evening primrose for arthritis, and chamomile for migraines. A variety of alternative approaches that may be used include acupuncture, magnet therapy, and biofeedback.

NURSING MANAGEMENT

ACUTE PAIN EVIDENCED BY REPORT OF MODERATE PAIN, CHANGES IN AUTONOMIC NERVOUS SYSTEM (INCREASED HEART RATE AND BLOOD PRESSURE), AND REDUCED ABILITY TO PERFORM ADLS RELATED TO SURGERY, INJURY, OR ILLNESS

Patient Outcomes

- Reports decreased pain levels
- Identifies previously successful pain-relief techniques to use now to decrease pain
- Identifies and minimizes factors that precipitate or aggravate pain
- Participates in assessment of pain and effectiveness of pain-relief methods
- Demonstrates increased mobility and activity

Interventions

- Perform a thorough pain assessment. Ask patient to rate pain on a consistent scale such as 0 to 10, with 0 being no pain and 10 being the worst possible pain. Be sure to determine the patient's perception of his or her pain, previous effective pain methods used, and any misperceptions the patient has about effective pain-relief methods.
- To reduce the patient's anxiety, explain the causes of pain, if known.
- Teach the patient and family about factors that may increase or decrease pain. Try to minimize factors that increase pain perception.
- Teach about any necessary painful procedures before they occur to reduce stress over anticipating the procedure. Patient teaching should include:

- Basic description of the procedure or test, its purpose, and equipment to be used
- A description of any sensations likely to be experienced
- Anticipated duration of procedure and discomfort
- Measures that can be used to reduce discomfort
- Provide accurate information about analgesics to reduce fear or misconceptions about addiction, tolerance, and physical dependence. Recognize that the patient or family may become anxious when medications are changed. Discuss any changes in medication, dose, or frequency with physician, and plan how to inform the patient about the pain control goals and parameters.
- Provide relief measures at regular intervals rather than on an as-needed basis, even when the pain is still tolerable. Do not expect patient to wait until pain is unbearable to administer the next dose:
  - Determine whether and when to give PRN medications.
  - Choose the appropriate analgesic when more than one is ordered.
  - Evaluate the effectiveness of administering medications at regular intervals.
  - Monitor responses to administered medications and report promptly any adverse reactions and when they are ineffective.
  - Suggest appropriate changes based on knowledge of the patient and previous response to pain-relief measures.
- Check with patient 30 minutes after administering a pain medication to assess its effectiveness. Include patient in rating level of pain before and after medication or other pain-relief method used. Use the same pain rating scale each time you assess the patient to ensure accurate evaluation.
- Encourage patient's participation in using alternative pain-relief methods such as relaxation exercises or use of heat or cold. Instruct the patient about rigid body position, which can increase pain, and techniques to reduce muscle tension:
  - Select a time when patient is relatively comfortable and able to concentrate so that teaching will be more effective.
  - Use pillows or other supports to splint and support body parts and reduce muscle tension.
- Discuss effects of stress, monotony, fatigue, and distraction on pain perception.
- Provide for privacy for pain expressions if the patient desires.
- Try to limit the number of caregivers interacting with patient and making decisions about pain management.
- Provide opportunities for rest and therapeutic use of distraction, such as visits or watching television, between uncomfortable treatments.
- If patient has a current or past history of drug or alcohol abuse, he or she still needs strong opioids to treat an acute pain problem. Putting this patient on an around-the-clock dosing schedule of analgesics is usually recommended to avoid euphoria. Other suggestions include long-acting analgesics and making a contract with the patient about what medications can be given.
- Consult with other staff members or the physician about increased medication at bedtime and before painful procedures to keep pain at tolerable levels throughout the day and to maximize patient's participation in required activities.

- Institute measures to reduce any adverse effects of narcotics. For instance, administer stool softeners and stimulant laxatives (e.g., senna-based products) to combat constipation, antiemetics for nausea, and mouthwashes for dry mouth.
- Help the patient to cope with the consequences of pain by encouraging discussion of fears, anger, and frustrations; acknowledge difficulty of situation; and praise and reinforce any efforts to handle pain.
- Consult with pharmacist and physician about alternative opioid and analgesic combinations.
- Consider using aspirin or acetaminophen simultaneously with opioid for maximal effect. Also consider use of nonsteroidal anti-inflammatory drugs (NSAIDs) for peripheral pain.

> **CHRONIC BENIGN PAIN** EVIDENCED BY ONGOING EPISODES OF PAIN, DIFFICULTY PERFORMING USUAL ACTIVITIES, AND OTHER EFFECTS OF CHRONIC PAIN, SUCH AS SLEEP DISTURBANCE OR POOR NUTRITION RELATED TO ILLNESS, SURGERY, OR INJURY MORE THAN 3 TO 6 MONTHS AGO.

Patient Outcomes

- Participates in assessment of pain
- Uses one or more alternative measures to manage pain
- Increases participation in activities
- Decreases use of pain behaviors for secondary gain
- Decreases dependence on narcotics for pain relief

Interventions

- Assess patient's previous and current pain behaviors.
- Encourage the patient to learn and use noninvasive pain-relief methods, such as muscle relaxation, deep breathing, guided imagery, distraction, TENS, and application of heat or cold.
- Incorporate family or caregivers in alternative pain-relief measures.
- Use analgesic medications in conjunction with alternative pain-relief measures to effectively control pain.
- Discuss with physician or pharmacist plan for weaning patient off opioids and onto non-narcotics. Titrate parenteral pain medications and switch to oral doses as soon as possible while ensuring adequate pain control.
- Teach patient and family that oral medication, when prescribed in appropriate dose and frequency, can be as effective as parenteral.
- Administer a loading dose and then maintain a therapeutic drug level of oral medications when first switching to gain the patient's confidence in new treatment.
- Ask patient to participate in evaluation of pain-relief methods by keeping his or her own pain diary.
- Help family or caregiver to recognize and decrease pain behaviors for secondary gain.

- Promote optimal mobility and meaningful activity in patient.
- Assess patient's nutrition and elimination functions related to use of medications and decreased mobility or activity.
- Assess patient's sleep pattern, levels of depression, or other psychologic reactions to prolonged pain. Consider use of adjuvant treatments, as indicated.
- Provide the patient and family with the opportunity to discuss fears, anger, and frustration in a private setting. Acknowledge the difficulty of the situation and any of the family's efforts to help the patient cope.
- As indicated, refer the patient for evaluation at a multidisciplinary pain clinic if problems are not improved before discharge.

ALTERNATE NURSING DIAGNOSES

> Altered Thought Processes
> Anxiety
> Self-Concept Disturbance
> Fear
> Ineffective Individual Coping
> Powerlessness
> Sleep Pattern Disturbance
> Spiritual Distress (Distress of the Human Spirit)

PATIENT AND FAMILY EDUCATION

- Provide information about all pain-relief methods available to the patient. Keep the patient and family informed about changes in treatment plan.
- Teach relaxation techniques (see Appendix A).
- Instruct the patient and family on the use of the pain rating scale.
- Allow the patient to make choices about relief methods used. Involve him or her in assessment of pain; teach how to use pain flow sheet or keep a pain diary, and select appropriate alternative pain-relief measures based on activities and effectiveness of relief methods.
- Initiate teaching with the patient, family, or caregiver related to pain-relief methods to be used after discharge. Review with them the ordered discharge medications, potential adverse effects and how to manage them, what to report to physician, and effective alternative pain-relief measures.

WHEN TO CALL FOR HELP

Pain-relief measures are ineffective.

Pain levels increase.

Patient or family is unwilling to learn about alternative methods of pain relief.

☐ Psychiatric problems are interfering with patient's use of prescribed pain-relief methods.

☐ There is increased frustration from dealing with the patient's or family's pain behaviors.

☐ Analgesics ordered are ineffective and physician refuses to make changes.

☐ Patient continues or increases use of pain behaviors for secondary gain.

☐ There are concerns over patient's or family's ability to manage pain after discharge.

☐ Evidence of abuse of opioids.

CHARTING TIPS

• Include the selected pain rating scale in the assessment and evaluation documentation. Besides the pain rating, document location and description of the pain.
• Use objective, nonjudgmental terms to describe pain behaviors and responses to pain relief measures. When possible, use the patient's own words to describe the pain.
• Document the response to all pain relief measures.
• Document any factors or activities that increase or decrease pain.
• Note all side effects of analgesics.

COMMUNITY-BASED CARE

• Review with the patient, family, or caregiver the patient's progress with pain management since admission.
• If patient is being discharged with prescriptions for opioids, give referrals for local pharmacies that carry these medications.
• Allow sufficient time for the patient to adjust to the change from parenteral to oral administration of pain medications and to practice alternative pain-relief measures before discharge.
• Consult with the physician if patient's pain is not controlled before discharge or if pain is expected to continue for some time thereafter. Obtain a home health referral to assess pain at home and follow up with medication compliance and monitor side effects.
• Instruct the patient, family, or other caregivers on how to use a pain flow sheet or maintain a pain diary at home.
• Suggest that the patient be referred to an appropriate pain treatment center where multidisciplinary treatment is offered.
• Include the selected pain rating scale in all assessment and evaluation documentation.
• Use objective, nonjudgmental terms to describe pain behavior and re-

sponses to pain-relief measures. When possible, use the patient's own words when describing the pain.

• Document patient's responses to all pain-relief measures used.
• Document any factors or activities that the patient or family can identify as an increase or decrease in pain tolerance or effectiveness of pain-relief methods.

Problems with Nutrition

THE PATIENT WITH ANOREXIA NERVOSA OR BULIMIA

LEARNING OBJECTIVES

➤ Describe the similarities and differences between anorexia nervosa and bulimia.
➤ Formulate nursing diagnoses and interventions for patients with anorexia nervosa or bulimia.
➤ Identify common nurses' reactions to the patient with anorexia nervosa or bulimia.
➤ Describe the complications of anorexia nervosa and bulimia.

GLOSSARY

Anorexia nervosa—A potentially life-threatening eating disorder characterized by self-starvation in a relentless pursuit of thinness, an intense fear of becoming fat, and delusional disturbance of body image.

Binge eating disorder—Recurrent episodes of binge eating that lead to feelings of distress. Not associated with purging.

Binge—Rapid consumption of large amounts of food in a short period of time (usually less than 2 hours).

Bulimia (bulimia nervosa)—An eating disorder characterized by consuming large quantities of food in a short time, terminating in abdominal pain, sleep, social interruption, self-induced vomiting, and/or laxative use.

Compulsive overeating—Consuming large volumes of food without purging.

Eating disorders—Gross disturbances in the patterns of ingesting food.

Purge—Planned or unplanned episode to undo damage of binge, including self-induced vomiting, laxative use, or diuretic use.

Dieting is a national obsession, especially with women. Numerous fitness clubs are filled with individuals trying to attain the idealized thin, muscular body. Cochrane (1998) reports that over 50 percent of American women are on a diet at any one time. Extreme thinness is increasingly common in models and actresses as the idealized image. It seems that it has become accepted behavior to be obsessed with body weight and shape and to view food as a source of stress. Self-esteem and happiness in young girls are often linked to weight and body shape. Adolescent girls may be rewarded for dieting with either increased social acceptance or praise from parents. When this social influence is combined with certain biologic, developmental, and family dynamics influences, it could be the beginning of an eating disorder. These disorders have little to do with simply not eating enough or overeating. Rather, they are psychiatric disorders with substantial emotional and physical consequences.

Anorexia nervosa and bulimia (sometimes called "bulimia nervosa") most commonly occur in young women, and the incidence of these disorders is on the rise. One to five percent of young women suffer from them (Wolfe, 1998). Women and girls are 10 times more likely to suffer from these disorders than men and boys. Patients with an eating disorder may be treated in psychiatric facilities, but are often admitted to an acute-care hospital for treatment of complications or for initial diagnosis to rule out other conditions. There are many similarities between these two eating disorders, and long-term anorexics may develop bulimia in later life (Table 16–1).

The term *anorexia* (as in anorexia nervosa) is really a misnomer because this condition has very little to do with appetite. It has more to do with the person's morbid fear of obesity causing obsessive fear of losing control of food intake. In fact, the person is often hungry and views the discomfort of hunger as a reminder of the deprivation he or she needs to inflict on himself or herself. Only in the late stages is appetite actually lost. The distorted body image causes the patient to view himself or herself as fat even though appearing emaciated. No amount of weight loss relieves the anxiety, causing this deadly cycle to continue. Complications can continue for years, even after successful treatment.

The death rate from anorexia nervosa ranges from 5 to 18 percent (DSM-IV, 1994). Poorer prognosis is associated with an older age of onset, a lower minimum weight, and vomiting. Purging, which promotes electrolyte imbalance and arrhythmias, is usually combined with compulsive exercise,

TABLE 16–1. COMPARING ANOREXIA NERVOSA AND BULIMIA

	Anorexia Nervosa	Bulimia
Epidemiology	• Over 95% female	• 90% female
	• Younger adolescent onset	• Young adult onset more likely
	• Fairly rare	• 2–3 times more frequent than anorexia
Appearance	• Emaciated	• Normal or overweight
	• Below normal weight	• Weight fluctuations
Family	• Rigid, perfectionistic	• More overt conflict
	• Overprotection	
Behavior	• Introverted	• Impulsive
	• Socially isolated	• More histrionic, acting out
	• High achiever	
	• Excessive exercise	
Signs	• Cachexia	• Dehydration
	• Hair loss	• Chronic hoarseness
	• Amenorrhea	• Chipmunk facies (parotid gland enlargement)
	• Dry skin	
	• Pedal edema	
Prognosis	• 5–18% mortality rate	• Death is rarer
	• Frequent lifelong problems with food	• Lifelong problems with food
	• Bulimia	
	• Depression	

making a most lethal combination. Successful treatment is measured by weight gain, return of menstruation (usually absent in anorexic women), and reduced number of compulsive behaviors.

Bulimia was officially designated as a psychiatric disorder in 1980 and is harder to diagnose than anorexia. It is more common than anorexia and effects a larger cross-section of the population. As with anorexia, bulimia is mainly a condition of younger women; however, some studies show that about 10 percent of bulimics are male (DSM-IV-TR, 2000). Men with bulimia tend to be older at onset. Both men and women often demonstrate difficulties with impulse control, associated with higher incidence of drug abuse and acting-out behavior such as petty crime. The long-term prognosis is unclear because the relapse rate remains high.

Unlike the patient with anorexia, the one with bulimia uses food as a temporary relief of stress, which leads to binge eating. The resulting sense of shame and disgust then causes the patient to purge by induced vomiting or use of laxatives. The cycle of bingeing and purging may begin as a way to lose weight but can become a compulsive behavior.

Bulimia is associated with fewer life-threatening complications than anorexia, but can lead to chronic conditions including sore throat, dental erosion, and/or parotid gland enlargement from chronic vomiting. A bulimic individual can consume thousands of calories in a short time.

A third eating disorder recently listed in the DSM-IV-TR (2000) is binge eating disorder, which involves eating large quantities without purging. People suffering from this disorder are most often obese or exhibit fluctuations in weight. Weight-loss programs report seeing more clients with this disorder.

ETIOLOGY

Individuals with eating disorders report a premorbid history of dieting and attempts to control their weight. What makes this progress to anorexia nervosa or bulimia is unclear, but most likely genetic, biologic, psychologic, and family factors are all involved. There are many similarities in etiologic theories between these two conditions. Both disorders are also significantly associated with depression and family dynamics, in which food plays a large symbolic role.

Anorexia nervosa may have *genetic* influences because there is an increased incidence of its occurrence among daughters and sisters of anorexics. The *biologic* influence may be multi-factoral. Research suggests that there is an interrelationship between multiple neurotransmitters, including dopamine that regulate appetite, body size, and fat distribution. Dysfunction of the hypothalamus has also been implicated. Because the symptoms usually begin in adolescence, hormonal changes may be an important contributor.

Psychoanalytic theory suggests that the core of anorexia can be a child's fear of maturing and unconscious avoidance of developmental tasks. By not eating, the person forestalls sexual development and maintains his or her role as child in the family. Other dynamics include perfectionist tendencies developed through demanding, overachieving parents. Anorexia gets out of control as the person tries to achieve the perfect image. Many family therapists believe that anorexia symptoms represent a dysfunctional family situation. The patient tries to present a "perfect good girl" image, trying to meet the family's distorted view of perfection. Also, the eating disorder gives the patient a sense of control that counteracts the feelings of loss of control, anxiety, and need to avoid conflict. Some reports indicate that a mother's preoccupation with weight and food can be a source of conflict between mother and child, and the eating disorder becomes a means of control for the child. An overwhelming sense of worthlessness in the child may also be responsible. Comorbid psychiatric disorders include major depression and obsessive-compulsive disorder.

Specific theories on the cause of bulimia are limited. *Biologic* views regard low levels of the neurotransmitters norepinephrine and serotonin as associated with bulimia. Low serotonin is known to increase the need for intake of carbohydrates and are also associated with depression. Bulimia may be related to impaired satiety mechanism.

Family dynamics in bulimia are often characterized by a high degree of conflict, marital discord, and acting out. This may contribute to the patient's developing increased anxiety with intimate relationships and a fear of abandonment and conflict surrounding parental authority. Low self-esteem contributes to feelings of inadequacy and a deep-rooted sense of shame and guilt. Some studies have noted an increased incidence of family members with a history of alcoholism and/or presence of physical or sexual abuse. These individuals are more likely to have comorbid psychiatric disorders, including borderline, panic disorder, and major depression.

RELATED CLINICAL CONCERNS

Anorexic and bulimic patients may have a history of being overweight when young. Anorexics have been noted to weigh more at birth. Bulimics may have a history of anorexia when younger, as well as a tendency for obesity within the family.

Life-threatening complications from anorexia include cardiac arrhythmias, electrolyte imbalance, and cardiomyopathy. Serious bulimia complications can include electrolyte imbalance and erratic blood sugars.

LIFE SPAN ISSUES

CHILDREN AND ADOLESCENTS

Anorexia and bulimia remain a condition of adolescence and young adulthood. Children as young as 8 years old often admit to preoccupation with diet and atypical eating habits. A sense of self-consciousness and insecurity with the body is a normal part of growth and development; however, children whose self-esteem becomes more closely tied to satisfaction with their body size tend to become more prone to eating disorders. This is often influenced by the way in which adult caregivers perceive and respond to them. Children who are overweight may experience increased criticism and demands made upon them, leading to low self-esteem. In adolescence, awareness of cultural ideals becomes even stronger. Adolescents may notice that thinner contemporaries have more friends or dates.

POSSIBLE NURSES' REACTIONS

- May feel shocked or disgusted by patient's behavior or appearance.
- May resent the patient because of the belief that the disorder is self-inflicted. This may make it difficult to express empathy, which in turn may make the patient feel rejected.
- The nurse may feel helpless to change the patient's behavior, leading to anger, frustration, and criticism.
- The nurse may inadvertently re-create family power struggles with patient by trying to make the patient eat by nagging, cajoling, arguing, or even tricking. This will inhibit a trusting nurse-patient relationship.
- The nurse may feel overwhelmed with the patient's problems, leading to feelings of hopelessness or to the setting of rigid limits to feel more in control of the patient's behavior.
- Many nurses become embroiled in power struggles with these patients, which may trigger angry responses in the nurses.

ASSESSMENT

ANOREXIA NERVOSA

Behavior and Appearance

- Emaciated
- Tends to cover up body with large clothing in attempt to hide appearance, though some may exhibit thinness with a sense of pride
- Avoids being weighed; may try to manipulate weight by putting weights in pocket
- High achiever in school and work
- Ritualistic behavior surrounding food (such as eating every third bean)
- Spends time with food-oriented activities, such as cooking or shopping for others
- At mealtimes, tries to hide not eating by:
  - Cutting up food to give appearance of less food present
  - Moving food around plate
  - Hiding pieces of food in pockets or under plate
- Exercising obsessively (possibly in secret)
- Using laxatives or foods with a laxative effect excessively
- Not giving a realistic picture of his or her eating patterns

Mood and Emotions

- Has high anxiety associated with mealtimes, weight gain, being weighed, and especially any control issue
- When under stress, may feel need to starve self more
- Experiences feelings of sadness and low self-esteem
- May feel need to punish self for feelings of pleasure
- Denies feelings of sadness or anger and often appears pleasant and compliant

Thoughts, Beliefs, and Perceptions

- Distorted attitude toward appearance, weight, and food that overrides hunger and reason
- Distorted body image: sees self as fat despite others saying that the opposite is true
- Perfectionist, compulsive, rigid
- Seeing self as helpless and dependent; great difficulty making decisions
- Possible mental status changes from malnutrition such as memory lapses, poor attention span, poor judgment, and bizarre behavior
- Denying seriousness of low body weight

Relationships and Interactions

- Introverted; avoids intimacy and sexual activity
- Secretive
- Fears trusting others; needs to be in control

Physical Responses

- Extreme weight loss; weight less than 85 percent of that expected for age and height
- Cachexia
- Fatigue
- Amenorrhea
- Hair loss; presence of lanugo (fine body hair covering)
- Low pulse rate, low blood pressure, low body temperature
- Chronic constipation
- Dry skin
- Altered lab values including low hemoglobin and hematocrit (or high if dehydrated), hypokalemic (especially if using laxatives or diuretics), high BUN and serum creatinine
- Insomnia
- Consuming large volumes of fluid to distend stomach, which may lead to hyponatremia
- Pedal edema related to malnutrition
- In late stages, may exhibit arrhythmias and congestive heart failure
- Pathologic fractures caused by bone loss from estrogen deficiency and ovarian dysfunction

Pertinent History

- Involved in activities in which small size is important, such as ballet or gymnastics
- Uses food-oriented coping mechanisms, such as stopping eating or excessive eating, to deal with stress
- Family history of depression, eating disorders

BULIMIA

Behavior and Appearance

- Weight is normal, slightly overweight and/or fluctuating.
- Routinely goes into the bathroom shortly after meals.
- Eats normally or sparingly when with others, and binges in private. Purging behaviors may follow, including self-induced vomiting, laxative or diuretic misuse, fasting, or excessive exercise.
- May appear normal without obvious problems.
- Functions normally.
- Behavior is sometimes histrionic or impulsive.
- Tends to act out.

Mood and Emotions

- Binge triggered by some emotional stress; initially some relief of anxiety during the binge but tension slowly increases as feelings of remorse and guilt build
- Purge in response to feelings of remorse and guilt

- Anxiety over appearance and weight
- Anxiety around mealtimes as patient fears loss of control
- Feelings of anxiety, depression, self-disgust

Thoughts, Beliefs, and Perceptions

- Perfectionist
- Preoccupied with appearance, weight
- Self-critical
- Very aware that own behavior is abnormal
- Feels powerless over binge-purge cycle
- Believes he or she is unable to change
- Suicidal thoughts

Relationships and Interactions

- Overt conflict within family
- Goes to great lengths to keep binge-purge behavior a secret from others
- Generally social and gregarious, with a strong need to be accepted by others
- Sexually active

Physical Responses

- If bingeing: abdominal pain, malaise, fluctuating blood sugars.
- If vomiting: chronic hoarseness, parotid gland enlargement causing chipmunk facies, dental caries, loss of enamel on teeth, skin changes over dome of the hand (if use finger down throat to induce vomiting). Use of ipecac to induce vomiting can induce cardiac symptoms including palpitations, chest pain.
- If abusing laxatives: abdominal pain, diarrhea.
- Other symptoms may include dehydration, hypokalemia, and cardiac arrhythmias.

Pertinent History

- Anorexia nervosa as a teenager
- Drug or alcohol abuse (especially cocaine as a way to control appetite)
- Involvement in activities in which weight must be kept down such as modeling, ballet, athletics

COLLABORATIVE MANAGEMENT

Pharmacologic

Medications have had some success in treating eating disorders. Antidepressants, particularly fluoxetine (Prozac), and other selective serotonin reuptake inhibitors (SSRIs) have been used in patients with clinical depression. They may reduce the incidence of bulimic behavior as well. Some antidepressants also cause weight gain as a side effect. Antipsychotic and/or tricyclic antidepressant clomipramine medications may be used in patients who are extremely obsessive-compulsive. Cyclopheptadine (Periactin) has been used with some success in anorexics to help them gain weight as well as exerting an antidepressant effect. It is an appetite stimulant, antihistamine, and serotonin antagonist. Antianxiety medications have also been useful. Bulimics have also been treated with lithium and phenytoin (Dilantin). Anorexics may resist taking medication just as they do food, and it becomes another part of the power struggle to get the patient to comply.

Individuals with eating disorders may be using stimulant medications or herbal products such as "herbal Phen-fen" with ephedra to promote weight loss. This practice needs to be carefully assessed because of the serious side effects of some of these stimulants.

Dietary

The dietary regimen for the anorexic patient generally involves a slow, steady weight gain of no more than 2 pounds per week. Too-rapid weight gain can put undue stress on the heart and precipitate complications. Management by a clinical dietitian or nutrition support team is essential. These patients need careful assessment of their nutritional needs. In severely ill patients, malnutrition must be treated before any improvement from psychotherapy can be expected. For life-threatening situations, aggressive nutritional interventions are required. This may include enteral feedings with nasogastric or gastrostomy tubes or total parenteral nutrition. Some patients do well with these aggressive measures because they are relieved that they do not need to make decisions about food. Others may react with resentment and feel an increased loss of control, causing the patient to take more drastic control measures such as increasing exercise, using laxatives, or changing the drip rate or solution being infused. Bulimic patients need dietary education and supervision to control weight.

Psychiatric

Individual and group psychotherapy is essential in treating patients with bulimia and anorexia nervosa. Because patients with both conditions also commonly exhibit troubled family relationships, family therapy is also needed. The treatment plan for anorexia nervosa may include a behavior modification program. Patients are given rewards for any weight gains and increased restrictions for any weight loss or self-destructive behaviors. To increase the chance of success, patients should participate in developing the treatment plan. Written contracts that clearly explain the patient's behavioral expectations have been effective. Electroconvulsive therapy has also been used.

Bulimics may also benefit from keeping a diary of their food intake, feelings, and binge-purge behaviors. Patients who are hospitalized in the acute setting may benefit from evaluation by a psychiatrist.

NURSING INTERVENTIONS

ALTERED NUTRITION: LESS THAN BODY REQUIREMENTS EVIDENCED BY WEIGHT LOSS, AVOIDANCE OF FOOD, EXCESSIVE EXERCISE, HIDING FOOD, SELF-INDUCED VOMITING RELATED TO SELF-STARVATION, BINGE-PURGE CYCLE.

Patient Outcomes

- Increased oral intake (anorexia nervosa)
- Weight gain at rate of no more than 2 pounds per week or per prescribed treatment plan (anorexia nervosa)
- Reduced incidence of strenuous exercise and/or purging (bulimia)

Interventions

- Recognize that patient may be very defensive about eating behavior and attempts to keep it secret. Mealtimes may be very stressful. Create environment of acceptance to encourage a trusting nurse-patient relationship.
- If personnel are available, stay with patient during meals to be sure food is actually eaten. Create a social atmosphere rather than a supervisory one.
- Give patient as much control as possible around eating behavior. Encourage him or her to select some foods. Set limits, however, on length of mealtimes. Lengthy mealtimes tend to increase anxiety and acting-out behaviors.
- Monitor food and fluid intake. Measure urinary and fecal output. Assess skin turgor. Do this in a matter-of-fact manner. Avoid power struggles or criticism. For example, note what patient has eaten without scowling or making demands. Recognize that telling a patient, "You have to eat more" will create tremendous anxiety and probably lead to defiance. For the patient at home, recognize that monitoring food intake and controlling bingeing may be more difficult and require a commitment from family members.
- Weigh patient regularly, using same scale. Treatment plan may include setting a minimal safe weight range that must be maintained. This can remove the power struggle from mealtimes because patient knows what is expected.
- Set limits on dysfunctional behaviors such as strenuous exercise and use of bathroom after eating.
- Set limits on time spent alone in the bathroom after meals. Also insist that patient wait at least 30 minutes after eating before using bathroom.
- Present meals without threat, coercion, or criticism. Recognize that arguing about food will only increase the problem. In addition, avoid cajoling or tricking patient into taking more calories.
- If you suspect that patient is trying to sabotage the treatment plan, talk openly with patient about your concerns. Be aware that patient may have a need to hide food to give impression that he or she is eating.

- Reinforce the idea that patient can avoid more aggressive interventions, such as tube feedings, by meeting acceptable minimal weight standards, per treatment plan. For example, patient may need to gain 2 pounds a week. This can be a way for patient to maintain control because he or she can decide how to accomplish it.
- Obtain specific information from a patient who purges, including method of self-induced vomiting, laxative, or diuretic use.

> **BODY IMAGE DISTURBANCE** EVIDENCED BY INACCURATE PERCEPTION OF APPEARANCE AND MORBID FEAR OF OBESITY RELATED TO DISTORTED THOUGHTS AND INABILITY TO PERCEIVE BODY SIZE AND PHYSICAL NEEDS REALISTICALLY.

Patient Outcomes

- Verbalizes more realistic perception of his or her body
- Refers to body in a more positive way

Interventions

- Encourage patient to express feelings, especially about the way he or she thinks about or views himself or herself.
- Avoid overreacting to self-deprecating comments patient may make about his or her body. Recognize that these feelings and images are very real to the patient. For example, the patient may dwell on having "fat" legs even though they may be very normal or even emaciated looking. Listen to patient, and explore how the fear of fat creates distress. For example, "I understand you see yourself as fat; however, I do not see you the same way." Avoid responding to patient's self-deprecating remarks by minimizing the patient's statements.
- Encourage discussion of positive personal traits, especially regarding patient's body image.
- Encourage patient to dress attractively and to use makeup and jewelry, as appropriate.
- Avoid insincere compliments about patient's appearance.

> **INEFFECTIVE INDIVIDUAL COPING** EVIDENCED BY BINGEING-PURGING BEHAVIOR, OBSESSIVE BEHAVIOR AROUND FOOD RELATED TO DISTURBANCE IN IMPULSE CONTROL.

Patient Outcomes

- Verbalizes feelings to others while in care of the nurse
- Demonstrates reduced number of behaviors that would sabotage treatment plan
- Demonstrates more adaptive coping mechanisms while in care of the nurse
- Participates in decision making

Interventions

- If patient is panicked over personal feelings or behavior, remain calm and help patient focus on ability to remain in control. For example, patient may feel panicked over a weight gain and want to exercise or purge. Help patient focus on short-term goals that he or she can achieve. Identify one area over which the patient has some control. Reinforce coping abilities.
- Communicate support and empathy to patient. Be nonjudgmental to encourage sharing of feelings and coping mechanisms. Demonstrate acceptance by use of support and concern to help the patient feel lovable and accepted.
- Recognize the importance of developing a trusting relationship with patient. One or two staff members who attempt to develop a therapeutic alliance with patient can be particularly helpful. Recognize that patient may be very angry about entering treatment program. Developing a trusting relationship will take time. Show acceptance by use of touch, and if appropriate, talking about interests. Avoid just focusing on food.
- Be consistent in treatment plan. All staff members need to be aware of how to handle sabotaging of plan, such as hoarding food or self-induced vomiting.
- Listen for signs of perfectionist thinking and explore ways to challenge unrealistic expectations. Recognize that patient may have very rigid, fixed beliefs.
- Encourage patient to make small decisions. This tends to empower the patient and assists in imparting a sense of control and accomplishment.
- Assess patient for depression, suicidal risk, and substance abuse, and intervene as appropriate.
- Be aware of the family's role in patient's behavioral responses. Patient may need help in seeing himself or herself as a capable person outside the family unit.

ALTERNATE NURSING DIAGNOSES

Altered Thought Processes
Anxiety
Ineffective Family Coping: Compromised
Fluid Volume Deficit
Ineffective Denial
Knowledge Deficit
Powerlessness
Risk for Self-Mutilation
Sexual Dysfunction

WHEN TO CALL FOR HELP

Patient expresses suicide thoughts or makes a suicide attempt.

There is evidence of psychotic thinking, hallucinations, or severe obsessive-compulsive behavior including repetitive obsessive thinking.

> There are signs and symptoms of severe malnutrition or serious complications including cardiac symptoms, hypokalemia, or renal impairment.
>
> Patient demonstrates signs of substance abuse.
>
> Staff is in conflict over treatment plan.

PATIENT AND FAMILY EDUCATION

- Provide information on the long-term effects on the body of anorexia nervosa and bulimia.
- Involve family in what symptoms to identify and report. Review with them how to deal with self-destructive behaviors so as not to reinforce them.
- Provide information on the 12-Step Program as in Overeaters Anonymous for dealing with addictions if appropriate. This is helpful for some people with eating disorders.
- Review nutritional information and recommended dietary program.
- Teach stress management and relaxation techniques to reduce anxiety, especially at mealtimes or when feeling need to binge-purge.
- Educate patient and family on the need to continue long-term treatment.
- For patients who use self-induced vomiting, encourage adequate dental care.
- Reinforce need for close medical supervision.
- Teach central line care and tube feeding administration, as appropriate.
- Provide education on health effects of laxative and diuretic abuse.

CHARTING TIPS

- Document intake and output.
- Describe behavior at mealtimes, purging behaviors.
- Describe interactions with family.
- Describe patient's verbalization about his or her body image.
- Document all self-destructive behavior.
- Document assessment of potential complications, for example, cardiac status.

COMMUNITY-BASED CARE

- Psychiatric follow-up is essential, including family therapy. Referrals need to be made for appropriate treatment.
- Refer for adequate nutritional support follow-up if appropriate, including management of enteral feedings and central line care. If patient is being followed by a home health agency, encourage referral to dietitian. Home health agency social work and/or psychiatric home health referral may

also be helpful to encourage compliance with psychiatric care, for family support, and for behavioral management.
- Refer patient and family to support groups if available.
- Refer patient to dental care follow-up if patient is vomiting.
- Refer patient to Overeaters Anonymous if appropriate.

THE MORBIDLY OBESE PATIENT

LEARNING OBJECTIVES

➤ Differentiate obesity from morbid obesity.
➤ Identify potential lifestyle restrictions and prejudices faced by morbidly obese persons.
➤ Describe effective interventions to enhance self-esteem for these patients.
➤ Identify common emotional reactions of nurses to the morbidly obese patient.

GLOSSARY

Body mass index (BMI)—describes body weight relative to body fat. It is calculated by dividing weight in pounds by height in inches squared, then multiplying by 704.5.

Chronic obesity—Lifelong overweight condition with few fluctuations.

Developmental obesity—Obesity that began in childhood or adolescence and is often associated with problems of self-concept.

Ideal body weight—Standards based on actuarial tables of height and weight.

Morbid obesity—A condition in which an individual is 100 pounds or 100 percent over his or her ideal body weight or body mass index of greater than 40.

Obesity—Having an excess of adipose tissue and being at least 15 percent over ideal body weight or body mass index of greater than 30.

Pickwickian syndrome—Extreme obesity in which demands of body size on a small chest wall lead to cardiovascular and respiratory changes, including hypoxemia, cyanosis, reduced vital capacity, and pulmonary edema.

Reactive obesity—Obesity that starts later in life and is the result of maladaptive coping styles at times of stress such as death of a loved one or leaving home.

The cultural ideal of the thin body has no greater dichotomy than the image of those with extreme obesity, also known as morbid obesity. Although aesthetic preferences for body size and shape vary from culture to culture, today the thin, fit body is idealized for both women and men in America. Prejudice against the obese has a significant impact on anyone with a serious weight problem, but morbidly obese people often face outright discrimination.

The American population has been steadily gaining weight over the last 30 years. Currently 55 percent of people are classified as overweight and 22 percent as obese (National Institute of Health 1998 Federal Obesity Clinical Guidelines). Extreme or morbid obesity is seen in only a small percentage of the population, but its impact on healthcare is great because of the multiple medical complications caused by this condition. Body mass index (BMI) is now the standard used to determine obesity because it is more reflective of body fat percentages than the older ideal body weight tables.

Morbid obesity affects all ages and races, although it is much more common in lower socioeconomic groups. Obesity is equally distributed between men and women. Potential health problems include a wide range of chronic conditions, including hypertension, cardiac problems, diabetes, respiratory insufficiency, and joint and back disorders. Risk of death increases with a BMI greater than 30. Nutritional deficiencies are also extremely common because the obese person may lack a well-balanced diet or experience protein deficiencies related to crash dieting.

Society often views these individuals as undesirable. They may be abused by strangers and treated with contempt by family members. Even healthcare professionals may view them as emotionally disturbed, even though there is no increased incidence of psychopathology in morbidly obese people. Others may view these individuals as lazy, unkempt, and lacking in self-control. Many experts promote viewing these individuals as having a chronic illness rather than a cosmetic problem.

Morbidly obese people face discrimination particularly in the workplace because they are viewed as less healthy, less diligent, and/or less intelligent than their thinner peers. Certainly, with this kind of reaction, it is no wonder that these people often experience poor self-esteem, feelings of isolation and helplessness, and loss of control.

Morbidly obese individuals often have subjected themselves to many weight-loss strategies, only to regain the weight, which increases the stress on the body. Some studies suggest that individuals whose obesity has persisted for more than 5 years have very limited success with treatment.

Obesity is a complex issue, and any weight-loss program needs to include a multidisciplinary approach. Successful weight-loss programs need to include medically supervised diet and exercise programs and emotional and social support. When these measures have been unsuccessful, some people pursue surgical interventions, called bariatric surgery. Although many types of surgery for obesity have been tried, the most successful today is the vertical-band gastroplasty, in which a smaller stomach pouch is created through gastric stapling. This is generally considered only for people with a BMI greater than 40 or those over 35 with serious medical complications related to weight.

Some educators have noted that fewer than 50 percent of healthcare professionals advise obese patients to lose weight (Goldsmith, 2000). Some reasons for this low percentage include discomfort about addressing the subject, lack of time to talk with the client, and a belief that this recommendation will not make any difference. Yet a client is three times more likely to try to lose weight if he or she is advised to by a healthcare professional. However, extremely obese people may avoid regular medical care because of shame about their weight.

ETIOLOGY

Extreme obesity is a complex problem, and its etiology is probably multifactoral. Most often it begins early in life.

The *biologic* view considers that early onset is related to childhood development of large-size adipose or fat cells. The cellular hypertrophy results from increased food intake and decreased energy expenditure. Other factors may include impaired hunger-satiety mechanism in the hypothalamus and endocrine disorders leading to slower metabolism or changes in insulin or cortisol production. The set point theory focuses on the body as being programmed to maintain a certain level of fat stores. This could explain why some people gain weight so easily. *Genetic* studies have found that 60 percent of obese subjects have at least one or both obese parents (Galzis and Kempe, 1989). A protein called leptin has been identified to contribute to delayed satiety in some people.

Psychoanalytic theory views obesity as an expression of an intrapsychic conflict that occurred during the oral stage of psychosexual development. Unmet needs and stress in an infant can lead to overeating to decrease anxiety, express hostility, and compensate for lack of love. Unmet oral needs may contribute to behaviors such as being demanding and impatient. Weight can provide a shield against intimacy. This can explain why individuals who lose large amounts of weight without adequate psychologic support may experience intense anxiety and feelings of vulnerability. *Learning theory* looks at how overeating occurs in response to tension, stress, or boredom. This can be a learned behavior from childhood, when parents used food as a source of reward and attention. Increased obesity has also been found in people with a history of sexual trauma. Large size can be an unconscious mechanism for defense against an abuser. Binge-eating disorders may also be present. These individuals may use food as escape from stress and depression. Problems with bingeing are the most common reason for seeking counseling associated with being overweight.

Sociocultural factors must be included because food and eating are such important parts of our society. Social customs are often centered on food. Mealtimes may be an important part of family life and family traditions.

RELATED CLINICAL CONCERNS

Sedentary lifestyle, possibly related to a medical condition that limits mobility, is a significant factor in developing morbid obesity. In addition, treatment regimens for some conditions may increase the risk of severe obesity. Steroids can quickly contribute to increased adipose tissue development, and some antidepressants, antipsychotics, and estrogens can cause weight gain.

Obesity is particularly associated with heart disease, hypertension, and increased total cholesterol.

LIFE SPAN ISSUES

CHILDREN AND ADOLESCENTS

Ten percent of prepubertal children and 15 percent of adolescents are obese (Tunnessen, 1999). Obesity in childhood is linked to obesity in adulthood (developmental obesity). In addition, obesity in adults in the child's life contributes to childhood obesity. The child may learn to use food for comfort, solace, reward, and love. Some other contributing factors include more sedentary lifestyles with emphasis on television and computers, fast foods high in calories and fat, and reduction in sports programs in schools. Obese children are often seen by others as sloppy, less intelligent, lazy, and less likeable. Obese children are often victims of teasing and social isolation, adding to poor self-image and causing these children to retreat to food as a coping mechanism. Poor self-image often remains throughout life regardless of the person's educational or vocational success. Childhood growth spurts may resolve some overweight tendencies, but other children go on to be morbidly obese. Weight loss in children must be approached cautiously to prevent nutritional imbalances.

ELDERLY PEOPLE

A past history of obesity is the major contributor to obesity in elderly people. An increased sedentary lifestyle as a result of failing health or medications, or poor nutrition because of low income, low energy, or depression also contribute.

POSSIBLE NURSES' REACTIONS

- May view patient as sloppy, lazy, weak, lacking impulse control, mentally ill
- May feel overwhelmed and hopeless with patient's problems
- May resent the demands placed on the staff with the increased workload created by patient's size and need for special equipment
- May tend to focus on patient's size rather than view him or her as an individual with unique feelings
- May feel guilty for these negative feelings

ASSESSMENT

Behavior and Appearance

- Binge eating, secretive night eating, hoarding food
- Repeated dieting
- Dressing in large, oversized clothing
- Sedentary lifestyle, may avoid chance to exercise

- May exhibit night eating syndrome with cycle of insomnia, increased hunger, eating large amounts, morning anorexia

Mood and Emotions

- Depression
- Difficulty being assertive
- Guilt, shame associated with overeating
- Strong emotions that trigger need to eat
- May feel hopeless, overwhelmed, out of control
- Unrealistic expectations, leading to disappointment

Thoughts, Beliefs, and Perceptions

- Finds many powerful meanings in food, such as comfort, love, and security
- Distorted body image
- May see self as thinner, possibly indicating denial, or larger than true self
- May respond to external cues and thoughts rather than hunger in deciding what and when to eat
- If weight is lost, possible fears of success or intimacy on an unconscious level when patient can no longer hide behind the weight

Relationships and Interactions

- May lack social skills
- May avoid social situations for fear of rejection
- May cover feelings of rejection by joking

Physical Responses

- Hypertension
- Diabetes
- Arthritis, trauma to joints and back
- High serum cholesterol
- Cardiac disease
- Malnutrition
- Fatigue
- Dyspnea on exertion
- Pickwickian syndrome: includes sleep apnea, daytime somnolence related to carbon dioxide retention, and symptoms of congestive heart failure

Pertinent History

- Multiple attempts at weight loss
- Childhood obesity
- Chronic illness
- History of obesity and sedentary lifestyle

COLLABORATIVE INTERVENTIONS

Pharmacologic

The drug traditionally used in weight-loss programs is amphetamine. It is included in many over-the-counter "diet pills" even though they have been of limited benefit in suppressing appetite. In addition, they frequently have adverse side effects, including hypertension, stroke, and renal failure. Antidepressants such as sertraline (Zoloft) and fluoxetine (Prozac) have a side effect of anorexia and have been used with success in long-term weight-loss programs. They also reduce irritability associated with depression.

New weight loss drugs include sibutramine (Meridia), which suppresses appetite by blocking serotonin and norepinephrine; and orlistat (Xenical), which reduces absorption of 33 percent of dietary fat. Both drugs have significant side effects that limit their use. Overweight individuals may also be using over-the-counter weight-loss products and herbal products such as herbal Phen-fen (ephedra). These stimulants must be used with caution in the presence of heart disease.

Administering any medications to morbidly obese people requires extra caution because some may require dose adjustments. Some medications may need to be given in higher doses because of the increased body weight, whereas other drugs, such as theophyllines, may need to be administered in lower doses because the metabolism of the drug is affected by the patient's lower protein or higher fat stores. Check with the pharmacist for specific information on the chosen drug. The route of administration can also affect absorption and distribution of the drug. Drugs administered intramuscularly may not be absorbed if the needle does not reach the muscle. If the medication is deposited in fat tissue, its absorption is slowed, and onset of action may be delayed. Intravenous administration may be the most effective route. Because IV access is often difficult, central line insertion may be the most efficient.

Dietary

Beginning and maintaining a weight-loss program in morbidly obese people requires close medical and dietary supervision. It must be remembered that even large persons can still be malnourished, and proper balance in the diet must be addressed. A complete nutritional assessment needs to be done. Patients with medical problems require very close supervision to maximize outcomes.

NURSING MANAGEMENT

SELF-ESTEEM DISTURBANCE EVIDENCED BY NEGATIVE SELF-IMAGE, FEELINGS OF POWERLESSNESS RELATED TO FEELINGS OF SELF-DEGRADATION AND RESPONSE OF OTHERS TO THE OBESITY.

Patient Outcomes

- Verbalizes positive traits about self
- Verbalizes concerns to nurse
- Demonstrates fewer self-critical remarks
- Participates in self-care
- Does not let self-consciousness about weight interfere with care needs

Interventions

- Avoid preaching or criticizing about need for weight loss; these approaches will only increase patient's negative feelings and sense of hopelessness and powerlessness.
- Provide privacy and treat patient with modesty. Be aware that patient may be extremely sensitive to having body parts exposed.
- Have extra help available before turning or ambulating a patient to prevent falling and help patient feel more secure.
- Have adequate-sized and reinforced equipment such as wheelchairs and beds to avoid embarrassment of squeezing patient in to accommodate your equipment. Check to see if patient has own custom wheelchair. Have family bring clothing from home if hospital gowns are inadequate.
- Recognize that patient may feel very anxious about being stared at by strangers, particularly in a hospital situation. Prepare other departments for patient's appearance and needs.
- Listen for cues as to how patient views self and appearance. If patient makes self-deprecating remarks, explore these feelings. Focus on positive traits other than body size. Patient does not need to be reminded of his or her large size.
- Give patient the opportunity to share feelings. He or she needs to be viewed as an individual and encouraged to identify feelings.
- Explore use of makeup, hairstyle, and dress, as appropriate, to increase feelings of self-esteem.
- Encourage the patient's participation in treatment plan to avoid passivity. Provide encouragement to make decisions about all aspects of care. Work with patient to problem-solve ways to maintain participation.
- Assess patient's support system and encourage his or her involvement.

ALTERED NUTRITION: MORE THAN BODY REQUIREMENTS
EVIDENCED BY MORBID OBESITY RELATED TO EXCESSIVE INTAKE, EMOTIONAL FACTORS, OR ALTERED HEALTH MAINTENANCE.

Patient Outcomes

- Begins to identify feelings or thoughts that contribute to overeating
- Demonstrates changes in eating patterns
- Identifies one short-term goal to attain
- Demonstrates non–food-related coping mechanisms

Interventions

- Assess patient's condition and priorities of care before assuming that treatment plan should include weight loss. Patient must be involved in deciding if weight loss is a realistic objective at this time. Patient motivation is essential to the success of a weight-loss program.
- Obtain baseline weight. Identify scales adequate to handle patient's weight beforehand. Also, consider using two scales or, in the hospital setting, use a bed with adequate built-in scales.
- Assess the patient's eating patterns and typical daily intake. Provide a supportive environment so that patient can feel secure to be honest. Recognize that patient may feel need to minimize his or her intake.
- Assess patient's knowledge level about eating patterns. Be alert to beliefs held about weight and weight loss by patient and family. For instance, patient may say that the entire family is "fat" or "it's genetic."
- Assess skin and mobility. Patient may be prone to skin breakdown and complications related to poor mobility or hygiene.
- Identify coping mechanisms to deal with stress and anger that do not involve food, such as taking a walk, deep breathing, or talking to a friend. Give patient feedback on alternative coping mechanisms and identify the link between stress and desire to eat.
- Focus on short-term goals to identify successes in weight loss or improved mobility. Help the patient identify nonfood rewards when goals are met.
- For the patient at home, explain that removing easily accessible high-fat and high-calorie foods from the house will lessen temptation.
- Assess family involvement. Recognize that family can consciously or unconsciously sabotage weight-loss plans by exposing patient to old eating habits. Encourage the family to eat foods similar to those eaten by the patient for shared meals.

ALTERNATE NURSING DIAGNOSES

Activity Intolerance
Altered Health Maintenance
Body Image Disturbance
Impaired Gas Exchange
Ineffective Individual Coping
Noncompliance

WHEN TO CALL FOR HELP

Patient experiences serious complications from diabetes, hypertension, or heart disease.

Patient expresses desire to start a potentially dangerous quick weight loss program.

Patient exhibits signs of severe depression or self-destructive behaviors.

 Patient demonstrates signs of substance abuse.

PATIENT AND FAMILY EDUCATION

- Provide information on starting an exercise and weight-loss program.
- Strongly encourage patient to maintain medical supervision for any weight-loss or exercise program.
- Provide information on behavior techniques for weight loss, such as eating slowly and serving smaller portions.
- Teach patient to become more aware of body signals of hunger and satiety.
- Teach appropriate exercises within patient's ability. Explain that even minimal exercise, such as short walks several times a day, can help reduce weight and promote health.
- Teach patient how to monitor for possible complications such as diabetes and cardiac problems.
- Give family information on weight loss, nutrition, and ways to support patient's health.
- Consider focusing education on reducing medical complications and increasing activity rather than just weight loss.
- Teach coping mechanisms to reduce anxiety that do not involve food.
- Encourage patient to continue in psychosocial support program after weight loss is achieved to learn skills to deal with new image.

CHARTING TIPS

- Document baseline weight, mobility, and skin condition.
- Document response to activity.
- Document eating patterns.
- Note coping mechanisms in response to stress.
- Note indications of motivation regarding treatment.

COMMUNITY-BASED CARE

- Provide referral information to support groups such as Weight Watchers or Overeaters Anonymous as appropriate.
- Encourage nutritional and medical follow-up.
- Assess whether patient needs assistance with transportation to medical care.
- Provide information to home health agency or other healthcare providers on patient's special equipment needs and other concerns.

Problems Within the Family

FAMILY DYSFUNCTION

LEARNING OBJECTIVES

➤ Differentiate between traits of functional and dysfunctional families.
➤ Discuss the role of systems theory related to the family.
➤ Describe the signs of caregiver role strain.
➤ Identify effective nursing interventions to help the family cope with the illness of one of its members.

GLOSSARY

Dysfunctional family—A family that develops ways of interacting with one another that leads to impaired functioning, both among the members and outside the family boundaries.

Extended family—Family network beyond family of origin, including stepparents, grandparents, aunts and uncles, and others.

Family—A small social system made up of people held together by strong reciprocal affections and loyalties and living in a permanent household that persists over time.

Family of origin—Family into which one is born or adopted.

As the basic unit of society, the family is the most important influence on shaping whom we become. The traditional nuclear family, with two parents and child or children, has undergone tremendous changes in the last few decades, and some of these changes will affect generations to come. According to the most recent U.S. census data available, less than 25 percent of all U.S. families fit the description of a traditional nuclear family. This number continues to decline with each census. Single-parent households represent the single biggest change in U S. family life (Bianchi, 1995). The 2000 U.S. census showed a 25 percent increase in female single parent households and a 62 percent increase in male single parent households since the 1990 census. Changing economic needs, changes in women's and men's roles, and a decreased tendency to accept unsatisfactory relationships have contributed to a high divorce rate and significant changes in family structures. Single-parent households, stepfamilies, childless couples, and a variety of combinations of cohabiting individuals are increasing. Friedman (1998) notes that these new family constellations are increasingly accepted in our society.

Stresses caused by relationship adjustments can influence one's health status. Also, a change in the health of any member of the family can create family disorganization or even a crisis when roles, patterns, or routines must be restructured. Anger, guilt, and denial may all occur as the members try to adapt.

Even in families that function satisfactorily, an illness may cause a tremendous crisis as the family shifts life patterns to meet the demands created by the illness. A family member may need to take on the added demands of being a caregiver to an ill person at the same time as he or she is handling other major family responsibilities. Even the healthiest functioning family may enter a crisis period in response to a devastating illness or death. Relatives may need to move in, which changes the social structure of the family, or the family may need to outlay large amounts of money to provide extended care, affecting the family's future goals. Changes in health of parents and siblings from one's family of origin and extended family may require helping with caregiving.

Because of the impact illness has on the family and the family members have on the patient's recovery, members need to be involved in the patient's treatment plan. Family response can represent a major source of stress to the nurse as family conflicts and dynamics are acted out. Family members' own fears, lack of sleep, conflicts with each other, and loss of emotional support can all contribute to their sense of isolation and possible mistrust of healthcare professionals.

ETIOLOGY

Bowen's *family system theory*, developed in the 1950s, views the family as a homeostatic system of relationships. A change in functioning of one member results in compensatory changes in the other members in an attempt to maintain equilibrium. For example, when a family member becomes ill, other members will adapt to fill the roles of the ill member while he or she is sick. The family system is always changing as it adapts to internal and external stimuli in its attempt to remain stable.

All families have unwritten, covertly expressed rules, such as "conflict is wrong," and roles, such as "Dad makes the final decision." These covert roles are often more obvious as the family is coping with stress and often requires an enormous amount of adjustment when roles must be reversed. For example, if the father, who makes all the decisions, becomes ill, a normally dependent member may accept more of the decision-making responsibilities, reversing the established roles. If past relationship problems do not support the changes, family members may exhibit unhealthy behaviors such as anger (possibly directed at the hospital staff) and guilt. The illness can also exacerbate any relationship problems among other family members.

In stressful situations, family members may exhibit behaviors that seem to temporarily help the relationship while they focus on the current crisis reducing the anxiety and intensity of existing relationship problems. Some of these attempts at solutions can create more stress for a family member. At times, one member is identified as the "problem" and the rest of the family focus attention on that member and his or her problem. This is called scapegoating and allows the family to avoid confronting the real conflicts within the family. For example, parents with marital relationship problems may focus their attention on their child's behavior problems rather than their own.

RELATED CLINICAL CONCERNS

The family can play a key role in how a person responds to illness. Support and love from family may encourage a patient to concentrate on healing and strengthen his or her will to survive. In some families, however, the sick individual may be viewed as dependent and unacceptable, reducing his or her will to survive and remain a burden to the family.

LIFE SPAN ISSUES

CHILDREN

The family represents the young child's whole world. The family ideally gives the child a supportive environment in which a sense of trust and seeing one's self as a separate, competent person is developed. As the child grows, the world expands outside of the family, exposing him or her to new ideas, conflicts, and inconsistencies. Separation from this comfort can create an enormous amount of stress for both child and family.

Other outside factors may influence this separation anxiety. As more and more children are being cared for by babysitters or in day care, adjustment to an environment outside the home may be less stressful. However, if the child has experienced a loss of a loved one, such as by death or divorce, separation may be even more stressful.

The great increase in the number of stepfamilies has created new, complicated relationships. Children must adapt to new family members, yet maintain relationships with parents, siblings and others.

ELDERLY PEOPLE

With today's longer life expectancies, elderly people are more likely to become incorporated into new families as they remarry, cohabitate, or maintain some type of group living situation. Adjusting to a new spouse's family at an advanced age can be a challenge because adult children may be ambivalent, or even resentful, about their parent's new relationship. These new relationships can create some major relationship problems within the families and may result in very difficult situations when the parent becomes ill.

The need to care for sick elderly relatives is also a source of family relationship problems. Today, because many families do not have one member who stays at home and has the ability to care for an ill parent, caregiving can become a tremendous burden, both physically and financially. The caregiver may be faced with overwhelming guilt and, possibly, anger. An ill parent may be viewed as an intrusion into a family already overwhelmed with caring for their children with both parents working. If an elderly person with a chronic illness is admitted to the hospital, it is essential to assess how well the family is coping with the situation and how well they are able to care for the elderly person. In the home, be aware of what family members are trying to verbalize. Sometimes they would like more assistance but hesitate to ask for it because they are too afraid or feel guilty.

POSSIBLE NURSES' REACTIONS

- May anticipate problems with all families because such problems are so common
- May resent the disruption in routine that may result when family members want to be involved in patient care
- May feel uncomfortable in the presence of family members acting out their conflicts
- May resent the family's criticisms, which may be their attempt at maintaining control of the situation
- May relate patient's situation to personal family conflicts, possibly causing uncomfortable feelings
- May become overinvolved with a patient's family and experience the emotional highs and lows related to patient's progress and family response
- May incorrectly view a family as dysfunctional if their relationship styles differ from the nurse's past experience in a family
- May feel overwhelmed with dysfunctional family's problems

ASSESSMENT

Each family exhibits unique behaviors related to the normal roles established within the family. Some of the common problem behaviors are listed on the following page.

Behavior and Appearance

- May exhibit behaviors that isolate others from family interactions.
- Change in behavior patterns when in the presence of various family members.
- May exhibit a defensive response to staff members.
- May consistently place blame on others.
- May exhibit a lack of empathy toward the ill family member.
- May exhibit a lack of congruence between verbal and nonverbal communication.
- Some family members may be open and realistic about diagnosis, treatment, and prognosis, and others may deny any problem, blame the staff members for the problem, or avoid the patient altogether.

Mood and Emotions

- May exhibit contradictory, confusing, or inappropriate reaction to the situation
- May be unable to express or display feelings
- May avoid emotional situations

Thoughts, Beliefs, and Perceptions

- Family may indicate inaccurate or unrealistic beliefs about the patient's condition or prognosis or one's ability to provide adequate care.
- Family may be operating on the basis of myths or inaccurate beliefs that impede care.
- Family may think it is wrong to share concerns with others.
- Family may focus on personal reactions to the patient rather than objectively viewing the patient's needs.

Relationships and Interactions

- Roles among family members may be rigid.
- Individual family members may do anything to placate others to prevent an angry response or rejection.
- Family may have difficulty managing conflict.
- Family may be in a state of constant conflict.
- Family may pay undue attention to the ill family member.
- Family may appear to get along well when the history suggests that relationship problems have existed in the past.
- Family members may evade opportunities for communication.
- Family may avoid visiting or having contact with the patient.
- There may be inappropriate or miscommunication among family members. Communication may be unclear, nonspecific, or indirect.
- One family member may take the lead in defining the needs of the patient and family, or several members may jockey to assume the lead role.

Pertinent History

- History of child abuse, domestic violence, elder abuse, or family conflict
- History of psychiatric illness or substance abuse
- Recent losses or deaths in the family and past significant losses or trauma

COLLABORATIVE MANAGEMENT

Family Therapy

Family therapy can be an important treatment to assist the family under stress. When problems such as a psychiatric disorder, abuse, marital conflict, and/or substance abuse are present, a therapist can assist the family in dealing with the current stressor and finding more long-term solutions to their relationship or adjustment problems. Therapists may meet with all the family members or limit meetings to a few key members. Young children can also be included.

Social Services

Social service agencies can investigate needed support services for families in distress on either a long- or short-term basis. They can direct the families to agencies that may provide additional finances or extra help, such as Meals on Wheels.

NURSING MANAGEMENT

> **ALTERED FAMILY PROCESSES** EVIDENCED BY INABILITY TO MEET DEMANDS OF ITS MEMBERS, AVOIDANCE OF MAKING DECISIONS, INAPPROPRIATE COMMUNICATION BETWEEN MEMBERS RELATED TO IMPACT OF ILL MEMBER ON FAMILY SYSTEM, DYSFUNCTIONAL FAMILY PROCESSES.

Patient and Family Outcomes

- Participates in treatment planning and care of ill family member
- Identifies resources available to assist family in coping
- Acknowledges diagnosis and prognosis of ill family member

Interventions

- Identify the family constellation, patterns of family interactions, and family leader(s). Assess the ways in which the family members interact with each other and the patient's response to family involvement. Determine from patient whom he or she considers closest family and recognize that this could be close friends rather than relatives. Avoid making assumptions about whom the patient wants involved.

- With a large family, consider asking them to identify one member who will get the information on the patient's condition and take the responsibility to share it with the rest of the family. This avoids the need for multiple calls for information.
- As appropriate, ask the patient whom he or she wants to be involved.
- Involve these family members in treatment plan. Inform them of what is happening according to patient wishes. Take the time to orient family to agency routines and visiting hours.
- Identify family support systems within the family.
- If family members exhibit disruptive behaviors, evaluate the underlying reasons. Talk with patient and family to determine the cause.
- Analyze the family's ability to care for the patient and what they need to know when caring for the patient at home. Encourage family involvement in basic care needs if acceptable to patient. Involving the family in the care can help the patient accept his or her condition. For example, having the spouse care for a condition such as a colostomy can give the patient a sense that he or she is not disgusted by patient's body.
- If patient does not want family informed of his or her condition, talk with patient to identify reasons and fears. Not including the family may be a way of maintaining denial. Respect the patient's wishes, but continue to talk regarding the risk of social isolation. If patient is seriously ill, one person will need to be identified who knows his or her wishes.
- If family wants information withheld from the patient, discuss their fears. Point out that hiding the truth is not helpful to the patient. Dishonesty inhibits future trust and communication. Help family acknowledge their fears. However, recognize that certain cultures have strict rules concerning sharing bad news with loved ones, especially a parent. Avoid becoming angry at this situation and alienating the family. The family could distrust the healthcare team and block communication channels.
- Regularly assess the family's awareness of patient's condition and expectations for recovery and future treatment. Avoid use of medical jargon.
- If the family seems to avoid involvement in the patient's care or treatment plan, determine the reason. Consider giving them one task to do at a time to encourage their involvement without being overwhelmed.
- Encourage the family to verbalize their feelings about the illness. Respect their need for privacy to express emotions. Encourage family to leave patient's room to discuss areas of conflict. Use open-ended questions to promote sharing of feelings and concerns about problems with family interactions.
- Allow flexibility in visiting, if possible. Recognize the need for family members to spend the night and for young children to be allowed to visit. As needed, set clear limits on disruptive behavior, and limit the number of visitors to reduce stress and fatigue on the patient. Encourage visitors to coordinate who will visit on certain days and times.
- As needed, organize a care conference with family members to discuss patient's care needs and any conflicts the family and staff may be having. Avoid having too many staff members in attendance as this could intimidate family. Focus on reassuring the family of the care and concern of the

staff for the patient. Consider involving physician, social worker, or clinical nurse specialist to help intervene if conflicts continue.
- Acknowledge and facilitate family strengths. Promote self-esteem of individual family members by acknowledging their skills and influence on patient ("Your spouse really perks up when you visit").

> **CAREGIVER ROLE STRAIN** EVIDENCED BY DIFFICULTY PERFORMING CAREGIVING ACTIVITIES, INABILITY TO MEET OTHER FAMILY RESPONSIBILITIES, DEPRESSION, AND ANGER RELATED TO MULTIPLE LOSSES AND BURDENS ASSOCIATED WITH CAREGIVING RESPONSIBILITIES.

Patient and Family Outcomes

- Expresses frustrations assertively
- Provides safe care to patient
- Maintains personal needs along with caregiver needs
- Identifies resources available for assistance

Interventions

- Assess caregiver's ability to meet the demands of the patient's care. Identify coping mechanisms and support systems available.
- Allow caregiver the opportunity to share feelings and concerns away from the patient. Reinforce the need to express concerns and emotions. Give caregiver permission to express negative feelings, such as anger and resentment. Provide supportive, safe setting to do this. Reinforce the idea that negative emotions are normal to reduce feelings of guilt.
- Encourage caregiver to be assertive in asking for assistance. Reinforce that others may not know what caregiver's needs are. This is especially important if the caregiver tends to demonstrate martyr behavior.
- Be aware of outside stressors on family members influencing their reactions. Fatigue and working long hours with an ill family member can contribute to ineffective coping mechanisms. Talk with them about possible resources to reduce stress, including enlisting other family members to help, reducing expectations, and hiring outside help.
- Assess caregiver's expectations. Encourage caregiver to have realistic expectations of what he or she can do.
- Remind the family that past conflicts do not disappear even when someone is ill. When family members must spend long hours providing care, resentments can increase. Encourage the family to concentrate on dealing with the immediate stressor while taking steps to work on unresolved conflicts once the situation has resolved sufficiently.
- Encourage the caregiver to develop a routine to care for his or her own needs of sleep, eating, and socializing to effectively care for the patient. Enlisting other family members or hiring outside help can provide the needed break. If the caregiver is unable to get out, help him or her identify ways of maintaining contact with friends by regular phone calls, letter writing, and e-mail.

- At times families "promise" a loved one they will never put him or her in a nursing home, so caregivers hide their feelings. Talk openly about how these promises are sometimes made without realizing the full scope of the situation.
- Give caregivers recognition for the good job they are doing.
- Be alert to caregivers' signs of increasing distress including depression, suicidal risk, hopelessness, and signs of potential physical and/or emotional abuse of the patient.

ALTERNATE NURSING DIAGNOSES

> Anticipatory Grieving
> Ineffective Family Coping: Compromised
> Knowledge Deficit
> Noncompliance
> Sexual Dysfunction
> Sleep Pattern Disturbance

WHEN TO CALL FOR HELP

☐ Indication of family not acting in the best interests of the patient, such as taking patient out of hospital against medical advice or pushing inappropriate treatments.

☐ Any indication of abuse within the family must be reported per agency policy and state law.

☐ Indications that patient is not being cared for adequately include poor hygiene, pressure ulcers, poor nutrition, and dehydration.

☐ Be alert for destructive behavior within the family such as substance abuse, attacking each other, or demoralizing patient.

PATIENT AND FAMILY EDUCATION

- Provide specific information about patient's illness and care needs, such as pamphlets, videos, and other patient education materials. Make sure these materials match family members' reading level and language.
- Review with family members what to expect from patient's illness and how it may affect communication and coping within the family. Let them know that family problems can get either worse or better during this time of stress.
- Reinforce the need for family members to maintain own self-care routines and to be aware of signs of stress that may lead to them being sick.
- Provide information on support groups and group education programs as well as appropriate Web sites.

- Work with caregivers to develop routines that will make the care as easy as possible. For example, setting up the patient's room at home on the first floor of a two-story house will reduce the caregiver's need to go up and down stairs all day.
- Prepare family for possible course of the illness and anticipated changes in care.
- If the family is planning to hire help, provide suggestions on identifying and managing possible problems, such as the attendant not showing up for work on time or not caring for patient appropriately.

CHARTING TIPS

- Describe which family members visit the patient and the interactions that occur.
- Document information on family structure, which family members patient lives with, and care resources available.
- Document teaching given to family and include their response to any education given.
- Describe caregiver's ability to provide patient care.
- Document family awareness of the patient's condition and diagnosis.

COMMUNITY-BASED CARE

- Involve family in the discharge plan early in the treatment.
- Consider a home health referral after patient is discharged from the hospital to assess caregiver's ability to provide care.
- Provide specific referrals for additional help in the home or alternate care options.
- Provide specific information on appropriate support groups, such as for family members of people with Alzheimer's disease, stroke, or drug abuse. Also give information on hotlines or other agencies that may be useful.
- Make sure social worker is involved; consider social work evaluation in the home as well.
- Refer family to a family therapist, if appropriate.
- Identify appropriate equipment that will be needed in the home to provide care (for example, oxygen, hospital bed, and wheelchair). Assist in making arrangements for delivery or refer to social service.
- Communicate with home health agency regarding family communication problems and conflicts that may affect care.

LEARNING OBJECTIVES

➤ Identify suspicious signs of child abuse, domestic violence, and elder abuse.
➤ Discuss common traits of victims of any type of abuse.
➤ Discuss common traits of abusers.
➤ Identify common nurses' reactions to abuse.

GLOSSARY

Abuse—Willful infliction of physical injury or mental anguish or the deprivation by the caregiver of essential services.

Domestic violence—Intentionally inflicting or threatening physical injury or cruelty to one's partner.

Economic abuse (fiduciary)—Using another's resources for one's own personal gain without permission or making the victim financially dependent on the abuser.

Incest—Any type of exploitive sexual experience between relatives or surrogate relatives before a victim reaches 18 years of age.

Neglect—Deliberate deprivation of necessary and available resources, such as medical or dental care.

Physical abuse—Deliberate violent actions that inflict pain and/or nonaccidental injury.

Psychologic abuse—Deliberate and willful destruction or significant impairment of a person's sense of competence by battering the victim's self-esteem and inhibiting normal psychosocial development.

Sexual abuse—Using the victim for sexual gratification when the victim is unable to resist or consent. This includes rape and developmentally inappropriate sexual contact, incest, and using a child for prostitution or pornography.

Family violence may be America's number one public health issue, yet many nurses caring for victims of this type of violence are often unaware that it is occurring within the families of their patients. Child abuse, domestic violence, and elder abuse can lead to lifelong emotional and physical problems for the victims and tears away at the very fabric of society as a whole.

Victims are often too fearful or ashamed to report abuse, become adept at hiding the signs, or use massive denial to convince themselves that the abuse is not that bad, so that a violent family situation often goes unnoticed by outsiders. Healthcare professionals must be vigilant to recognize the overt and covert signs of abuse. Every state mandates that suspected child abuse be reported, and some states are enacting similar laws for domestic violence and elder abuse. The Joint Commission on Accreditation of Healthcare Organizations (JCAHO) now also requires that standards for identifying and providing services to victims of child abuse, domestic violence, and elder abuse be in place (2001). Nurses in all settings must be alert to signs of abuse. Home health nurses in particular are in a key role to identify abuse within a patient's family.

Child abuse includes physical and emotional abuse, neglect, and sexual abuse, and occurs at all socioeconomic levels. Although statistics are difficult to attain, it is estimated that at least 1 million American children are victims of abuse and neglect each year (1997 Health and Human Services). The youngest children (under 3) are the most vulnerable and the most likely to die from abuse or neglect. Reported cases of child abuse have steadily increased over the last few years, but many cases are not reported. Children are a most vulnerable segment of the population because they depend on others for all their needs. Parents are the most common abusers.

Victims of child abuse are at an increased risk of becoming abusers as adults. Even though the child may hate the abusive situation, he or she never gets an opportunity to observe healthy parenting or to learn adaptive coping mechanisms to deal with frustration without violence. Other long-term effects include low self-esteem, high risk for substance abuse, tendency toward depression, difficulty trusting in close relationships, and violent lifestyle including crime. An early sign of child abuse in the victim can be abuse of family pets by the child. Children may try to deal with the situation by controlling another being or seeking an outlet for their anger through a more vulnerable victim.

Girls are the most frequent victims of sexual abuse. Eighty percent of sexually abused children know their abuser, and about 50 percent of cases involve a parent or caregiver (Mulryan, Cathers, & Fagin, 2000). Long-term effects of sexual abuse include fear of intimacy, sexual problems, eating disorders, and an overwhelming sense of powerlessness. Victims may block out the memory of these incidents until later in life, when a major event or trauma triggers memory recall.

Domestic violence most often refers to men abusing their female partners. However, women abusing their male partners or abuse within homosexual couples does occur. This is an enormous societal problem. Like child abuse, domestic violence is found at all socioeconomic levels. It accounts for 22 to 35 percent of emergency department visits for women (Shea, Mahoney, & Lacey, 1997). Victims of abuse may endure physical, emotional, and sexual abuse. The abuse may increase when the woman becomes pregnant if the abuser perceives competition from the baby. The battered woman syndrome refers to the common personality characteristics of these victims. These women are often economically dependent on their spouse or partner, exhibit very low self-esteem, and believe that they somehow deserve the abuse. Pediatricians may be the first to identify this victim because the woman often will not seek medical attention for herself but will seek it for her children. In addition, many times when there is domestic violence in the home, the children are victims of abuse or neglect. Fifteen percent of all homicide victims are spouses (Novello and Soto-Torres, 1992). The victim of the abuse may be the killer in retaliation for past abuse.

One of the most frequently misunderstood factors in domestic violence is why these women remain with the abusers. It is important to understand that they often feel trapped and have little money, resources, or support, and fear being killed or losing custody of or potential injury to their children. Permeating all these factors is the overwhelming sense of powerlessness.

Elder abuse includes neglect as well as physical, sexual, and emotional abuse. Exploitation of the person's financial reserves by family, hired help, or strangers is also considered abuse. This can occur in the home or in residential facilities. Gray-Vickrey (2000) notes that elder abuse effects 10 percent of the geriatric population. This problem is greatly underreported and will continue to increase as the population grows older. One problem in reporting it is the inconsistency of laws defining elder abuse. Some states do not include neglect or psychologic abuse in their definition, so it is essential to be aware of how elder abuse is defined in the state where you are working or reside. Because the abuser is often the victim's caregiver, even including the elderly spouse, victims rarely report the abuse. They fear reprisals or abandonment because they are dependent on the caregiver. Society's lack of interest in elderly people may add to the underreporting. Elder abuse can also be difficult to detect by professionals because common signs such as bruising and skin tears may be common in older populations. The patient with dementia is particularly vulnerable because he or she is unable to speak up or will not be believed because of his or her intermittent confusion.

ETIOLOGY

There are similarities in all types of family violence (Table 17–1). A family history of abuse remains a common thread, particularly in child abuse and domestic violence. Childhood exposure to abuse increases a general sense of low self-esteem and reduced ability to deal with frustration, as well as lack of role models to learn to interact in a healthy relationship. Another similarity is the presence of a vulnerable victim.

Various theories examine what causes a person to abuse another.

Psychologic theory suggests that abuse provides the abuser with a sense of power and prestige that boosts his or her self-image. The abuser hates the vulnerable powerless feelings within himself or herself and is able to block them out by creating (transferring) these denigrated feelings in others.

TABLE 17–1. CHARACTERISTICS OF VICTIMS

Type of Victim	Characteristics

Child
All ages, with greatest
  risk under age 5
  (including infants)
  and for fatalities
  under 2 years of age
	• Incest generally begins after 9 years of old
	• Self-blame for family conflict
	• Low self-esteem
	• Fear of parent or caretaker
	• Cheating, lying, low achievement in school
	• Signs of depression, helplessness
	• One child sometimes singled out in family due to being labeled as "difficult," product of unwanted pregnancy, reminds the parents of someone they dislike or even themselves, prematurity (inhibited parent-child bonding)

Spouse	• Low self-esteem • Self-blame for batterer's actions • Sense of helplessness to escape abuse • Isolation from family and friends • Views self as subservient to partner • Economic dependence on abuser
Elder	• Over 75 years old • Mentally and/or physically impaired • Isolated from others

Sociocultural views examine the role of violence in our society. With easy access to weapons and the frequent exposure to violence from the media, potential abusers can identify violence as a socially acceptable coping mechanism. Another contributing factor is that abusers are often isolated with limited resources for assistance. Alcohol and substance abuse by the abuser also contributes by lowering impulses and inhibitions and reducing sensitivity to the impact of their behavior.

Additional traits that contribute to child abuse include a parent who sees himself or herself in the child, the child not meeting parent's expectations, and the parent's viewing the child as being there to satisfy the parent's needs. At times, a parent has no tolerance for normal child behaviors, such as crying, because of the past experience of being unable to express these needs in childhood. So the child's normal behavior reminds the parent of his or her own unmet childhood needs and unresolved anger toward his or her own parents. There is also a very high correlation with drug and alcohol abuse in this parent. The other parent is usually aware of the abuse but remains unable or unwilling to intervene. That parent may unconsciously deny the existence of abuse and is often a victim of spousal abuse. Stepparents may also be abusers as hostility toward the new mate or previous spouse is projected on the child. Incest in the family may be related to sexual problems between husband and wife. Long-term effects for child abuse victims include low self-esteem, difficulty trusting others, anxiety, anger, phobias, depression, and eating disorders.

Domestic violence tends to escalate when the abuser is intoxicated. He or she often displays tremendous jealousy and fears losing the partner. At the same time, the abuser may blame the partner for his or her own problems. Inflicting injury on the woman gives the male abuser a temporary sense of power and esteem. Other factors contributing to domestic violence include the victim's lack of financial support, belief that the children need both parents, and lack of a social support system.

As noted earlier, elder abusers are often caregivers. These abusers often have limited coping mechanisms and limited support, and are emotionally and financially dependent on the elderly person. Most often they live with the elderly victim. At times, family members can become abusers as resentment toward the elder's dependency increases, or as retribution for the elder's perceived failures as a parent when younger.

Walker (1979) identified the *cycle theory of family violence*. This theory includes the following stages:

1. *Tension building stage:* Minor incidents of pushing, shoving, and verbal abuse occur.
2. *Acute battering stage:* Built-up tension is released by the abuser on the victim, leading to more brutal and uncontrollable abuse. Afterwards the abuser often does not remember the intensity of the incident. The victim is often able to remember the incident in detail without the emotion.
3. *Honeymoon stage:* The abuser has a sense of remorse that leads to a period of apology, and attempts to make up for the abuse by presents, special treats, and affection. The victim is finally receiving the love and attention she or he so wants and desperately desires to believe there will be no further abuse. This may allow the victim to forgive the abuser and even drop legal proceedings or plans to report the abuse. Unfortunately, this stage is usually short-lived and, without intervention, becomes even briefer over time. The intensity and frequency of the cycle and severity of injuries tend to increase over time.

RELATED CLINICAL CONCERNS

Neurologic impairment and substance abuse can trigger the abuse cycle by disinhibiting impulse control in the abuser. Illness may be a risk factor to becoming a victim. Resentments may build from caregiving responsibilities when the potential victim is dependent on the potential abuser. In addition, more violence may be inflicted on the developmentally challenged child.

POSSIBLE NURSES' REACTIONS

- The most common reaction is anger and disgust directed at the abuser. These strong negative feelings can cloud the nurse's assessment and judgment and interfere with selecting appropriate interventions for the abuser.
- The nurse may feel great sympathy for the victim.
- The nurse may also feel anger toward the battered woman who displays powerlessness. May blame her for staying with the abuser or being helpless and become angry if she does not take advice offered.

- The nurse may feel overwhelmed with the family's problems and helpless to change them, especially if the possible victim denies abuse.
- The nurse may feel intense sadness and distress, which could lead to the wish to save or "rescue" the victim. The nurse may act out these feelings by making promises to the victim that in reality cannot be met or could create an unsafe situation for both of them. This could isolate the victim even more.
- Because abuse may be so upsetting, the nurse may deny evidence or refuse to believe it, especially sexual abuse.
- The nurse may fear reporting abuse because of fear of getting involved, possible legal implications, or reprisals from abusers. The nurse may not want to be responsible for displacing the victim from the family. (Note: most states have Good Samaritan clauses in abuse laws that protect health-care professionals from liability in reporting.)
- Abuser may intimidate the nurse.
- The nurse may identify with the victim or abuser if he or she has had personal experience with abuse.
- May participate in a conspiracy of silence with others to avoid addressing potential problems.

ASSESSMENT

CHILD ABUSE

Child Behaviors and Symptoms

- History of injury inconsistent with child's developmental level (for example, baby turning on hot water)
- Failure to thrive; dull or inactive demeanor
- Signs of malnutrition, poor hygiene, or lack of health care
- Fears discussing how injuries occurred
- Lack of reaction to frightening events (for example, being given an injection) as child has learned to hide fear
- Unusual injuries such as cigarette burns, rope burns, spiral fractures from twisting injury, bite marks
- Unexplained retinal hemorrhage, subdural hematoma—can be a sign of "shaken baby syndrome"
- May demonstrate magical thinking that doctor or nurse will know family secret
- Fear of returning home
- Apprehension when hearing a child cry because thinks another child is being hurt
- Antisocial behavior, such as lying and stealing
- Wearing inappropriate clothing that covers bruises
- Bruises or bleeding in external genitalia
- Torn, bloody underclothing
- Pain on urination or frequent urinary tract infections
- Abnormal discharge or odor in genital area, indications of sexually transmitted diseases

- Pregnancy in adolescent
- Sudden onset of sexually related behavior, such as excessive masturbation, age-inappropriate sex play, or overseductive behavior
- Child being given a variety of gifts or privileges
- Change in behavior including depression, anxiety, regression, running away from home, substance abuse, decline in school performance, inflicting abuse on family pets or other animals

Parental Behaviors

- Exaggerated or absent reaction to child's injury
- Failure to show empathy for child
- Inconsistent explanations of injuries
- Care sought for child's minor complaints but not for more obvious illness
- Demands to take child home if pressured for answers or refuses hospitalization
- Explanations not matching injuries; attempts to blame the child
- Nonabusing parent refusing to acknowledge even obvious abuse (Box 17–1)

DOMESTIC VIOLENCE

Victim

- Injuries to head, abdomen, breasts, genitalia
- Injuries while pregnant
- Patterns left by item used to cause injury such as rope or teeth
- Frequent urinary tract infections
- Mother of abused child

BOX 17–1. General Warning Signs of Abuse

- Delay in seeking treatment for injuries, minimizing injuries
- History of being accident prone
- Pattern of injuries not accidental looking, for example, identical burns on bottom of feet, identical injuries on both sides of head
- Multiple injuries in varying stages of healing
- Conflicting stories from victim and abuser about cause of injury
- Inconsistency between history and injury
- Unusual, even bizarre explanation for injuries
- Repeated visits to emergency rooms or clinics
- Previous report of abuse
- Patient reporting abuse
- Patient fearful of caregiver or partner
- Visits variety of doctors, emergency rooms for treatment

- History of rape
- Lack of care for own chronic illness
- Demonstrates guilt for seeking treatment
- Use of alcohol or tranquilizers to cover hurt
- Indicates acceptance of violence as a way to maintain family
- Socially isolated with limited financial resources and family support
- Implies a sense of deserving abuse
- Stress-related complaints of headaches, insomnia, nervousness
- Wearing clothes and makeup to cover bruises
- Denies abuse or gives explanations that do not match injury

Abuser

- Minimizes injuries even when they become life threatening
- Speaks for victim or doesn't let him or her speak
- Controlling, angry
- Does not want victim to be alone with healthcare providers
- Tends to isolate victim by eliminating his or her social support system
- Insists on taking patient back home even if inappropriate
- Criticizes or humiliates victim in front of others
- Access to guns, other weapons
- Abuses family pets
- Rationalizes actions ("she deserved it")

ELDER ABUSE

Victim

- Evidence of malnutrition, dehydration, poor hygiene, pressure ulcers, not receiving needed medical care
- Unusual injuries such as twisting fractures, cigarette burns on face or back, perforated eardrums from being slapped
- Evidence of sexually transmitted diseases, unusual genital injuries
- Deterioration in mental status including confusion and depression
- Sudden lack of funds in person who previously had resources
- Frail, dependent, possible mental impairment requiring care from family member or hired help
- Extreme dependency, attachment to new caregiver
- Evidence of inappropriate use of restraints

Abuser

- Often lives with victim, lacks resources to live elsewhere
- Refusal to allow diagnostic tests, hospitalization
- Much younger than patient
- Cashes victim's social security and/or pension checks
- Sudden, intense involvement with patient with little input from other family members

- Evidence of drug or alcohol abuse or mental illness
- Expects dependent elder to meet his or her needs
- Caregiver overwhelmed with patient's care needs, demonstrates frustration and resentment, isolated with limited assistance
- Elderly spouse with dementia
- Coerces senior to change will to his or her benefit
- Shows no guilt or rationalizes actions

COLLABORATIVE MANAGEMENT

Psychotherapy

Individual and/or group psychotherapy are often used to treat both victims and abusers. For the victim, individual therapy may focus on the damage done to self-esteem and facing and resolving intense emotions toward the abuser, as well as toward others who may have tolerated the abuse (often the other parent in child abuse). The victim should be removed from living with the abuser before entering treatment to reduce the fear of retaliation. In domestic violence, therapists often recommend that the couple separate for a period of time before starting treatment.

Children who are suspected victims of sexual abuse need to be evaluated by therapy professionals in this specialty. Repressed, traumatic events of the past, such as childhood sexual abuse, may also be uncovered during therapy as an adult. This repressed abuse could be influencing the patient's current life without his or her knowledge. However, this is very controversial because repressed memories have been found to be inaccurate. Group therapy may also allow the victim to learn from other victims and develop assertive skills.

More intensive psychotherapy or psychiatric treatment may be required for the abuser if psychopathology is suspected.

Because family violence is a symptom of family dysfunction, family therapy is often part of the overall treatment plan. When children are in the home where abuse has occurred, they must be part of the healing process. In addition, support group programs are available for both victims and abusers.

NURSING MANAGEMENT

> **INEFFECTIVE FAMILY COPING: DISABLING** EVIDENCED BY CHILD ABUSE RELATED TO HISTORY OF ABUSE IN THE FAMILY, LACK OF RESOURCES, ISOLATION.

Child Outcomes

- Remains free from injury or neglect
- Seeks comfort and assistance from nurse

Parent Outcomes

- Seeks assistance for abusive behavior
- Demonstrates nurturing behavior toward child
- Refrains from abusive behavior

Interventions

- Establish a trusting relationship with child and parents. Avoid threatening behavior or criticizing parents in front of child. See Table 17–2, Interviewing Abuser or Abuse Victim.
- Observe parent-child interaction closely, especially when both are under stress. Observe caring and feeding behavior. In the home, observe sleeping arrangements and environmental conditions.
- Recognize that the child very often will not betray his or her parents. Even in the worst situations, the child may fear losing the only security he or she knows and consequently, will deny any problems.
- Involve the child in treatment plan to increase his or her sense of control.
- Demonstrate support, acceptance, and affection of the child. Reinforce child's self esteem by positive feedback and recognition.
- If child needs discipline, discuss punishment, and clarify that no physical abuse will be used. Consider referral for psychiatric or play therapy evaluation to better understand what is being expressed.

TABLE 17–2. INTERVIEWING AN ABUSER OR ABUSE VICTIM

Do	Don't
Conduct the interview in private.	Conduct the interview with a group of interviewers.
Be direct, honest, and professional.	
Be understanding.	Try to prove abuse by accusations and demands
Be attentive.	
Inform the patient before making the referral to child or adult protective services and explain the process.	Display horror, anger, shock, or disapproval of the abuser or the situation.
	Place blame or make judgments about the abuser or the victim.
Assess for risk of danger and help reduce that risk before discharge.	Allow the victim to feel "at fault" or "in trouble."
	Probe or press for answers the victim is not willing to give.
For Children	
Tell the child that the interview is confidential.	Force the child to remove clothing.
Use age-specific language.	
Ask the child to clarify his or her meaning or words you do not understand.	
Tell the child whether any future action will be required.	

Source: Reproduced with permission. Smith-Dijulio, K, and Holzapfel, SK: Families in crisis: Family violence. In Varcarolis, EM (ed): Foundations of Psychiatric-Mental Health Nursing. WB Saunders, Philadelphia, 1994.

- Encourage play. Be aware that child may be better able to express feelings through play.
- Reinforce parent's strengths, and acknowledge importance of continuing medical care for the child.
- Reinforce positive parenting behavior. Role-model caregiving behaviors for them.
- Avoid hostility toward the parents. At the same time, maintain the child's safety. If child is at risk for being taken inappropriately by parents, have staff remain in attendance with security nearby and inform the parents of your reasons for doing so.
- If sexual abuse is suspected, child needs to be evaluated by appropriate professionals, including psychologist, pediatrician, gynecologist.
- Be aware of agency policy and state laws on reporting suspected child abuse. Contact supervisor and/or social worker to implement appropriate reporting. Participate in collecting evidence, as indicated, and ensure that proper procedures are followed.
- Be sure that supervisors, physicians, and social services are informed when a suspected abuse is reported.

INEFFECTIVE FAMILY COPING: DISABLING EVIDENCED BY DOMESTIC VIOLENCE RELATED TO VULNERABLE VICTIM, ABUSER WITH FAMILY HISTORY OF ABUSE, ISOLATED, LIMITED RESOURCES, AND/OR INTENSE JEALOUSY.

Victim Outcomes

- Acknowledges the abuse
- Identifies options to escape abuser
- Remains in treatment even if pressured to not obtain care

Abuser Outcomes

- Seeks assistance for abusive behavior
- Refrains from harming others

Interventions

- Establish a trusting relationship with the victim. Avoid displaying shock or disgust at the story. Encourage victim to share fears and concerns. Ask specific questions to avoid a vague response.
- Assess the victim's safety. If there is a risk, implement agency security policies, as appropriate. If victim is in the hospital, restrict phone calls and visitors. Consider a pseudonym for the patient's name. For patients at home, determine need to involve the police and information on legal restraining orders. If there are children in the home, determine their risk of injury. Be aware of state and agency policies for reporting domestic violence.
- Reinforce victim's self-esteem. Identify positive traits and coping mechanisms. Encourage victim to talk about accomplishments and goals.

- Encourage victim's participation in treatment plan including follow-up with medical appointments. Help victim take control of some areas of his or her life and make some decisions.
- If possible, identify available support systems and determine their awareness of family's problems. Encourage patient to involve some people who can help. Support maintaining regular social contacts.
- Encourage realistically evaluation situation. Do not reinforce denial or avoidance.
- Be aware that during the "Honeymoon Stage" the victim may not be willing to discuss abuse. Describe the cycle of abuse to the victim. Give the victim written information on resources to use at another time.
- Encourage problem solving. Challenge him or her to identify realistic options, and reinforce all efforts to be assertive.
- Encourage talking about events that led up to the abusive event. Dispel any myths of guilt or responsibility for causing or deserving the abuse.
- Be sure that supervisors, physicians, and social services are informed when a suspected abuse is reported.

> **INEFFECTIVE FAMILY COPING: DISABLING** EVIDENCED BY ELDER ABUSE RELATED TO MULTIPLE STRESSORS ASSOCIATED WITH ELDER CARE.

Elder Outcomes

- Identifies resources available for assistance
- Remains safe and without injury
- Continues to receive adequate health care

Caregiver Outcomes

- Identifies resources available for assistance in patient care
- Demonstrates more effective coping mechanisms
- Provides safe care to the elderly patient

Interventions

- Assess the elderly patient's condition and determine the role of caregiver in providing adequate care. Patients with pressure ulcers, dehydration, lacerations, and bruises need to be evaluated; however, be aware that these may occur unrelated to abuse or neglect.
- If abuse is suspected, talk with patient and caregiver separately. With the patient, listen to his or her description of the caregiver and any complaints he or she may have. Then verify the information, if possible, with the caregiver, other family members, or healthcare providers. Establish a trusting relationship with the caregiver by acknowledging positive accomplishments, as well as the stress of caregiving.
- If signs of abuse occur in a long-term care facility, observe patient care routines and the care of other patients. Note the use of restraints and the qual-

ity of hygiene provided. In the home, if patient is being left alone while restrained, action must be taken immediately to stop this unsafe practice.

- Provide education to staff in long term care on identifying and preventing abuse/neglect.
- Recognize that patients with altered mental status may falsely accuse caregivers of abuse. However, every accusation must be evaluated.
- Encourage the patient to be as independent as possible by remaining involved with family and friends, having his or her own telephone, and having neighbors check his or her status regularly. Appropriate independence will also promote self-esteem and self-reliance. Even in the highly dependent patient, it is important to maintain the individual's sense of control.
- Encourage problem-solving skills in patient and caregiver. Promote their abilities to find alternate solutions under stress.
- If patient is in an unsafe environment, implement agency policies and state laws as appropriate to determine reporting mechanism and action. If patient refuses to leave environment, determine patient's ability to make decisions. Involve physician and/or social worker as needed. Consider psychiatric evaluation. Involve family and friends if needed to encourage patient action.
- Determine caregiver's stress level and determine if additional resources are available and would defuse the situation.
- Be sure that supervisors, physicians, and social services are informed when a suspected abuse is reported.

ALTERNATE NURSING DIAGNOSES

Altered Family Processes
Altered Parenting
Caregiver Role Strain
Risk for Violence
Knowledge Deficit
Noncompliance
Post-Trauma Response
Powerlessness
Rape-Trauma Syndrome

PATIENT AND FAMILY EDUCATION

- Teach effective parenting skills, including appropriate discipline. Abusive parents need skills in disciplining children without violence and often need to learn acceptable outlets for their frustration.
- Incorporate assertive skills to teach potential victims, including young children, to speak up when rights are violated and learn to say no.
- Teach family members the signs of abuse and how to report it.
- Family members need guidelines for hiring caregivers and selecting assisted living situation.
- Teach older adults how to avoid abusive situations by maintaining active social network, and to seek legal advice before allowing anyone to take their

possessions or manage their finances. AARP has written guidelines to avoid elder abuse. These can be accessed through the Web site www.aarp.org.

- Teach a victim of domestic violence to identify a plan in advance to leave home when needed. This plan should include having a place to go, setting aside money, and implementing security measures for victim and children.
- When children must be removed from their home, prepare them for the emotional grief response that may occur when they are separated from their parents. No matter how bad the home was, children will still grieve. Be sure they understand that they are not being punished.
- Suspected abusers need information on alternative ways to resolve conflicts. If appropriate, refer them to counselors who specialize in abuse who can educate them on the role of substance abuse and violence.
- Review with victims and abusers the need to involve family and friends for assistance.

CHARTING TIPS

- If abuse is suspected, carefully document, possibly with photos, any evidence of wounds, injuries, or poor hygiene. Follow institutional protocols carefully if called upon to participate in evidence collection.
- Document the nature of interactions between victim and abuser.
- Note victim's reaction to the abuser, especially when discharging patient.
- Document victim's report of abuse.
- Document interventions made, including reporting abuse and maintaining patient safety.
- Document any discrepancies between the victim and potential abuser's explanation of injuries.

WHEN TO CALL FOR HELP

Aggressive, belligerent behavior escalates to violence.

Presence of abuser leads patient to fear of violence or of being kidnapped.

Abuser is intoxicated.

Abuser intimidates patient or staff.

Victim leaves healthcare agency to return to unsafe environment.

COMMUNITY-BASED CARE

- Provide written information on appropriate resources, including: parenting support groups such as Parents Anonymous; parenting education programs; shelters; safe houses; 24-hour local crisis hot lines for abuse or National Child Abuse Hotline (1-800-4ACHILD); and National Organization

for Victim Assistance (800-TRY-NOVA). If abuse is suspected and patient denies it, provide the information, and encourage patient to keep it in a safe place. For elder abuse, contact the local Adult Protective Services.
- Web sites include www.preventchildabuse.org and www.acf.dhhs.gov/programs/cb/
- Provide information on legal referrals and security measures. If police are involved, reinforce information they give to patient.
- As appropriate, refer patient for counseling or family therapy.
- Refer for home health follow-up to assess home environment. Inform all referring agencies of concerns about abuse.
- Vocational counseling information may be helpful to the domestic violence victim.
- Anticipate caregiver needs in the home and provide adequate support and equipment.
- Discuss day-care options for children or elderly people.

Problems with Spiritual Distress

THE PATIENT WITH SPIRITUAL DISTRESS

Margaret L. Mitchell, RN, MN, MDIV, MA, CNS

LEARNING OBJECTIVES

➢ Define spiritual distress.
➢ Identify some life event and physical changes that may precipitate spiritual distress.
➢ Differentiate between religion and spirituality.
➢ Identify effective interventions for dealing with an individual experiencing spiritual distress.
➢ Describe common nurses' reactions to patients' spiritual distress.

All people have a spiritual dimension, regardless of whether or not they participate in formal religious practices. Spirituality allows us to transcend the self and connect with people, our surroundings, and powers outside of ourselves. Spirituality can give meaning to life and impact the ability to trust, love, and forgive. Religion is different from spirituality, although it is complementary. Religion gives us tradition, ritual, and a specific doctrine. Spiritual distress is an existential crisis in which the beliefs or values around which the person has organized his or her life are threatened. Parents' belief system may be shaken when they learn that their child has an incurable illness or will not recover from an accident. For individuals, it can be learning of a life-threatening illness. When people are faced with these situations, you may hear them say, "Life will never be the same" or "How can I go on living?" The very foundation of their life as they know it is threatened. They may no longer feel safe and able to go about their everyday activities. Some may question their belief in God.

Spiritual distress may manifest itself in many different ways. Individuals are a complex combination of biologic, psychologic, sociocultural, and spiritual parts, all interacting and affecting all other aspects of the individual's life. With the restraints of managed care and with a further concern for cultural diversity, it is important to keep in mind that an insult to one's spiritual dimension can affect every other dimension of the individual and influence the patient's experience of illness.

Spiritual distress occurs when a person believes that life no longer has meaning or purpose, or experiences a sense of hopelessness. Like many other entities that can be viewed on a continuum, spiritual distress may be a temporary, transient phenomenon in a response to a specific stressor or it may be a longer-reaching event prompting the individual to question or reexamine assumptions and priorities. In a few rare instances, extreme spiritual distress may indicate psychopathology.

In many ways, spiritual distress can follow a similar pattern to the grief response. Grief over small losses may be short term, and with proper support, recovery will be rapid. Great losses affect the individual more profoundly and can be seen in changes in the person's mood, affect, energy level, interest in life, and somatic condition. In the most extreme pathologic grief, in which individuals are not recovering, their ability to carry out activities of daily living is greatly reduced and may sometimes require psychiatric hospitalization.

Both grief and spiritual distress deal with loss. The major difference is that spiritual distress disrupts the meaning that governs a person's life. There may be a perceived or real deterioration or collapse in his or her relationship with a divine Supreme Being, or with persons who represent the Supreme Being.

The presence of stressors does not necessarily predict or cause spiritual distress. The Chinese character for crisis, which is a combination of the symbols for danger and opportunity, helps one to understand this. For some individuals, a stressor or crisis, such as a life-threatening illness or tragedy, can ultimately become the source of a tremendously positive experience. Although they readily acknowledge that they would have never chosen such events, they ultimately view them not as traumatic events but as opportunities for growth. In some ways, it parallels a wilderness experience. The arduous physical demands allow an individual to transcend his or her immediate surroundings and experience a sense of empowerment that results in the person being better equipped to handle the challenges of life.

Nurses may feel uncomfortable or experience conflict when providing spiritual support if the patient is religious and the nurse is not or if the patient's expression of spirituality differs from that of the nurse. In addition, nurses may experience conflict with a patient's belief system, as with a Jehovah's Witness patient who refuses a life-saving blood transfusion. These are normal responses to the unknown. How one responds to a patient's spiritual needs depends both on one's education and background. It is important, however, not to evaluate the patient's value system by personal standards.

Patients' responses to illness have been found to influence nurses' own spiritual beliefs. In a 1994 study by Taylor, Amenta, and Highfield, oncology nurses ranked their patients as a major source of spiritual nurturing. Nurses, however, may have difficulty providing spiritual care because of lack of skill, time constraints, or fear of being criticized by co-workers. The Joint Commission for Accreditation of Healthcare Organizations (1999) has added a standard on determining spiritual support services for patients on their admission to healthcare institutions. Certain settings, such as hospices, require incorporation of a spiritual assessment and offering of chaplaincy services. Nurses who work or have worked in this type of setting are often more comfortable responding to spiritual distress.

ETIOLOGY

Spiritual distress occurs when particular stressors or life events threaten the individual's belief system and affect biologic, psychologic, sociocultural, and spiritual aspects of life. These stressors may be unique to the individual, or they may be similar to reactions experienced by others after certain events.

The crisis may have a variety of causes, including loss of a significant person, employment, position, or status; financial reversal; major illness or loss of a body part, or a change in self-image. In some cultures it may also result from shame. However, what is lost is not as important as the value that the individual ascribes to it.

Cognitive theory looks at the effect of beliefs on feelings, and *psychodynamic* theory helps one understand the underlying process of spiritual distress. For instance, a great deal of spiritual distress can be experienced, even to the point of affecting physical health, when a person believes that he or she can never be forgiven. A person's belief in the ability to be forgiven may be associated with his or her perception of how others show approval. The individual may accept forgiveness from God or a higher power in the same manner as forgiveness was accepted from parents because the relationship with God or a higher power is often similar to the relationship with one's parents.

Psychologic theories look at the various dynamics that can result in spiritual distress. A person with a high degree of inner strength, or ego functioning, may experience less spiritual distress in response to a loss than one who has a lower level of ego functioning. The way in which one normally adapts to crises and changes will also influence the risk of spiritual distress. Persons who are inflexible may have more difficulty accepting major changes. Similarly, individuals who are prone to anxiety may feel overwhelmed in the face of major change and have difficulty dealing with it.

Crisis theory considers not only the normal changes in life and life event stressors, but also looks at the impact of disaster or massive crisis on the individual. Faith or a belief system may help a person to cope with a crisis, but if the crisis is of a high magnitude, the person may feel that his or her belief system is challenged or inadequate and may be of little help.

One of the hallmarks of a disaster or massive crisis, such as a devastating hurricane, earthquake, or crash of an airplane, is the enormous sense of an individual's loss of control and extreme feelings of vulnerability. There may be a sense of betrayal, and the events may be expressed as not being "right." The individual may reveal a sense of how things "should" be, his or her expectation of the world. The sense of betrayal and anger may be expressed in spiritual terms such as "How could God let this happen?"

A sense of mastery over one's environment, highly prized in American culture, is threatened when a major crisis occurs. When an individual no longer feels safe in usual activities, a feeling of unease can spread to other areas of life.

RELATED CLINICAL CONCERNS

Although identifiable traumatic events may precipitate spiritual distress, it is important to be aware of physiologic conditions that may exacerbate the situation. Illnesses associated with increased sense of vulnerability and the possibility of death (particularly cancer) may lead to heightened spiritual awareness. Pain, suffering, and severe side effects may affect spiritual life. Patients may also have a reduction in the energy they need for their usual means of spiritual coping, such as praying and attending religious services.

Although there is no clear relationship between specific disease entities and spiritual distress, a spiritual state can be influenced by biologic changes, such as changes in neurotransmitters, endocrine levels, or blood chemistry. Just as there are differences in coping mechanisms, there are differences in the way in which the individual as an organism responds to illness. Even when an event appears to be a precipitant for spiritual distress, biologic factors could also be at work. A complete physical assessment and supporting tests can help determine these biologic factors.

Psychoactive substances can influence mood and, consequently, the way in which the individual perceives the situation and how well he or she functions in responding to it. Nurses need to be aware of the many prescription drugs that have such effects, such as beta-blockers, steroids, antihypertensives, immunosuppressants, and chemotherapy.

LIFE SPAN ISSUES

CHILDREN

Because the belief systems of young children are not as developed as those of adults, children may not be able to adequately verbalize their sense of spiritual distress. Instead, they may present with such physical symptoms as weight loss, failure to thrive, and reversal of developmental milestones. Most frequently their stress is in response to loss of a parent or caretaker or a major change affecting a parent or caretaker. The child can sense the distress of the parent. For example, a young child may not fully understand the impact of death, but he or she can sense, and be negatively affected by, the tremendous distress the loss of a child or spouse can cause his or her caretaker. The child often responds by being more clinging or dependent at times of crisis.

Signs of distress in older children may be subtler. Some children experiencing depression may act out in different ways. Behavioral problems may be exacerbated. It is important to pay attention to subtle changes in a child, such as a lack of interest in usual pursuits, withdrawal or isolation, or a decrease in school performance. One of the most traumatic events for children is loss of parents or siblings by death or divorce. Children may mistakenly believe that they personally caused the loss of the parent and may not comprehend other dynamics at work. Children's spiritual and/or religious beliefs are strongly influenced by those of their parents. More questioning of parental values tends to occur when the child becomes an adolescent.

ADOLESCENTS

Adolescents are generally more able to articulate distress, but they may be hesitant to confide in an adult. More aware of the complexities of life and often having a strong personal moral code, they may be traumatized by the failings of an idealized parent. Loss of parents, siblings, classmates, or acquaintances by death, divorce, or relocation can be tremendously stressful events for the adolescent. Youths whose sexual orientation differs from parental or societal expectation may either act out or experience their crisis in secret. Another traumatic event includes sexual exploitation by peers or adults. Even though pregnancy during teen years is rising, it may be exceedingly traumatic for the individual. Teens, especially girls, must deal with the dilemma of pregnancy and the changes it will make in their lives and those of their parents. Teens are also vulnerable to life's tragedies such as the death of a parent, which can lead to questioning of spiritual beliefs and loss of hope.

Because adolescents are so impressionable and idealistic, they are very vulnerable to the influence of cults and religious conversions. The beginning recognition that life is not as ideal and perfect as they once believed may cause individuals to lose hope and question their former spiritual beliefs.

ELDERLY PEOPLE

Later life is a period characterized by extremes. There is tremendous variety in functioning. For some, a significant change in physical or sensory functioning may affect their view of self and their spiritual beliefs. Many individuals experience the death of a spouse and friends and changes in residence. Some may depend more on their spiritual life as their acquaintances diminish and limitations grow. Spiritual distress in elderly people often includes questions regarding the afterlife, values, and reflections on the satisfaction and accomplishments of their lives. Forgiveness related to past wrongdoings by themselves or others may become more important.

Religious teachings from childhood may become more important in later years as people face changes and losses. However, sometimes attending worship services and participating in religious practices may be more difficult to accomplish because of illness and fatigue.

POSSIBLE NURSES' REACTIONS

- May not feel comfortable or adequately prepared to help patients with spiritual concerns.
- May be influenced by their own background, beliefs, values, and experiences, which may differ from those of the patient.
- May react negatively or judgmentally, or distance themselves from patients whose beliefs, practices, lifestyles, or cultures differ from their own.
- May focus attention on religious content rather than assessing other issues that may be the cause of anxiety.
- May attempt to change or argue with religious content of patient's beliefs.
- May confuse religious with spiritual beliefs.
- May feel powerless when unable to help patients with spiritual concerns. Nurses may distance themselves from patients to cope with their own feelings of inadequacy.
- May not understand the meaning of the loss from the patient's spiritual

perspective and may try to reassure the patient in ways that are not effective or meaningful.
- May resent clergy because of their closeness and ability to meet some patients' needs.
- Conversely, out of feelings of fear and inadequacy, may refer patients to the chaplain too quickly rather than attempt to deal with the concerns.
- May reassure patients based on their own knowledge of illnesses and fail to hear the patients' concerns.
- May feel judgmental about individuals expressing spiritual concerns or practices, especially if those concerns are unfamiliar to the nurse.
- May feel anxious when encountering unfamiliar practices.
- May feel so stressed, overworked, or overwhelmed by the physical needs of the patient or their own workload that they do not consider the spiritual dimension.
- May have trouble setting personal limits on the role of the nurse and spiritual beliefs.

ASSESSMENT

Behavior and Appearance

- Often has religious items or literature at bedside
- Frequently quotes from the Bible or other spiritual literature
- May display exaggerated religious rituals or behavior such as reading the Bible excessively rather than talking
- May appear withdrawn and preoccupied with own beliefs, unable to focus on conversations and events in immediate environment
- Makes constant reference to religious themes in conversation
- Asks frequent questions such as "Is this God's will?" or "Why is God letting me suffer?"
- Lethargic; may exhibit a lack of interest in surroundings
- May be overtly or passively suicidal
- Frequently questions others about their spiritual beliefs
- States that spiritual beliefs are no longer comforting
- Behavior changes, such as increased alcohol use or acting out

Mood and Emotions

- Highly anxious
- Denies emotions or concerns
- Expresses bitterness or anger over perceived abandonment by God or belief that God is causing the suffering
- Appears depressed
- Expresses feelings of helplessness or hopelessness
- Does not derive enjoyment and satisfaction from formerly pleasurable activities

Thoughts, Beliefs, and Perceptions

- Believes that nothing can help
- Exhibits global, all-or-nothing thinking
- Believes that life is overwhelming and that he or she cannot continue living
- Questions long-held beliefs and may doubt his or her faith
- Believes that he or she has committed sins that cannot be forgiven
- Is self-absorbed in own belief system
- Views self as guilty and in need of punishment
- Views self as spiritually superior to others
- Believes that a higher power requires suffering and pain and therefore refuses pain control measures
- Views self as having a great mission to accomplish
- Claims to hear voices of God, Moses, or other religious figures
- Holds omnipotent view of self—a specialness that rests in the inability to be forgiven by God or higher power

Relationships and Interactions

- Feels isolated and alone even in the presence of others
- Withdraws from others who do not share similar beliefs
- May experience change in relationship with family or friends who are involved with religious beliefs
- May seek out members of similar religious group for support, caregiving

Physical Responses

- Reports increased discomforts
- Change in eating or sleeping patterns

Pertinent History

- Involved in specific religious groups, cults, or a variety of different religious groups (Box 18–1)
- History of emotional disorders or emotionally charged previous situations, such as abortion or catastrophic events

COLLABORATIVE MANAGEMENT

CHAPLAINCY/CLERGY

Some healthcare agencies may have full-time chaplains on staff. Others may have volunteer chaplains or links to clergy in the community. Chaplains provide spiritual counseling and are often knowledgeable about community support resources that may be useful for the patient. Working with the social workers, they can help in making funeral arrangements or locating needed services or volunteers. Chaplains can help both patients and staff members to find ways to cope with the problem situation. However, not all patients

---

BOX 18–1. Assessing for Spiritual Beliefs

Initial Assessment

1. What is your source of strength and hope?
2. What is your religious affiliation, and how important is this in your life? Any recent changes?
3. Is there a clergy person available to you while in the hospital?
4. Are there any religious or spiritual practices that are important to you while in the hospital?
5. Are there any religious or spiritual articles that are important to you while in the hospital?
6. Is there any spiritual literature that is important to you while in the hospital?

Advanced Assessment

1. Has being sick or in the hospital made any difference in your feelings toward God or in your beliefs?
2. What has bothered you the most about being sick or in the hospital?
3. What helps you the most when you are afraid or in need of special help?
4. What religious or spiritual idea or concept is most important to you?
5. What did your family believe? What was meaningful and important to them?
6. What exposure, if any, did you have to religious or spiritual beliefs as a child? Has that changed? How?
7. Have your religious interests arisen gradually or out of a crisis?
8. Do you have special religious leaders? How do you view them?
9. What would help you maintain your spirituality?
10. Does prayer provide comfort for you? If you pray, about what do you pray? When do you pray?
11. What happens when you pray or meditate?

---

hold clergy in high regard. Some can talk about spiritual concerns more effectively to a nurse. Others may view clergy negatively or with suspicion or fear that they are associated only with bad news, depending on previous life experiences. Also, depending on the situation, the patient may prefer to share concerns with a chaplain other than the one associated with the place where he or she worships.

Clergy are restricted as to what information they can share with nursing staff and others. Like mental health professionals and lawyers, clergy are bound by professional ethics and law regarding what they may reveal of anything told to them in confidence.

NURSING MANAGEMENT

SPIRITUAL DISTRESS EVIDENCED BY QUESTIONING BELIEFS, DESPAIR, HOPELESSNESS, OR INABILITY TO PRACTICE BELIEFS RELATED TO SUFFERING, ILLNESS, OR HOSPITALIZATION.

Patient Outcomes

- Verbalizes "I feel better," "I feel relieved," "I feel at peace," or similar statements
- Demonstrates increased social interaction
- Reports feeling rested and comfortable
- Demonstrates reduced crying or other signs of distress

Interventions

- Empathize with patient's degree of pain or despair.
- Recognize that your own personal values and beliefs may not be effective for others. Be willing to set aside your own beliefs when analyzing the patient's spiritual needs.
- Become familiar with the patient's beliefs and practices.
- Use self-disclosure of own spiritual beliefs only to foster patient's therapeutic goals.
- Use questions to determine the role that religion and spirituality play in the patient's life. For example, "The chart says you are Catholic. Are there any religious practices that are important to you during your illness?"
- Seek assistance of or referrals to hospital chaplain or other resources when you feel uncomfortable or unable to meet the patient's spiritual needs. Recognize the role that members of the patient's church or temple can play in providing support.
- Involve chaplains in team meetings and patient care conferences to collaborate on treatment plan.
- Promote use of prayer and scripture when appropriate if within patient's belief system (Box 18–2).
- Become familiar with agency policy regarding praying with patients.
- Provide supportive, private environment to meet spiritual needs.
- Substitute supportive response for prayer when the setting or timing is inappropriate.
- Work with patient and staff to adapt patient's schedule or activities to incorporate religious rituals whenever possible.
- Allow patient to ventilate thoughts and feelings. Explore what precipitated the feeling of loss. Help patient clarify any underlying feelings of guilt. Help the patient explore and evaluate whether the source is rational or distorted.
- Help patient explore previously held false assumptions and, as indicated, refer to spiritual passages affirming hope, if within the nurse's comfort and knowledge.
- Allow family to participate in religious rituals such as ritual body care after death or baptism of a critically ill child.
- Be open to patient's expression of spiritual concerns. Avoid dismissing practices as inappropriate or pathologic.
- If the patient shares fears, remember that acceptance and listening are more important than having the answers.

BOX 18–2. Guidelines for Use of Prayer and Religious Literature

1. Prayer combined with therapeutic use of self can be used to meet the patient's spiritual needs and show empathy. A therapeutic relationship must already be established with the patient before engaging in prayer, a more intimate form of communication.
2. Prayer can consist of simply sharing a few brief sentences to express an immediate need or can be taken from a formally written source.
3. The request for prayer and religious literature should be initiated by the patient. If you are not comfortable, discuss with colleagues other alternatives.
4. Ask the patient to define the specific needs for which he or she is requesting prayer.
5. Ask what passages the patient wants to read and how they are significant.
6. Validate expressed feelings such as pain, fear, anxiety, stress, helplessness, or anger at God.
7. Know that prayer can be an affirmation of God's presence and hope for the patient.
8. If reading from religious literature, select passages carefully. Consult with chaplain or other staff if in doubt. Some passages may be misinterpreted, be interpreted literally, or be beyond the level of this patient.

SPIRITUAL DISTRESS EVIDENCED BY RELIGIOUS DELUSIONS OR OBSESSIONS RELATED TO IMPAIRED THOUGHT PROCESS.

Patient Outcomes

- Demonstrates improved reality orientation
- Verbalizes concerns and conflicts
- Verbalizes improved sense of well being
- Demonstrates appropriate social interactions

Interventions

- Become familiar with the norms of the patient's particular religious group to assess the patient's deviation from standard practice.
- Be aware that delusions may represent areas of personal conflict or concerns. For example, the Messiah complex may reveal that patient has a need to feel special, and dwelling on past sins may show that patient feels badly about self. Focus on feelings the patient is having rather than on content of delusion.
- Use great caution in reinforcing religious beliefs with psychotic patients because this may perpetuate reality distortions. Seek assistance from available mental health resources as well as chaplain or clergy.
- Set limits on time spent talking about obsessions and performing ritualistic behavior with the patient. Make a contract regarding time when you will listen. Be consistent.

- Encourage patient to discuss concerns other than religious issues. Bring patient back to recent specific experiences or events.
- Avoid arguing with the patient about the validity of his or her beliefs. Rather, acknowledge the feelings these beliefs may evoke, such as fear or sadness.
- Recognize that reducing obsessional thoughts or compulsive behavior may result in increased anxiety or possibly even a panic reaction (see Chapter 7, Problems with Anxiety, for interventions). Discuss with the physician the need for evaluation by a mental health professional and appropriate medication.

> **HOPELESSNESS** EVIDENCED BY DEPRESSION, APATHY, WITHDRAWAL, REJECTION OF SPIRITUAL BELIEFS RELATED TO LOSS, IMPENDING DEATH, INCURABLE DISEASE, LACK OF MEANING; SPIRITUAL CRISIS.

Patient Outcomes

- Verbalizes phrases like "I hadn't thought of it that way" or "I feel better"
- Demonstrates increased social interactions
- Able to identify one or more future goals

Interventions

- Encourage patient to share feelings and concerns and talk about what has triggered the sense of hopelessness.
- Maintain a concerned yet positive attitude around patient, but avoid an overly cheerful approach that may inhibit communication.
- Focus on short-term, concrete goals; identify specific things the patient can do now. For instance, focus on the pleasure of visiting with granddaughter today rather than the hope to be playing tennis next year. Make a plan with patient for achievable goals, such as sitting up in chair for 5 minutes longer today than yesterday. Often a patient may feel less hopeless and depressed if progress in one area can be achieved.
- Recognize that pain, fatigue, and other stressors will affect ability to maintain hope. Use interventions to deal with these stressors.
- Seek out chaplain to discuss patient's beliefs to help challenge hopelessness and support a more hopeful view.
- Recognize that, with time to work through a loss or crisis, the patient may be able to focus on the future. Allow the patient time to work through the grieving process.
- Be aware of your own anxiety around patient. Patient could sense your tension and think that his or her issues are unacceptable.

ALTERNATE NURSING DIAGNOSES

Potential for Enhanced Spiritual Well-Being
Altered Thought Processes
Anxiety
Dysfunctional Grieving

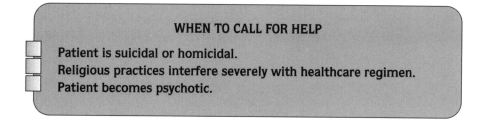

PATIENT AND FAMILY EDUCATION

- Educate patient and family on ways to incorporate religious practices into the treatment plan for the specific illness. For instance, the patient can adapt dietary restrictions and fasting requirements around specific beliefs.
- Educate the family on the importance of patient's spiritual beliefs if the family is not supportive of them.
- Encourage family to not impose their beliefs on the patient if they are different.
- Encourage family to bring in Bibles or religious articles, as appropriate.

CHARTING TIPS

- Document patient's beliefs, especially as they relate to patient's illness.
- Document conflicts between patient and family.
- Document patient's response to visit with clergy.
- Document nursing interventions and patient responses to spiritual interventions such as prayer, scripture reading, or meditation.

COMMUNITY-BASED CARE

- Refer to clergy or agency chaplain, as appropriate.
- Encourage attendance at religious or health-related support groups, such as Reach for Recovery.
- Encourage participation in patient's own house of worship as indicated.
- Utilize members of patient's religious community to assist with home care when appropriate.

Nursing Management of Special Populations

THE PATIENT WITH SLEEP DISTURBANCES

LEARNING OBJECTIVES

➤ Differentiate between mild, moderate, and severe sleep pattern disturbances.
➤ Identify factors leading to poor sleep and fatigue.
➤ Select appropriate interventions for dealing with sleep pattern disturbances.

GLOSSARY

Fatigue—An overwhelming, sustained sense of exhaustion or lack of energy and decreased capacity for physical or mental work.

Insomnia—Abnormal wakefulness, an inability to fall asleep easily or to remain asleep during the night.

Narcolepsy—An infrequent but serious disorder consisting of recurrent episodes and uncontrollable sleep.

Obstructive sleep apnea—A serious sleep-related breathing disorder manifested by daytime sleepiness or excessive loud snoring. Frequently associated with cardiac dysrhythmias.

Sleep apnea—Sleep-induced respiratory impairment.

Sleep deprivation—Periods without normal sleep pattern, resulting in irritability, fatigue, difficulty concentrating and memory, poor muscle coordination, and sometimes hallucinations and illusion with delirium.

Sleep disorders—Chronic disturbance of sleep patterns affecting the amount, quality, or timing of sleep or events occurring during sleep, such as nightmares.

Sleep drunkenness—Exaggerated transition from sleep to waking, with confusion state lasting 1 to 2 hours or longer, during which perception and judgment are compromised.

Somnolence—abnormal drowsiness or sleepiness during usual waking hours.

Sleep is unconsciousness from which a person can be awakened by sensory stimuli such as sound, light, and touch. Sleep disorders put an individual at risk for experiencing a change in the quantity or quality of rest and sleep as related to biologic and emotional needs. Adverse physical, mental, and emotional changes may occur if normal rest and sleep patterns are interrupted. Most people have suffered from at least transient sleep disturbances. Many factors lead to poor sleep, such as the environment of the sleeping area (levels of sound, light, and temperature), the age and general physical and psychologic condition of the patient, and recent stressful events.

Sleep was considered a homogeneous quiet period with minimal brain activity until the discovery of the electroencephalographic (EEG) record. With this technology, the description of rapid eye movement (REM) and non-rapid eye movement (NREM) periods during sleep and their association with dreaming has provided better understanding of sleep physiology and sleep disorders.

Sleep research has shown that there are two types of sleep during a sleep period: sleep when the brain is very active (REM) and sleep with slow brain waves (NREM). The reason why these two types of sleep exist is unknown. The sleep center is located in the pons and the medulla. Most sleep at night is NREM sleep; it occurs when a person first falls asleep and is a deep and restful sleep.

On the basis of EEG studies, sleep is divided into five distinct stages: REM sleep and four stages of NREM sleep.

Stage 1 NREM: Transition from wakefulness to sleep; about 5 percent of time spent asleep in adults; person feels very drowsy; musculature relaxes.

Stage 2 NREM: Characterized by specific EEG waveforms; occupies about 50 percent of sleep time; muscles relax further; cerebral activity decreases.

Stage 3 NREM: Physiologic changes evident; vital signs decrease; gastrointestinal functions and venous dilation increase to facilitate cellular metabolism and exchange.

Stage 4 NREM: Known as slow-wave, deepest level of sleep with lowest level of body function. Stages 3 and 4 together occupy about 10 to 20 percent of sleep.

During NREM sleep, pulse and respirations drop 20 to 30 percent, blood pressure decreases, muscles relax, skin vessels dilate (increasing heat loss), metabolic rate decreases by 10 to 30 percent, and body temperature decreases. NREM stages 3 and 4 tend to occur in the first half of the night and increase in duration in response to sleep deprivation.

REM sleep occurs cyclically throughout the night, alternating with NREM sleep about every 80 to 100 minutes, lasts about 5 to 30 minutes, and is associated with dreaming that is remembered. REM sleep increases in duration toward the morning. During REM sleep, heart rate and respirations often become irregular and metabolism and temperature increase.

The need for sleep decreases with age: Newborns should sleep 18 or more hours a day, school-age children and teens about 10 to 12 hours, adults 7 to 9 hours, and elderly people about 6 hours per night with additional napping during the day. Sleep needs increase during illness. Lack of sleep results in progressive deterioration of mental functioning, physical fatigue, discomfort, and emotional instability.

More than 100 different disorders of sleeping and waking have been identified. Both the American Psychiatric Association (2000) and the Association of Sleep Disorders have developed a system for classifying sleep disorders into four main categories (Box 19–1).

The term "sleep hygiene" is used to describe a holistic approach to sleeping that encompasses many behaviors. Everyone should practice good sleep hygiene to prevent or relieve insomnia, or simply to safeguard sleep, making it more restful and pleasurable (Box 19–2).

BOX 19–1. Classifying Sleep Disorders

DSM-IV-TR Classification

- Dyssomnias—primary insomnia, primary hypersomnia, narcolepsy, breathing-related sleep disorder, circadian-rhythm sleep disorder (jet lag, shift work)
- Parasomnias—nightmares, sleep terror, sleepwalking
- Sleep disorder related to another mental disorder such as anxiety, grief, depression, psychosis
- Sleep disorders caused by a medical condition and substance-induced sleep disorder

Association of Sleep Disorders Centers Classification

- Problems with falling and staying asleep
- Problems with staying awake (excessive sleepiness)
- Problems with adhering to a regular sleep-wake schedule
- Sleep disruptive behaviors (parasomnias) such as sleepwalking

BOX 19–2. Sleep Hygiene

Suggestions for Increasing Adequate, Restful Sleep

- Establish a regular time for going to bed and getting up in the morning and stick to it, even on weekends and during vacations.
- Use the bed for sleep and sexual relations only, not for reading, watching television, or working; excessive time in bed seems to fragment sleep.
- Avoid naps, especially in the evening.
- Exercise before dinner. A low point in energy occurs a few hours after exercise; sleep will then come more easily. Exercising close to bedtime, however, may increase alertness.
- Take a hot bath about an hour and a half before bedtime. The body temperature then begins dropping rapidly, which may help sleep after that time. (Taking a bath shortly before bed increases alertness.)
- Do something relaxing in the half hour before bedtime. Reading, meditation, and a leisurely walk are all appropriate activities.
- Keep the bedroom relatively cool and well ventilated.
- Do not look at the clock. Obsessing over time will just make it more difficult to sleep.
- A light snack before bedtime can help sleep, but a large meal may have the opposite effect.
- Avoid fluids just before bedtime so that sleep is not disturbed by the need to urinate.
- Avoid caffeine in the hours before sleep.
- Quitting smoking not only brings many health benefits to any smoker, it also eliminates the effects of nicotine that contribute to sleep loss.
- Patients who cannot sleep after 15 or 20 minutes should get up, go into another room, and read or do a quiet activity using dim lighting until they are sleepy again. (Don't watch television, which emits too bright a light.)
- Sleeping alone may be more restful than sleeping with another person. If a person with insomnia is distracted by a sleeping bed partner, moving to the couch for a couple of nights might be useful.
- Take a nap in the early afternoon if needed to stave off drowsiness. But remember that naps can disrupt nighttime sleep. If you must nap, do so for no longer than 30 minutes in the late afternoon.

ETIOLOGY

Many medical and psychiatric conditions may affect the patient's ability to maintain normal sleep pattern. Patients with respiratory conditions, Alzheimer's disease, and chronic pain frequently complain of sleep problems. Anxiety, depression, mania, and delirium are also often accompanied by inability to sleep satisfactorily. Stress and acute grief often cause short-term insomnia.

Before a sleep disorder diagnosis can be made, the patient should have a thorough physical examination; review of all medications (prescribed, illicit, and over the counter); and the person's spouse or bed partner should be asked about the person's sleeping habits. Evaluating a sleep-wakefulness complaint requires a thorough history that considers medical, toxic, and environmental conditions, as well as drug and alcohol use. If tolerance to or excessive use of drugs or alcohol is the likely cause of the insomnia, the patient must undergo withdrawal under careful supervision. Sleep problems are associated with a long list of drugs, including stimulants and alcohol. Hypnotics used over a long period of time can also cause insomnia because of the development of tolerance and suppression of REM sleep.

Sleep lab studies reveal that some patients with obstructive sleep apnea have about 30 episodes of upper airway obstruction each night, resulting in inability to achieve a deep sleep state because of hyperventilation, carbon dioxide retention, and severe hypoxemia. Treatment possibilities include weight loss for obese patients and positive-pressure respiratory treatments to keep the airway open. Surgical intervention (a procedure to remove excess tissue in the pharynx or a tracheotomy) may be required for more serious cases.

Narcolepsy is sometimes accompanied by cataplexy (partial or complete loss of muscle tone), presleep hallucinations, and sleep paralysis. These symptoms are more debilitating than the sleepiness. Specific treatment includes short daytime napping and prescription of a central nervous system stimulant.

Conditions most frequently associated with excessive daytime sleepiness include:

- Regularly sleeping 10 to 14 hours
- Psychophysiologic causes: Transient and situational sleepiness caused by stress, boredom, or depression
- Nocturnal myoclonus, also known as "restless legs" or leg jerking
- Idiopathic CNS hypersomnolence not caused by head trauma
- Sleep drunkenness
- Menstrual cycle-associated syndrome: Increased daytime sleepiness around time of period
- Self-induced insufficient sleep: Related to increased work hours, pressured deadlines, or other self-imposed behavior.

RELATED CLINICAL CONCERNS

Hospital routines and policies, such as how late sleeping medication may be given or how late patients can watch TV, can actually restrict nurses in effectively intervening with the more common sleep disturbance problems. Patients often complain that hospital rules and routines are disturbing to their normal sleep patterns. After just a few days in an unfamiliar environment with multiple sleep interruptions, a patient's usual sleep routine can be almost totally reversed, with the patient sleeping most of the day and awake most of the night (Redeker, 2000).

If the patient's physical condition requires intense nursing care, sleep needs will be secondary until physical stability is achieved. However, the need for sleep and its role in a patient's care plan must not be overlooked, even during acute care periods. Sleep deprivation is a major contributor to ICU psychosis. Anything that can be done by the staff, patient, or family to attain and maintain a better sleep pattern will be beneficial to the patient (Kahn, et al., 1998; Freedman, Kotzer, & Schwab, 1999).

Many medications used to treat medical conditions can contribute to sleep problems, including many asthma medications, cortisone, levodopa, thyroxine, and some chemotherapies. An occasional sleeping pill may be beneficial to patients with a short-term sleeping problem. However, chronic use of sleeping medications is ineffective for most insomniacs (Beck-Little & Weinrich, 1998: Ford & Kamerow, 1989).

LIFE SPAN ISSUES

CHILDREN

Sleep terrors, enuresis, and bedtime fears are more common in toddlers and in children 7 to 12 years old. Sleepwalking and tooth grinding (bruxism) are considered childhood sleep disorders because they are probably developmentally related and usually disappear before or during adolescence.

Children can develop distress at bedtime because of fears of separation and other anxieties. Providing a calm, reassuring routine is important.

ELDERLY PEOPLE

Age is the single most powerful determinant of a person's sleep physiology. As a person ages, sleep becomes more fragmented; a 60-year-old awakens on average 22 times each night compared to about 10 times for a younger person. Sleep disturbances increase with age and change in type during the aging process. Elderly people typically have more trouble falling asleep and awaken frequently throughout the night and early in the morning. They are more easily awakened by noise or other stimuli and are especially prone to drug toxicity with hypnotics because of reduced renal function. Antihistamines are frequently used as safe alternatives. Insomnia is more common in women than men, although older men have more disrupted sleep than older women (Schnelle, et al., 1999).

POSSIBLE NURSES' REACTIONS

- May experience patient-staff conflict because patient states that he or she was awake all night and the nurses reported that the patient had slept.
- May be unwilling to or feel incapable of doing anything about patients' sleep problems.
- May feel that hospital rules cannot be changed and patients will just have to tolerate frequent interruptions.
- May become frustrated because patients who are awake all night require more care. This problem is compounded when staffing is short.

ASSESSMENT

Behavior and Appearance

- Tired, lethargic, depressed, agitated, even delirious, depending on cause and duration of sleep disturbance
- Drawn and pale, with puffy dark circles under eyes
- Frequent yawning, dozing during the day
- Forgetting appointments or responsibilities
- Minor accidents, such as dropping things, hitting self on cupboard or table corners, not being able to complete or misdoing routine tasks

Mood and Emotions

- Changes in mood
- Less tolerance for even minor problems
- More frustrated at difficult tasks
- Severe anxiety
- Irritable
- Angry and hostile
- Depressed

Thoughts, Beliefs, and Perceptions

- Minor errors in memory or ability to calculate
- Confusion
- Inability to retain information
- Inattention and lack of concentration
- Hallucinations, paranoia, or psychotic thinking

Relationships and Interactions

- Spouse or partner complaints about patient's sleep problems
- Changes in sexual relationships
- Change in relationship caused by patient's irritability and fatigue

Physical Responses

- Decreased energy for usual activities
- Daytime sleepiness and napping
- Increased fatigue
- Sleep apnea
- Cardiac dysrhythmias
- Low arterial oxygen levels
- Morning headache
- Less pain tolerance
- Injuries as a result of sleepwalking, narcolepsy, or sleep deprivation

Pertinent History

- History of sleep disturbance
- Medical diagnosis associated with sleep disturbances
- Situation or lifestyle events that affect sleep pattern
- Immobility as a result of casts or traction
- Pain, illness
- Pregnancy
- Anxiety
- Depression
- Lifestyle disruptions, such as changes in occupation, finances, or relationships
- Environmental changes, such as hospitalization or travel
- Use of medication or other chemical substances, such as alcohol, caffeine, tranquilizers, sedatives, hypnotics, antidepressants, antihypertensives, amphetamines, anesthetics, barbiturates, or steroids
- Alternative work schedules such as evening or night shift work

COLLABORATIVE MANAGEMENT

Pharmacologic

Pharmacologic treatment of insomnia generally includes hypnotics and sedatives used for short periods of time. Effective management of pain and other symptoms will enhance sleep also. Using sedatives to induce sleep confounds the sleep stages and may actually lead to worsening of the sleep disturbance and to depression if used for more than a few days or weeks. They inhibit other mental and physical activities, such as respiration, cognition, circulation, digestion, and elimination.

Tricyclic antidepressants, MAO inhibitors, and diazepam, all used at times to enhance sleep, may cause sleep disturbances when discontinued or reduced. With antidepressants and some hypnotics, REM sleep is actually suppressed and, when these medications are discontinued, the REM rebound can cause agitation and frightening dreams.

Herbal remedies include chamomile, kava kava, and St. John's wort. Some herbal products, such as ephedra and ginseng, can contribute to insomnia.

Nonpharmacologic

Cognitive-behavioral therapies, such as relaxation techniques, hypnosis, massage, guided imagery, and even aromatherapy, can break the self-perpetuating nature of some insomnias—"the less you sleep, the more you worry about losing sleep."

Exercise is one of the best ways for persons of all ages to achieve healthy sleep. Light therapy has proven effective for delayed sleep syndrome and jet lag. Shift workers can adjust well by working in bright light and sleeping in a completely darkened room.

Sleep restriction therapy, along with light meals, one-hour exposure to sunlight, and exercise, has been shown to have a long-lasting effect on some patients. A person incrementally decreases the amount of time allowed for sleep until he or she stays asleep 85 percent of the allowed time, after which he or she incrementally increases the allowed sleeping time.

Psychotherapy

Many people are reluctant to seek nonmedical therapy for sleep-related problems. Yet insomnia is commonly caused by emotional stress and mental disorders that can be successfully treated. For those who follow through with treatment, about three-fourths benefit from psychotherapy (DSM-IV-TR, 2000).

NURSING MANAGEMENT

SLEEP PATTERN DISTURBANCE EVIDENCED BY DIFFICULTY FALLING ASLEEP, FREQUENT AWAKENINGS, AND/OR EARLY MORNING RISING RELATED TO SLEEPING IN UNFAMILIAR ENVIRONMENT, POSTOPERATIVE CARE, OR HOSPITAL CARE ROUTINES THAT INTERRUPT SLEEP PATTERN.

Patient Outcomes

- Able to sleep a satisfactory amount of time and awaken feeling rested
- Able to rest between disturbances for required care
- Has enough rest to participate in activities ordered, including pre- and postoperative care and rehabilitation

Interventions

- Assess the patient's sleep for quantity and quality. Ask about patient's normal sleep habits. Determine what is promoting or inhibiting patient's sleep in the new environment.
- To help establish a sense of security, familiarize patient with environment; walk around unit, and describe building.
- Establish a sleep routine for the patient using familiar sleep habits if possible, such as special activities in preparation for sleep, fixing the bedding, or playing music.
- Allow the patient some personal comfortable bedding and pajamas and other personal possessions if available.
- Encourage the use of presleep relaxation measures including back rub, meditation, prayer, soft music, reading, or bedtime snack if patient desires.
- Position patient comfortably; assist in turning and using bathroom as needed.
- Minimize use of caffeine or other stimulants in afternoon and evening.

- Provide a quiet, undisturbed period of sleep with comfortable room temperature and nonglaring, dim lighting if needed.
- Use hypnotics or sedatives only as a last resort or if patient is experiencing unusually stressful events. Do not use more than a few days because sleep patterns can be further disturbed by frequent or chronic use of sleep medication.
- Teach the causes and interventions for sleep disturbance provoked by new environment. If sleep-rest pattern continues to be disturbed after a reasonable amount of time for adjustment, reassess for other possible problems, such as depression or anxiety.
- If possible, assess patient's sleep habits before and after surgery and observe for behavior changes that may indicate sleep deprivation, such as confusion or agitation. Plan nursing care activities with patient to limit number of disturbances and to increase sleep periods within patient safety and postoperative care requirements
- Have staff members on night shift provide the patient with feedback on his or her sleep pattern.

IMPAIRED REST-ACTIVITY PATTERN EVIDENCED BY PACING, AGITATION, INABILITY TO REGULATE ONE'S OWN BEHAVIOR RELATED TO HYPERACTIVITY, HALLUCINATIONS, AND OTHER PSYCHOTIC SYMPTOMS.

Patient Outcomes

- Remains awake during the day
- Sleeps at least 4 hours every night
- Demonstrates appropriate nighttime behavior

Interventions

- Identify factors that increase stimulation to patient and attempt to reduce or eliminate these factors.
- Provide a calming environment.
- Limit coffee and other caffeine-containing foods and drinks such as tea, cola, or chocolate, especially after 4:00 p.m. Encourage use of decaffeinated products.
- Establish a contract with the patient to lie down and remain quiet for a specified period of time at night.
- Discourage daytime naps. During the day, encourage patient to keep drapes open and remain active. Provide structured activities during the day if needed.
- Avoid reinforcing behaviors that encourage being awake at night such as not allowing eating, television, or socializing.
- Administer ordered medications as indicated. Discuss with physician and pharmacist the changing of doses or timing of medications.

ALTERNATE NURSING DIAGNOSES

Anxiety
Fear
Hopelessness
Impaired Gas Exchange
Ineffective Breathing Pattern
Ineffective Individual Coping

WHEN TO CALL FOR HELP

☐ Increased complaints of inability to rest or sleep to the point of physical or mental fatigue affecting patient's ability to participate in treatment or rehabilitation or safely perform daily activities

☐ Onset of delirium, paranoid thinking, or hallucinations related to sleep deprivation

☐ Long-term or episodic misuse or abuse of sedatives or hypnotics

☐ Idiosyncratic response to sleep medication

☐ Evidence of serious complications of sleep apnea, such as chest pain, shortness of breath, cardiac dysrhythmias, or dyspnea

PATIENT AND FAMILY EDUCATION

- Teach patient and/or family about improving sleep hygiene.
- If the patient is using sleep medications, review the potential adverse effects and problems with long-term use.
- Review negative effects of poor sleep habits, especially irregular bedtimes and use of stimulants before bedtime.
- Review the role of diet and exercise in helping enhance sleep.
- Educate patient that sometimes short-term insomnia during times of grief or stress is normal and will usually resolve.

CHARTING TIPS

- Document the patient's reports of poor sleep, increased tiredness, or fatigue.
- Make note of the patient's sleep history and bedtime routines to enhance continuity of care.
- Document the patient's response to sleep interventions.
- Document the use of and response to sleep medications.

COMMUNITY-BASED CARE

- Educate the patient and family about general benefits of a regular sleep schedule and offer suggestions for better sleep.
- Provide referrals, as indicated, to sleep disorder center for patients with obstructive sleep apnea, narcolepsy, or other serious disorders.
- Encourage the patient to minimize use of sedatives and/or hypnotics.
- Provide information about sleep problems to other staff members if patient is transferred to another unit or facility.

THE CHRONICALLY ILL PATIENT

LEARNING OBJECTIVES

➢ Describe some important tasks that a person needs to accomplish to adapt to chronic illness.
➢ List common nurses' reactions to the chronically ill.
➢ Describe appropriate interventions for chronically ill patients with self-care deficit, alteration in self-concept, and impaired social interactions.

GLOSSARY

Acute illness—A condition caused by a disease that produces symptoms and signs soon after exposure to the cause, that runs a short course, and from which there is usually a recovery or an abrupt termination in death.

Chronic illness—A condition not cured by medical intervention and requiring periodic monitoring and supportive care to reduce the degree of illness and to maximize the person's functioning and responsibility for self-care.

Disability—Any long- or short-term reduction of activity that results from an acute or chronic condition.

Exacerbation—Resumption of pronounced symptoms from an illness.

Remission—Period during which the disease is controlled and symptoms are not obvious.

Even though more Americans are affected by chronic illness than acute illness, the U.S. healthcare system focuses more money and research on treating acute illness. In 1995 there were 99 million Americans living with one or more chronic illnesses including arthritis, hypertension, diabetes mellitus, respiratory disease, visual impairments, and mental illness (Robert Wood Johnson, 1996). In addition, heart disease, cancer, and stroke, which are the leading causes of death in adults, can cause major disability and have significant impact on long-term care. Though the highest incidence of chronic illness is in the over-65 population, all ages are affected. By 2005, it is estimated that the number of Americans with chronic illnesses will increase to 112 million. The increase in the chronically ill population is a result of increased life expectancy, new technologies and pharmaceuticals that prolong life with chronic illness, and breakthroughs in treating acute illnesses such as myocardial infarctions and infections.

Unlike acute illness, which is time limited, chronic illness is often permanent, with no definite timetable to give the person a frame of reference to plan for the future. Most chronic illnesses require major adjustments in the individual's lifestyle. The periods of uncertainty, remissions and exacerbation, and in some cases, a slow, steady decline in health can significantly strain the coping mechanisms of the individual and his or her family. Whether the individual and family can continue to cope effectively with the anxiety this creates depends on how long the individual's normal routine can be maintained, how frequently medical crises require treatment, and how easily treatment can be incorporated into the individual's normal lifestyle. In addition, changes in family routines such as caregiver responsibilities, role changes, financial strain, and changes in socializing patterns and sexual relationships significantly influence the psychosocial response to chronic illness.

ETIOLOGY

Chronic illness requires facing a numbers of losses and changes that affect the patient and family. Many psychologic theories address the process of adapting to a chronic illness. *Grief* theory is one of the most significant. During the grieving process, the individual can experience denial, anger, depression, and finally, acceptance.

Denial can occur at the time of diagnosis or during remissions and/or exacerbations as a protective mechanism against the distress and fear created by the disease. Anger occurs as the individual struggles with giving up dreams and hopes because of the illness. Anger can energize the person to try to gain control over the illness. There may be a need to obsessively seek second or third opinions, call information hotlines, use the Internet, talk to others with the condition to gain information on new treatments, and go to extremes to implement lifestyle changes such as diet or giving up smoking. Depression occurs when the individual feels the pain of giving up his or her former healthy self. Experiencing fear, sadness, and discouragement and reminiscing about the past can occur as part of the grieving process. Acceptance occurs gradually and may come and go as the illness changes. If the individual is unable to come to some acceptance, each new limitation will feel like a fresh emotional injury and the person will experience ongoing demoralization.

Poor adaptation to chronic illness can cause noncompliance, dependency, loss of self-esteem, and depression. Noncompliance may be the result of denial, used to protect one's self from having to acknowledge the illness; anger, used to maintain control over the situation; or fear of dependency.

Most patients with chronic illness need to accept a dependent role at some point in their illness, even if it is for a short time with dependence on medication or equipment. However, people who view themselves as weak and vulnerable may become dependent for longer amounts of time, possibly for the rest of their lives.

Because our society values independence so much, adjusting to chronic illness can be a blow to self-esteem when the individual must face relying on others for help. For those individuals who have pre-existing low self-esteem, physical or lifestyle changes such as becoming dependent on medical equipment can negatively affect body image and, ultimately, lowers self-esteem even further. These patients may reject others because they feel unlovable. As they become more isolated, they are at a higher risk for depression.

Miller (2000) identifies 4 factors that influence adjustment to chronic illness:

1. Knowledge of the illness and therapies
2. Coping resources
3. Problem-solving skills
4. Personal mastery as well as motivation

CLINICAL CONCERNS

Chronic illnesses can influence an individual's response to an acute illness and the potential for recovery. For example, persons with chronic pulmonary disease may have difficulty surviving major surgery. The presence of more than one chronic illness often adds to the demands made by even a relatively minor illness.

LIFE SPAN ISSUES

CHILDREN

Up to 20 percent of children have a chronic illness, with the most common being asthma (Copeland, 1993). How the child responds to the illness depends on the child's developmental stage and the parent's response. Under stress the child may regress to a previous developmental stage. Denial, overprotectiveness, rejection, and overcompensating are examples of poor parental responses and can significantly influence the child's adaptation response. The child's illness can cause dysfunction within the family as frequent doctor's appointments, changing living arrangements, and financial stress cause disruption in family life and increase the child's anxiety. Siblings may experience jealousy and resentment for the increased attention to the ill child, embarrassment, shame, fear of becoming ill, guilt from believing they caused the illness, or an extreme sense of overprotectiveness. These feelings are influenced by the parent's response. The sibling may also regress to a previous developmental stage during times of stress.

ADULTS

Chronic illness can be a devastating blow in adulthood, a time when expectations are highest. Many illnesses can impede performance of an important role such as breadwinner or parent.

ELDERLY PEOPLE

The most common chronic illnesses in the over-75 age group include arthritis, hearing impairment, hypertension, heart disease, cataracts, and orthopedic impairment (Ebersole and Hess, 1997). Adapting to chronic illness depends on the resources available to the person, including caregiver availability, financial resources, and living arrangements. Spouses or other supportive people may be chronically ill as well. Advancing chronic illnesses may force elderly persons to move out of the home into unfamiliar surroundings, such as to a retirement home or nursing home. Also, treatment for multiple chronic illnesses can drain one's coping reserves, and the symptoms of one chronic illness such as reduced vision from cataracts affects the management of another one such as being able to give insulin to one's self. Elderly spouses who must be the primary caregivers provide an additional stress and can contribute to poor compliance because of their inability to cope with the illness.

POSSIBLE NURSES' REACTIONS

- May view caring for the chronically ill as depressing because of deteriorating patient health
- May have difficulty defining care goals as optimal maintenance rather than curative.
- May lack empathy and blame noncompliant patient as causing his or her own problems.
- May feel powerless to provide any hope to the patient for the future

ASSESSMENT

Behavior and Appearance

- Obvious disability or change in appearance caused by illness
- Unkempt, poor hygiene because of depression and lack of energy
- May require obvious assistive devices such as oxygen or a wheelchair

Mood and Emotions

- Depressed
- Angry
- May lack emotional reaction as a result of denial
- Guilt over burden created by illness
- Fear and anxiety caused by uncertain future or physical discomfort

Thoughts, Beliefs, and Perceptions

- Powerless to control condition, complications, or side effects
- May generalize view of self as weak and ineffectual into all areas of life
- May think obsessively about his or her health or physical condition
- May view body as unattractive or damaged
- May be able to maintain self-esteem and sense of competence

Relationships and Interactions

- May need to become dependent on others for care, transportation, financial support
- May have difficulty in maintaining personal relationships because of lack of energy, physical discomfort, or embarrassment
- May need to change living arrangements to facilitate care, causing the individual to develop new or changed relationships with others
- May experience changes in sexual relationships because of physical discomfort, loss of energy, or poor self-image
- May experience a sense of social isolation or rejection because friends and family may avoid patient if they are uncomfortable being around someone with a disability

Physical Responses

- These vary depending on specific illness.
- Symptoms must be reassessed frequently because they may or may not be related to the chronic illness.
- Ability to perform activities of daily living can be affected.

Pertinent History

- Past history of chronic illness, other conditions, or disabilities
- History of psychiatric disorders, especially depression and substance abuse

COLLABORATIVE MANAGEMENT

Pharmacologic

Because patients with chronic illnesses are often on multiple medications, there is an increased risk of interactions between medications or between medications and food. Each new symptom needs to be assessed carefully to determine if the cause is the illness or the treatment. For example, confusion and lethargy could be a sign of a deteriorating medical condition or the result of overmedication.

Individuals may utilize a variety of complementary or alternative approaches to deal with symptoms and/or treat the illness.

NURSING MANAGEMENT

IMPAIRED SOCIAL INTERACTION EVIDENCED BY INABILITY TO ESTABLISH AND/OR MAINTAIN STABLE, SUPPORTIVE RELATIONSHIPS RELATED TO LOSS OF BODY FUNCTION BECAUSE OF CHRONIC ILLNESS.

Patient and Family Outcomes

- Patient identifies behaviors that deter socialization.
- Patient demonstrates behaviors that encourage socialization.
- Family provides support to patient.

Interventions

- Assess the patient's support system, living arrangements, and care needs. Identify areas where patient needs assistance in his or her care routine.
- Identify types of behavior that may impede socialization, such as manipulative, dependent, hostile, depressed, or passive-aggressive behavior. As needed, help patient become aware of how these types of behaviors may discourage interactions with others. Explore ways to change these behaviors.
- Encourage patient to share worries and concerns with others, as appropriate. Also encourage patient to make an effort to provide support to family members as they learn to adjust. If the patient consistently focuses others' attention on his or her health problems, give the patient feedback on understanding others' responses.
- Encourage patient to accept help from others, as needed, while maintaining independence within the limitations of the illness.
- Patient may need assistance to express feelings and wishes to his or her caregiver in a nonthreatening way. Role-play with patient. This promotes independence and self-esteem in patient and caregiver.
- Encourage patient and family to be aware of communication patterns when under stress, and explain how these may negatively affect their relationships.
- Allow family to share their concerns and frustrations about the patient with you. Explore with the patient ways to resolve issues. If both agree to participate, consider bringing patient and family together to discuss these issues.
- Encourage patient to participate in activities and interests that do not involve his or her illness.
- Encourage patient to maintain contact with supportive people through phone calls, letter writing, e-mail, and tapes.
- Assist patient in identifying ways to establish new relationships.

> **SELF-CONCEPT DISTURBANCE** EVIDENCED BY SELF-DESTRUCTIVE BEHAVIORS, UNWILLINGNESS TO FACE EFFECTS OF ILLNESS, EXCESSIVE DEPENDENCY, DEPRESSION RELATED TO ALTERATION IN BODY IMAGE FROM CHRONIC ILLNESS.

Patient Outcomes

- Remains as independent as possible within limitations of illness
- Demonstrates acceptance of his or her body by such behaviors as talking positively about self, taking care of own physical needs
- Implements adaptive coping mechanisms

Interventions

- Develop a trusting relationship with patient to encourage sharing feelings with you. Providing privacy and respect for patient's feelings and body will enhance that trust.
- Encourage patient to express feelings and thoughts about the illness and the way the illness has changed self-image.
- Assess the effect of illness on the patient. Clarify misconceptions, myths about illness, treatment, and functional ability. For example, patient may believe the portable oxygen tank cannot be taken in the car, so he or she no longer goes out with friends.
- Help the patient begin to accept self with the new limitations. Involve the patient in own care, gradually increasing those areas for which the patient can take responsibility. Encourage expressing feelings about the illness and body image. As appropriate, involve the family.
- Be aware of what others' behavior communicates to patient. For example, if patient's wife puts on disposable gloves every time she is with patient, she is nonverbally communicating her discomfort being around him. She needs to be encouraged to examine how this behavior affects him.
- Explore the patient's strengths and interests. Provide encouragement to focus on these, not just on the illness. Explore ways to develop former interests that are within his or her functional abilities.
- Encourage participation in rehabilitation and education programs, as appropriate.

> **POWERLESSNESS** EVIDENCED BY NOT PARTICIPATING IN ACTIVITIES OF DAILY LIVING, ANGER, AND DEPRESSIVE BEHAVIOR RELATED TO THE IMPACT FROM CHRONIC ILLNESS.

Patient and Family Outcomes

- Demonstrates participation in care within limitations of illness
- Performs activities of daily living within limitations of illness
- Verbalizes one area in which he or she can have some control

Interventions

- Assess patient's ability to perform activities of daily living and to maintain medical regimen for chronic illness care.
- Identify some aspect of patient's care in which he or she can retain control. Then make sure all caregivers support this.
- Provide needed education and resources to enhance performing these activities to encourage independence.
- Involve family and caregivers in identifying ways to promote independence. Teach them ways to help patient without taking over completely.
- In areas in which patient must be dependent on others, promote patient participation in decision making and timing of care to promote some control.

- To successfully promote independence in an activity, you may need to break down each activity into small segments and then focus on one segment at a time.
- Explore the patient's feelings regarding activities that he or she is no longer able to perform. Encourage the grieving response to express feelings and encourage acceptance. Then explore activities of interest within the patient's functional abilities.

ALTERNATE NURSING DIAGNOSES

Grieving, Anticipatory or Dysfunctional
Ineffective Individual Coping
Noncompliance
Ineffective Family Coping: Compromised
Knowledge Deficit
Hopelessness

WHEN TO CALL FOR HELP

There are indications that the patient is not being cared for adequately, such as poor hygiene, pressure ulcers, poor nutrition, or dehydration.

Patient is not complying with treatment plan, which could lead to life-threatening complications—for example, the patient is not taking insulin or is refusing dialysis.

Patient is demoralized by destructive behavior within his or her family, such as substance abuse.

Severe depression, threat of suicide.

PATIENT AND FAMILY EDUCATION

- Provide appropriate education for the individual's chronic illness and medical regimen.
- Provide information on prevention of complications or progression of the illness.
- Involve family and/or caregivers in this education.
- Teach assertive and problem-solving skills to patient who is dependent on others for much of his or her care to gain a sense of control over health care.
- Review with family ways to promote independence and self-esteem in the patient.
- Teach relaxation techniques as a way to reduce anxiety (see Appendix A).
- Teach family the stages of grieving and ways to cope with these.

CHARTING TIPS

- Document patient and family response to health teaching.
- Note caregiver responses to patient. Use specific examples rather than a subjective opinion of the response.
- Document patient's reaction to illness, prognosis, and body image changes.
- Document patient's participation in treatment plan.

COMMUNITY-BASED CARE

- Involve patient and family in the discharge plan early in treatment.
- Provide specific referrals for additional help in the home or alternative care options as needed.
- Identify equipment patient will need in the home, such as hospital bed or wheelchair, to enhance independence and caregiving.
- Refer patient and family to support programs and self-help groups specific to patient's illness, such as ostomy or stroke groups.
- Refer to counseling as needed.
- Consider home health referrals to assess caregiver's ability to provide care and patient's compliance in the home.
- Communicate with all referring agencies regarding identified problems.
- Encourage seeking out information on the illness from the Internet or library.

THE DYING PATIENT

LEARNING OBJECTIVES

➤ Describe common fears faced by the dying patient.
➤ Describe common nursing staff reactions when caring for the dying patient.
➤ Discuss the role of hospice in the caring for the dying patient and family.
➤ Describe effective nursing interventions to help the dying patient and family.

GLOSSARY

Advance directive—A document prepared by an individual to provide guidance to the healthcare team in the event that the person is no longer capable of making decisions.

Euthanasia—The act by a physician or another person of administering a treatment with the specific intent to end a person's life.

Hospice—A philosophy of care and a program for the terminally ill that focuses on providing dignity, comfort, control, and choices at the end of life. At home or in a facility, hospice care is provided by an interdisciplinary team of specially trained professionals who coordinate services for the patient and family to enhance the quality of life for the time remaining.

Palliative care—Management of patients with active, progressive, far-advanced disease for whom the prognosis is limited and the focus is on care to enhance quality of life. Goals for interventions are generally focused on symptom management.

Physician-assisted suicide—Means provided by a physician to be used by the patient to end his or her life.

Facing the end of life, whether from a prolonged terminal illness, advanced age, or injuries remains the greatest and final challenge. For some people, facing this challenge may be a gradual process as a disease advances; for others it may come suddenly and unexpectedly. With advanced disease, some individuals may be preparing themselves all the way through the course of the illness while others maintain strong optimism or denial.

In the U.S, the acute hospital remains the most common location of death. The National Hospice and Palliative Care Organization reports that, as of 1999, 50 percent of deaths occurred in hospitals, 25 percent at home, and 25 percent in nursing homes. Home deaths are most associated with hospice care. Although most people report that they wish to die at home, the acute hospital remains the most common location at the end of life because some people still pursue aggressive treatment, their wishes about resuscitation are unknown, or the family is uncertain about what to do. Unfortunately, the hospital may not always be the best prepared for providing a peaceful, comfortable setting for patient and family because of the focus on aggressive interventions. More hospitals are now developing palliative care programs to address these issues. Policies need to be in place to address comfort care and provide adequate medications. Families and staff members need to be clear on the appropriate use of analgesics and sedatives at the end of life and that the use of these is different from euthanasia. Wherever the patient is, though, the nurse remains the key person to advocate for the patient's care and provide care and support at the end of life.

The National Hospice and Palliative Care Organization has developed three outcomes that embody quality end-of-life care and can be adapted to any setting:

1. Safe, comfortable dying—providing appropriate symptom management to achieve comfort
2. Self-determined life closure—patient autonomy and participation throughout the process
3. Effective grieving for survivors

These outcomes provide an effective model for healthcare professionals to use when providing care to dying patients.

ETIOLOGY

As a person faces the end of life, coping takes many forms. There are no consistent expected behaviors, although generally the person copes in the same way as he or she has at other times of crisis. For example, if a person has tended to be angry and isolated, it is common to see the same reactions during the dying process. The following are some of the common fears faced by the dying patient and family that influence how they will cope.

Fear of Pain and Suffering   This is often listed as the greatest fear of the dying. Images of loved ones who died in severe pain are particularly associated with cancer. These memories may cloud the perceptions of what the end of life will be like. Fear of pain and suffering has received more attention in the last few years because pain and hospice professionals are attempting to educate the public and healthcare professionals that the vast majority of pain can be treated by relatively simple means (Agency for Healthcare Policy and Research, 1994). Nearly all pain and suffering from end-stage disease can be effectively controlled with the knowledge and technology available today. The experience of pain and suffering can create isolation and depression for the patient and guilt for the family, so addressing this fear is essential to enhance physical and emotional comfort.

Fear of Abandonment   Increasing weakness and loss of control can increase anxiety and a sense of vulnerability in being left alone. This fear can be experienced in relation to the patient's physician, who is less involved once aggressive treatment has stopped. This can even be reinforced if a physician communicates, "There is nothing more to do". It is important for the physician to remain involved throughout the course of the terminal illness. Family members and physicians who feel helpless and anxious may inadvertently avoid the patient to escape distress or because they do not know what to say. It is important to realize how this affects the dying patient.

Loss of Control   Because our society values self-reliance and independence, loss of control is particularly frustrating. Weakness, fatigue, confusion, and distressing symptoms can all contribute to this fear. Individuals who value their independence may try to retain it as much as possible, even to their detriment. For example, a patient who lives alone may refuse to hire a live-in caregiver, even though he or she is no longer able to care for basic needs. Families often struggle to try to help their loved one maintain valued independence, yet provide for their safety. Loss of control can induce feelings of guilt as the patient needs to rely on others. Making the decision to stop aggressive treatment in the face of advanced disease can represent a major loss of control because the patient may feel that he or she is "giving in" to the disease.

Loss of Hope   Hope is a natural part of human existence, and as death approaches, it may be more and more difficult to retain. This can contribute to depression and loss of control. Hoping for a peaceful death and hoping to achieve a specific goal before death are examples of reframing hope at the end of life.

Fear of the Unknown   Death presents the greatest unknown to many people. Questions such as "What will happen to my family, my life plans, my body?" are difficult to face. They are also very difficult for others such as family members and even caregivers. Yet the patient may need to express them. Even though we may not have answers to these questions, providing an environment in which fears can be expressed is a great support. Spiritual support may also provide more comfort at these times.

The dying person also faces grief in facing the loss of his or her self, body, and loved ones. Family members may experience many of these same fears.

RELATED CLINICAL CONCERNS

The three leading causes of death today in the U. S. (U. S. Mortality Use Data, 2000) are:

1. Heart disease
2. Cancer
3. Stroke

All of these causes of death are most often associated with chronic, long-term illness characterized by exacerbations and progressive symptoms. Pain, suffering, and distressing symptoms are all associated with long-term illnesses. Uncontrolled pain is by far the greatest fear and a major contributor to patient wishes for hastening death.

Patients in the final weeks of life report fatigue and weakness as the most disturbing symptoms, contributing to emotional distress.

LIFE SPAN ISSUES

CHILDREN

Addressing the needs of dying children takes a dedicated team experienced in working with children and their families. Because of their young age, children are often medically treated very aggressively until the end, making preparation for death more difficult. Professionals may be ambivalent about when to bring up these issues. Parents, especially younger ones, may have little experience with death and will need special assistance in preparing for it.

Parents and professionals often struggle with how to prepare the child. Adults who do not want to face this may expend most of their energies denying the possibility of the child's death. Children are very sensitive to their parents' reactions and may very well realize what is happening without being told directly. The sick child needs to be approached according to developmental level as to how much he or she can understand. Adults need to stress a sense of comfort, security, and family closeness. A pediatric hospice can provide parental support and education in this area.

Siblings often need special attention at these times, yet their needs may be overlooked because of the crisis with the sick child. Siblings often struggle with many anxieties about their own health, jealousy for the sick child who gets special attention, and even feeling responsible for the illness. As with the sick child, the use of play and drawings can be used to help them express feelings that they are too young to verbalize. Siblings should also be included in the care of the ill child, but still be given permission to live a normal life. Seeking help from pediatric professionals is essential.

ELDERLY PEOPLE

The major developmental task of old age is to prepare for death. Life review, letting go of responsibilities and possessions, and adjusting to health changes are normal parts of the life cycle that elderly people must face. The death of close friends may occur much more frequently as one ages. Women in particular have a greater likelihood of losing their spouse and living alone. Death is not as feared in this age group. For many, a gradual giving up of plans, hopes, and dreams may provide preparation. Maintaining independence for as long as possible, along with respect, support, and good symptom management, are important contributions to good end-of-life care in this population.

POSSIBLE NURSES' REACTIONS

- May become detached from the dying patient to avoid the pain of losing him or her
- May have unrealistic expectations of how the patient should die (e.g., that family members will all get along)
- May fear losing control of own emotions around the patient and family, as well as co-workers
- May fear participating in hastening the patient's death when aggressive symptom management is ordered or when a patient requests that life-prolonging measures such as tube feedings be stopped
- May identify with a patient of similar age or circumstances, leading to more anxiety
- Facing the death of a patient may stir up past unresolved losses for the nurse, leading to feelings of sadness or anger
- May experience intense anger with family of a dying patient who are not providing the type of support the nurse thinks is appropriate

ASSESSMENT

Behavior and Appearance

- Crying, agitation
- Unable to concentrate
- No apparent reaction
- Extreme change in usual behavior patterns
- Life review
- Completing efforts for estate planning, mortuary arrangements, distribution of personal belongings

Mood and Emotions

- Shock, numbness
- Depression
- Anxiety, panic
- Mood swings

- No obvious emotional reaction
- Anger
- Guilt, remorse

Thoughts, Beliefs, and Perceptions

- Maintaining hope for a variety of things, including cure, more time, completion of goals
- Difficulty making decisions
- Denial, avoidance of preparation
- Reviewing one's life work and seeking validation for one's contribution
- Seeking the meaning of one's life
- Pursuing spiritual beliefs, especially regarding the afterlife

Relationships and Interactions

- Seeks support from others
- Fears being alone
- Withdrawal
- Projection of anger onto others
- Need to see loved ones to say good bye
- Wish to resolve past conflicts
- Wish to pass on thoughts, memories, stories to others

Physical Responses

- Disrupted sleep
- Confusion, agitation
- Pain, other symptoms that can be exacerbated by emotions
- Possibility that family may develop symptoms similar to those of patient

Pertinent History

- Unresolved or multiple past losses
- Ambivalent relationship with loved ones
- Tendency to isolate self
- History of psychiatric disorder or substance abuse
- Experiencing traumatic, painful death of a loved one

COLLABORATIVE INTERVENTIONS

Pharmacologic

Adequate pain and symptom management must be achieved before any psychosocial issues can be addressed. The vast majority of pain and other symptoms of end-stage disease can be controlled with analgesics, anxiolytics, antiemetics, and other drugs as needed. Fears about addiction need to be addressed to ensure that no one is allowing needless suffering to occur. Side effects of medications used must also be anticipated and measures used to treat them must be provided.

Because depression and hopelessness can affect the quality of life, antidepressants can be useful at the end of life, even in a patient with only weeks to live. The side effect profile needs to be carefully reviewed before selecting any medications.

Patient and family may use a variety of complementary and alternative approaches to treat the symptoms of advanced disease or even to retain hope for a cure. Shark cartilage, Laetrile, and other unproven methods are sometimes continued at the end of life. The nurse needs to become familiar with possible side effects to help patients and families weigh the risks and benefits of using these products. For example, inserting a nasogastric tube just to administer shark cartilage may be too great a burden given the poor prognosis. Other approaches for relief of pain and other symptoms may include magnet therapy, acupuncture, biofeedback, and hypnosis.

Palliative and Hospice Care

Palliative care provides symptom management and support for patients with life-limiting illnesses when the goal may be to try to prolong life but still focus on comfort. Patients may still be receiving aggressive treatments such as chemotherapy to control symptoms.

Hospice care provides an interdisciplinary approach to care of the dying patient and his or her family when the goal is comfort. Medicare has provided a model for hospice services for patients with less than 6 months to live that has also been adopted by Medicaid in most states as well as by most private insurance companies. The hospice benefit will provide multiple services to patient and family under the direction of a hospice-trained physician and nurse to enhance comfort and support of the patient, family preparation, education, support. and bereavement follow-up, along with the chaplain, social worker, hospice physician, and volunteers.

Spiritual Care

Some people seek out spiritual support when facing the end of life. They may wish to renew past religious ties, address personal suffering, and seek to find meaning to their life and perhaps their suffering. The role of religious leaders and particularly chaplains at the end of life can be an important intervention. Most hospitals, as well as hospices, offer these services.

NURSING MANAGEMENT

ANTICIPATORY GRIEVING EVIDENCED BY DISTRESS AT FACING OWN DEATH, INCLUDING DEPRESSION, ANGER, AND GUILT RELATED TO THE TERMINAL ILLNESS.

Patient Outcomes

- Acknowledges terminal illness
- Expresses concerns, feelings of grief
- Verbalizes feelings of being supported in the grieving process
- Identifies potential coping mechanisms, support systems

Interventions

- Accept grieving behavior. Recognize that responses to grief are highly individual.
- Use open-ended questions and reflection to give the patient the opportunity to share feelings and concerns. Listen for patient readiness to discuss issues concerning death. For example, a patient may say, "I don't think I'll be around much longer". The nurse can respond by saying, "Tell me what you're worried about."
- Recognize that your role may be that of listener if patient needs to vent feelings. Providing an accepting environment to share these feelings is extremely important. Let the patient determine what issues he or she needs to explore. The patient may feel more comfortable discussing his or her grief with a nurse because of not wanting to upset family and friends.
- Facilitate communication between family and patient, if appropriate. Ask patient if he or she would like you to share personal concerns with the family if communication has been blocked. Prepare family for some of patient's concerns if OK with patient.
- Be aware of the need to preserve hope. Recognize that hope may take on many faces in the dying process. It could move from hope for a miracle to hope for less pain to hope to live until a grandchild's wedding. Caution yourself and others not to promote inappropriate hopefulness based on your own needs or discomforts.
- Recognize that behaviors such as frequent demands, criticisms, and frequent questioning may be indicative of patient or family sense of loss of control. Provide those involved with a role in decisions and allow some control where possible. Acknowledge the family's important role as patient advocate.

> **KNOWLEDGE DEFICIT** EVIDENCED BY FREQUENT QUESTIONING, LACK OF KNOWLEDGE OF THE DYING PROCESS RELATED TO FACING THE DEATH OF A LOVED ONE.

Patient Outcomes

- Demonstrates increased awareness of what to expect in the dying process
- Able to identify resources available for assistance
- Expresses questions and concerns

Interventions

- Keep the family informed about the patient's condition. Provide information on what they can do for the patient and what the staff is doing. Discuss with family how they want to be informed about the patient's death. For example, some families want to be called at any sign of deterioration; others want to be notified only of the death.
- Assess family members' understanding of patient's prognosis and awareness that patient will die soon. Then tailor education based on their level of awareness and readiness to accept more information.
- Reassure patient and family about options available to maintain comfort without euthanasia or physician-assisted suicide.
- Support cultural and religious beliefs during the dying process. Recognize that mourners may have rituals that need to be carried out at a death such as chanting or lighting candles.
- Determine patient and family readiness to discuss issues around goals of care. Code status, hospice care, degree of sedation wished, and continuing life-prolonging measures such as TPN or dialysis need to be addressed. Families and patients may need more information on the risks and benefits of all decisions made.
- Talk to family members about what to expect throughout the dying process. Review the symptoms the family may be seeing. When the patient is very close to death, provide information to help them prepare for when death is likely to occur.
- If children are present, ensure that they are included in general discussion to prepare them for what will happen. Speak with the adults away from the children when reviewing some information. Assist them on how to prepare the child. Adults should be encouraged to inform the child's teachers of what is happening.
- Provide information on local hospice programs if appropriate. Give information on bereavement support programs available in the area.
- Remember that family members have other responsibilities such as child care and jobs. Talk with them about how they are managing and support their decisions about when to stay with the patient and when to leave. Assess whether they are getting adequate sleep and nutrition. They may need permission to take care of themselves.
- Once the patient has died, inform family members in private. Give them the opportunity to have some private time with the patient. Assist them in getting other family members to the bedside if possible to provide support. Provide information as appropriate on procedures regarding mortuary arrangements, organ donation, autopsy, and so forth.

ALTERNATE NURSING DIAGNOSES

> Anxiety
> Body Image Disturbance
> Ineffective Family Coping: Compromised
> Ineffective Individual Coping

Powerlessness
Self-Esteem Disturbance
Sleep Pattern Disturbance
Pain
Spiritual Distress (Distress of the Human Spirit)

WHEN TO CALL FOR HELP

- Long periods of depression
- Patient and family avoiding dealing with important issues around end-of-life planning, code status
- Family behavior that affects patient's comfort (e.g., withholding analgesics)
- Patient with suicidal thoughts, requests for physician-assisted suicide or euthanasia
- No emotional reaction to impending death

PATIENT AND FAMILY EDUCATION

- Prepare patient and family for normal stages of grieving.
- Review the role of hospice in end-of-life care.
- Provide information on issues around care such as code status, need for analgesics, side effect management, and so forth.
- Provide information on advance directives. Encourage patient to clarify his or her wishes and share these with loved ones.
- If appropriate, encourage the dying patient to make a videotape, audiotape, memory book, or other form of legacy for the family, especially for young children who might not remember the patient.
- Review the signs and symptoms of death with loved ones throughout the dying process.
- Review information on organ donation, mortuary arrangements, and so forth as needed.
- Educate caregivers on patient care needs.

CHARTING TIPS

- Document grieving behaviors.
- Document patient's pain and comfort level.
- Avoid documenting judgments about patient and family behaviors.
- Document patient and family awareness of prognosis, goals, and wishes.
- Document presence and content of an advance directive.

COMMUNITY-BASED CARE

- Refer to hospice care if patient is going home or to assisted living or a nursing home.
- Refer to support programs for patients with advanced disease as well as bereavement groups for the family.
- Refer to pain clinics, palliative care programs as appropriate.
- Provide legal referrals for completing wills, managing finances.
- Refer family to caregiver support group, education programs.

Psychopharmacology: Database for Patient and Family Education on Psychiatric Medications for Adults

Yoshinao Arai, RN, MN, CS

LEARNING OBJECTIVES

➢ Identify the indications and clinical uses for antianxiety, antidepressant, mood stabilizers, and antipsychotic medications.
➢ List safe administration practices for patients taking these drugs.
➢ Select the appropriate nursing interventions and patient education strategies for patients taking these drugs.

In most cases psychiatric medications do not cure psychiatric disorders, but they can alleviate the symptoms caused by the disorders. The medications can minimize the disturbing impact of mental illness on a patient's ability to function. The ideal treatment outcome is the removal of all the negative impact of the illness on the person's ability to achieve his or her goals in life. This is the purpose of psychopharmacological interventions when augmented with psychoeducation and rehabilitation. Both pharmacologic and nonpharmacologic interventions are effective because they work in the brain to adjust its biochemical brain activity. The resulting biochemical changes in the brain enhance the process of psychiatric rehabilitation in a similar manner to that of neurologic rehabilitation. To attain the best benefits from psychiatric medication, the patient must see how medications can help to eliminate roadblocks in his or her life. This is best accomplished by identifying specific, important target symptoms with each individual patient.

Because many patients are not aware of the difference between reality and symptoms, it is often difficult for them to see a need for the use of medication. If a patient is aware of his or her need for medication, it can be difficult for the patient to assess a medication's efficacy because he or she cannot clearly distinguish what is reality and what is a symptom. Medication education, which is provided only at the beginning of a particular treatment, is not sufficient. Giving written information about a medication may only make the patient feel more anxious. Psychoeducational support should be an ongoing process that helps to maximize the efficacy and safety of the patient's medication regimen. With this support, the patient will be able to value the pharmacological therapies in relation to his or her life goals.

Nonpsychiatric medications are also associated with psychiatric symptoms. Patients who are receiving multiple medications for medical conditions may start to present psychiatric symptoms after the drugs are begun. It is not possible to list all the drugs or drug combinations that could elicit or aggravate psychiatric symptoms, but some are listed in Table 20–1.

This chapter provides the essential information required to help patients understand the value of the medications in terms of the positive impact the medications can create in their lives. This information is presented in the following order:

- Basic Concepts
- Medications for Symptoms of Anxiety Disorders
- Medications for Mood Symptoms
  - Antidepressants
  - Mood Stabilizers
- Medications for Psychotic Symptoms
  - Typical Agents
  - Atypical Agents
- Managing Side Effects of Antipsychotic Agents
- Collaborative Management for Advocacy

TABLE 20–1. NONPSYCHIATRIC MEDICATIONS ASSOCIATED WITH PSYCHIATRIC SYMPTOMS

Type of Drug	Symptoms
Antihypertensive agents	Depression
Antiparkinson agents	Hallucinations, confusion
Anticholinergic/digitalis-like/Cimetidine-like agents	Delirium, confusion
Steroids	Delirium, paranoia, mania, depression, anxiety

- Charting Tips
- Community-Based Care

BASIC CONCEPTS

PHARMACOKINETICS AND PHARMACODYNAMICS

It is necessary to have some basic understanding on what the body does to medications (pharmacokinetics) and what medications do to the body (pharmacodynamics).

Pharmacokinetics

Once a medication is taken orally, intramuscularly, sublingually, transdermally, or intravenously into the bloodstream, it can be eliminated in many different ways. Plasma proteins bind part of the medication, making this part inactive, or not bioavailable. Some of the medication is carried to the kidney, where it may be excreted unchanged in the urine. Some of the medication is carried to the liver, where it is transformed into a more water-soluble, active or inactive metabolite. Once transformed by the liver, the medication may be excreted in the urine or in the bile (then in the feces) and out of the body. Individual differences in the biotransformation via known or unknown mechanisms contribute to the observed wide range of clinical responses to a standard dose.

Pharmacodynamics

Psychiatric drugs can produce clinical responses even when only a small portion of the medication can reach their sites of action, i.e., the receptors in the synapses. The drug molecules can facilitate or inhibit the effect of neurotransmitters by interacting with receptors on neuronal cells in different neurotransmitter systems. These systems are often described by the predominant neurotransmitter present. Examples include the dopamine, serotonin, norepinephrine, acetylcholine, histamine, and gamma-aminobutyric acid systems.

The dopamine system in the brain has been thought to play a major role in causing psychotic symptoms. Blockade of certain types of dopamine receptors has been associated with alleviation of psychotic symptoms. It is recognized that blockade of other types of dopamine receptors causes neurologic or endocrine side effects, as discussed later.

The serotonin system has been thought to be associated with symptoms of depression, anxiety, and hallucinations. It is also postulated that blocking of certain serotonin receptors may be associated with controlling negative symptoms of schizophrenia, as discussed later. However, blocking of other types of serotonin receptors is associated with such side effects as hypotension, sedation, and ejaculatory dysfunction.

The norepinephrine system may be associated with mood and motivation.

Some of the new antidepressants target this system. Blockade of certain norepinephrine receptors is thought to be associated with such adverse effects as postural hypotension, dizziness, tachycardia, and sexual dysfunction.

The acetylcholine system may be associated with memory and smooth muscle functions.

Different types of pharmacologic interactions with the muscarinic type of acetylcholine receptors have been associated with alleviating parkinsonian symptoms or causing such side effects as dry mouth, constipation, blurred vision, urinary retention, ECG changes, and memory impairment.

The histamine system is thought to be associated with the sedative effects of medications that interact with the histamine receptors. It is also postulated that postural hypotension and weight gain can be caused by pharmacologic manipulation of the histamine system.

The gamma-aminobutyric acid (GABA) system in the brain is an inhibitory network that lowers the activity levels of all other neurotransmission systems. The efficacy of the benzodiazepine (BZ) family of medications is associated with their effect of blocking the activity of this system.

MAJOR CATEGORIES OF COMMON PSYCHIATRIC MEDICATIONS

Major advances in psychopharmacology include discoveries of psychiatric uses of chloral hydrate (1860s), barbiturates (1900s), antipsychotic medications (1950s), nonselective (tricyclic) and monoamine oxidase inhibitor antidepressants (1950s), benzodiazepines (BZs) (1960s), lithium (1970s), selective serotonin reuptake inhibitors (SSRIs, 1980s), atypical antipsychotics (1990s), and selective BZ receptor agonists (1990s). Most of these categories of medications are currently in use except the barbiturates, most of which were replaced by relatively safer agents such as BZs.

Commonly used psychiatric medications for adults can be identified under the following conventional categories: antianxiety agents (anxiolytics, sedatives, and hypnotics), antidepressants (older and newer agents), mood stabilizers, antipsychotic agents, and medications to control side effects. The generic and trade names for the medications are listed in boxes in each section. The possible daily dosage ranges (usually in mg/day) are also provided for each drug.

TARGET SYMPTOMS

When the pharmacologic interventions are considered, the treatment team and the patient or family should specifically define the psychiatric symptoms that the drugs of each category are treating.

Refer to the appropriate chapters to review common psychiatric symptoms as targets for pharmacologic treatment. After defining specific target symptoms with the patient or family, each symptom needs to be rated on a 10-point scale before the therapy is started and periodically afterward. This way, both you and the patient or family can keep better track of changes in reactions to medications over time.

PATIENT AND FAMILY EDUCATION

Educational needs of patients and their families should be assessed in the following areas in relation to psychopharmacologic treatments:

- Names of the medications
- When and how to take them
- Expected benefits, i.e., alleviation of target symptoms
- Skills to identify expected benefits
- Time it takes to be able to identify the beneficial effects
- Possible adverse effects
- What to do if the adverse effects are too disturbing to tolerate
- How long the medication(s) should be taken
- Possible drug interactions with alcohol, other medications, nutritional supplements, and so forth
- What to do if the target symptoms worsen

GENERAL CONSIDERATIONS FOR VULNERABLE POPULATIONS

Children

Children are generally more prone to serious disruptions by psychiatric medications that may interfere with development. Their livers and kidneys may not be developed enough to efficiently eliminate the drugs out of the body, although the opposite is generally the case when relatively higher doses are required for efficacy, partly because of children's faster metabolic capacity. Many medications have not been extensively researched in children. For example, even though haloperidol has been studied most of all psychiatric drugs, few controlled studies have been done to obtain data on the efficacy and safety of their use in children.

Elderly People

Elderly persons may be vulnerable to side effects of the medications in general for the following reasons:

- Decreased body water may lead to higher concentrations of the drug.
- Decreased plasma proteins may lead to more active drugs not being bound to proteins in the bloodstream.
- Increased portion of fat in the body may cause retention of very fat-soluble psychiatric medications and prolong elimination half-life.
- Decreased liver and kidney function may also prolong elimination half-life.

MEDICATIONS FOR SYMPTOMS OF ANXIETY DISORDERS

Certain clusters of anxiety symptoms can suggest various anxiety disorders (Table 20–2). However, anxiety symptoms are also common in most other psychiatric disorders such as schizophrenia, major depression, and bipolar disorders. In this case, the primary conditions need to be treated as well. The

TABLE 20–2. COMMON SYMPTOMS OF ANXIETY

Origin	Symptom
Physical symptoms of brainstem origin	Fatigue, cold chills, headaches, difficulty breathing, difficulty sleeping, dizziness, shaking, sweating, muscle tension, restlessness, GI disturbances, numbness in fingers and toes, and palpitations
Emotional symptoms of limbic system origin	Nervousness, fear, panic, apprehension, feeling detached from part of own body, or feeling that the surroundings are unreal
Cognitive symptoms of neocortical system origin	Intrusive thoughts or concerns about losing one's mind, losing control, frightening scenes, having physical illnesses, being inadequate, being disapproved, fainting, difficulty concentrating

same is true for anxiety symptoms that are secondary to other medical disorders such as mitral valve prolapse, hyperthyroidism, arrhythmia, inner ear disease, asthma, or to use of substances such as cocaine, caffeine, methamphetamines.

The most common antianxiety medications include anxiolytics, sedatives, and hypnotics. These include BZs and nonBZs (Box 20–1). Other categories

---

BOX 20–1. Most Common Antianxiety Medications

Benzodiazepines	Dosage
chlordiazepoxide (Librium)	15–100 mg/day
diazepam (Valium)	2–60 mg/day
lorazepam (Ativan)	0.5–6 mg/day
oxazepam (Serax)	30–90 mg/day
temazepam (Restoril)	7.5–30 mg hs
alprazolam (Xanax)	0.25–10 mg/day
flurazepam (Dalmane)	15–30 mg hs
clonazepam (Klonopin)	0.25–10 mg/day
Non-Benzodiazepines	
zolpidem (Ambien)	5–15 mg hs
zalepron (Sonata)	5–20 mg hs
Antihistamines and Anticholinergics	
diphenhydramine (Benadryl)	25–50 mg hs
Serotonin Antagonist	
buspirone (BuSpar)	15–60 mg/day

of medications for anxiety include antidepressants and beta blockers. In addition, some herbal products, including kava kava and valerian, are used.

HYPOTHESES ON MECHANISMS OF ACTION

The mechanisms of action of anxiety medications are unknown. However, two hypotheses on how medications alleviate anxiety symptoms involve the serotonin and GABA-BZ neurotransmission systems.

The serotonin system is supposed to be one of the mediators of a "fear network," which involves the brainstem, the hypothalamus, and the amygdala. The amygdala is a critical temporal lobe structure associated with the expression of anxiety and mammalian stress responses. It is hypothesized that medications influencing the serotonin system desensitize the "fear network" (Gorman, JM, et al, 2000).

The GABA system has an inhibitory function on the brain. When its function is enhanced by coupling of the BZs with the GABA-BZ receptors on surfaces of neurons, neurotransmissions are inhibited in most parts of the brain. Thus, some overexcitation can be leveled off to aid relaxation.

EFFICACY IN TREATING SYMPTOMS

Anxiety Symptoms

Anxiety symptoms respond well to BZs such as lorazepam (Ativan), clonazepam (Klonopin), chlordiazepoxide (Librium), diazepam (Valium), and alprazolam (Xanax). However, if it is expected that the symptoms will require treatment for more than several weeks, antidepressants or buspirone (BuSpar) will become the first drugs of choice. BZs can be used on a PRN basis or only for the first several weeks until the antidepressant or buspirone takes effect because of the possible development of dependence on BZs.

Among the antidepressants used for anxiety, serotonergic agents such as paroxetine (Paxil), fluoxetine (Prozac), sertraline (Zoloft), and fluvoxamine (Luvox) are thought to be the best choices as primary medications for long-term treatment of most anxiety symptoms. Other medications for anxiety include some beta-adrenergic blockers such as propranolol (Inderal) or anticonvulsants such as gabapentin (Neurontin) (Pollack, MH, et al., 1998).

Anxiety-Related Insomnia

BZs used as central nervous system (CNS) depressants reduce anxiety (anxiolytic effect) at lower doses and produce sedative effects at slightly higher doses. Most BZs also induce sleep (hypnotic effect) at higher doses. However, unlike the case with barbiturates, the central nervous system depressant effect of BZs does not increase to cause coma or death, even if the doses are further increased, as long as they are not used with other CNS depressants such as alcohol.

BZs generally have rapid onsets (i.e., 15–60 minutes after oral administration) except temazepam (Restoril) which may take 45 to 120 minutes to begin taking effect. The long half-life (48–150 hours) of flurazepam (Dalmane) is associated with morning hangover.

COMMON SIDE EFFECTS OF ANXIOLYTICS, SEDATIVES, AND HYPNOTICS

Disinhibition   BZs can cause behavioral dysfunction, including irritability and personality changes. Children, adolescents, and elderly people may be more prone to this paradoxical side effect.

Cognitive Deficits   High-potency BZs such as lorazepam (Ativan), clonazepam (Klonopin), and alprazolam (Xanax) are associated with memory impairment. These BZs may exacerbate preexisting cognitive impairment.

Dependence   The use of BZs as hypnotics for temporary insomnia should be for a maximum of 2 to 4 weeks only. Continued efficacy may last as long as 5 weeks, but there is no guarantee of efficacy afterwards. For persistent insomnia, regular or intermittent use of BZs as hypnotics should be reevaluated every 2 to 4 months. In the case of zolpidem (Ambien) or zaleplon (Sonata), the duration of use should be 7 to 10 days with reevaluation if the use exceeds 2 to 3 weeks. Rebound insomnia is unlikely except at doses higher than 20 mg of zolpidem or zaleplon.

Withdrawal Symptoms   Anxiety symptoms, delirium, seizures.

Overdose   Ataxia, hypotonia, nystagmus, coma.

Respiratory Depression   Use of BZs for sleep disturbance caused by sleep apnea can worsen the respiratory condition. Concomitant use with alcohol, tricyclic antidepressants, anticonvulsants, or clozapine (Clozaril) may increase sedative effects or cause respiratory depression.

RELATED CLINICAL CONCERNS

Children

Very few studies have been done to obtain data on the safety and efficacy of anti-anxiety medications for children and adolescents. The use of any kind of sedatives in sleep disturbances is not well investigated in controlled studies in children.

Elderly People

The best choices for anti-anxiety medications in elderly persons are short-acting, low potency agents without active metabolites, such as oxazepam (Serax). The minimum effective dose is 50 percent of the usual adult dose. This should be given PRN only for 1 to 2 weeks.

Pregnancy

The association of fetal damage with BZs is controversial (Barki, et al, 1998). However, it is recommended that BZs be tapered off sufficiently before delivery to minimize neonatal and infant withdrawal. Lorazepam (Ativan) and oxazepam (Serax) have less potential for accumulation in neonates. BZs at relatively low doses are not contraindicated in nursing mothers (Rubey & Lydiard, 1999).

Dual-Diagnosis Patients Who Have Both Psychiatric Disorders and Substance Abuse Problems

Avoid using BZs and tricyclic antidepressants (TCAs). Instead, use SSRI antidepressants, beta blockers (e.g., propraonolol) or anticonvulsants (e.g., gabapentin) for anxiety symptoms. BZs tend to be abused by this population. TCAs may have additive cardiotoxicity when they are taken with cocaine.

Use of SSRIs for Obsessive-Compulsive Disorder (OCD)

Higher doses of SSRIs such as fluoxetine (Prozac) 40 to 80 mg/day or paroxetine (Paxil) 40 to 60 mg/day) can be useful. Clomipramine (Anafranil) has not been the first choice of treatment because of its poor side effect profile.

PATIENT AND FAMILY EDUCATION

- Advise patient to avoid discontinuing BZs abruptly to avoid rebound or withdrawal symptoms.
- Advise patient to avoid adjusting dosing of BZs without consulting prescriber for the above reason.
- Teach patient that, unlike BZs, buspiron (BuSpar) has no tolerance or dependence effects.
- Teach patient that beta blockers can cause bradycardia or exercise intolerance.
- Tell patient not to take BZs with alcohol or OTC medications for insomnia.
- Teach patient to avoid making important decisions if BZs disturb concentration.

MEDICATIONS FOR MOOD SYMPTOMS

There are two categories of medications for mood symptoms: One is antidepressants, which are indicated for symptoms of depressive episodes; the other is mood stabilizers, which are indicated for symptoms of manic episodes.

ANTIDEPRESSANTS

The antidepressants include the older agents (tricyclic antidepressants and monoamine oxidase inhibitors), which were most used in the 1960s through the 1980s; and the newer ones (SSRIs and new agents), which are gradually replacing the older ones as the treatment of choice for various symptoms of depressive and anxiety disorders (Box 20–2). This change occurred because the newer agents have better side effect profiles than the older ones, as discussed later (Box 20–3).

Hypotheses on Mechanisms of Action

The exact mechanisms of action of antidepressants are unknown, but the following are hypotheses concerning the various types of antidepressants.

Tricyclic Antidepressants TCAs may work by affecting serotonin, norepinephrine, and dopamine neurotransmitter systems. Their side effects may be caused by interaction with muscarinic cholinergic receptors.

Monoamine Oxidase Inhibitors MAOIs potentiate neurotransmitters by inhibiting the function of the enzyme monoamine oxidase (MAO), which inactivates neurotransmitters. Inhibition of MAO, which is present in the central nervous system, gut, and platelets, may lead to increased absorption of tyramine, which can act as a false neurotransmitter and elevate blood pressure. Therefore, a tyramine-free diet is required with the use of MAOIs.

BOX 20–2. Target Symptoms of Depression

- **Apparent/reported sadness:** Sad mood reflected in speech, posture, and facial expressions. Depressed mood reported nonverbally regardless of the verbal messages (e.g., looks distressed but brightens up at times; appears miserable all the time).
- **Anhedonia or inability to experience pleasure:** Reduced interest in surroundings or activities that used to give pleasure (e.g., failure to feel any positive emotions).
- **Change in appetite:** Reduced desire for food or increased need to force oneself to eat (e.g., slightly reduced interest in food; eating because one has to).
- **Change in sleep pattern:** Reports experience of reduced duration or depth of sleep (e.g., slight dissatisfaction with sleep; sleep less than 3 hours a night).
- **Inner tension:** Feelings of vague discomfort, restlessness, or edginess leading to dread or panic (e.g., occasional edginess, irritability, restlessness; overwhelming panic).
- **Difficulty getting started:** Slowness initiating or performing daily activities (e.g., some sluggishness; unable to do anything without help).
- **Negative thoughts:** Representing thoughts of guilt, remorse, or inferiority (e.g., ideas of low self-esteem, failure, self-accusations; absurd and unshakable pessimism).
- **Poor concentration:** Representing difficulties in comprehending messages (e.g., difficulties in reading; inability to follow a conversation).
- **Thoughts on death:** Stating that a natural death would be welcome, that life is not worth living (e.g., weary of life; ending own life is considered as a possible option; active preparation for suicide).

BOX 20–3. Antidepressants

Older Agents

Tricyclic Antidepressants (TCAs) and their derivatives	Dosage
imipramine (Torfanil)	50–300 mg/day
amitriptyline (Elavil)	50–300 mg/day
clomipramine (Anafranil)	50–250 mg/day
doxepin (Sinequan)	25–300 mg/day
amoxapine (Ascendin)	50–300 mg/day
desipramine (Norpramin)	50–300 mg/day
nortriptyline (Pamelor/Aventyl)	25–150 mg/day

Monoamine oxidase inhibitors (MAOIs)

phenelzine (Nardil)	15–90 mg/day
tranylcypromine (Parnate)	10–60 mg/day

Newer Agents

Selective Serotonin Reuptake Inhibitors (SSRIs)

fluoxetine (Prozac)	20–80 mg/day
fluvoxamine (Luvox)	50–300 mg/day
paroxetine (Paxil)	10–60 mg/day
sertraline (Zoloft)	50–200 mg/day
citalopram (Celexa)	20–60 mg/day

Non-SSRIs

Serotonin and Norepinephrine Reuptake Inhibitor (SNRI)	
venlafaxine (Effexor)	75–375 mg
Serotonin 2A Blocker	
nefazodone (Serazone)	50–600 mg/day
trazodone (Desyrel)	200–600 mg/day
Serotonin 2A/C and Norepinephrine (alpha-2) Blocker	
mirtazapine (Remeron)	15–45 mg/day
Dopamine and Norepinephrine Reuptake Inhibitor	
bupropion (Wellbutrin, Zyban)	75–450 mg/day

Selective Serotonin Reuptake Inhibitors   SSRIs enhance serotonergic transmission, increasing serotonin in the synaptic clefts between neurons. This is caused by accumulation of serotonin in the cleft as the drug blocks the reuptake of serotonin back into the neuron.

Newer Agents (Non-SSRIs)   Bupropion (Wellbutrin) is thought to work by inhibiting norepinephrine reuptake in addition to its effect on dopaminergic transmission. Venlafaxine (Effexor) is a selective inhibitor of serotonin and norepinephrine reuptake. Nefazodone (Serzone) is thought to work by antagonizing serotonergic and alpha-1 adrenergic receptors.

Efficacy in Treating Symptoms

All antidepressants have equal efficacy on symptoms of depressive episodes. Improvement of mood may not be observed for 2 to 6 weeks. Selection of agents is based on the agents' different side effect profiles and the patient's tolerance to them. There is no reliable method to predict which patients will respond better to a specific agent. The factors to consider for agent selection include the patient's age, suicide potential, concurrent use of medications, and coexisting diseases. For example, SSRIs are safer in patients with a history of cardiac diseases or suicidal ideations. If the patient or a first-degree relative has had a good response to a certain agent in the past, another trial of the same agent is an option because the agent may be compatible with the individual's metabolic capacity.

Common Side Effects of Antidepressants

Tricyclic Antidepressants and Monoamine Oxidase Inhibitors   The major side effects of TCAs and MAOIs are lethargy, orthostatic hypotension, and anticholinergic symptoms (Table 20–3). These side effects tend to increase during the first month of treatment, but usually subside with time. The anticholinergic side effects include dry mucosa (mouth, nose, or vagina), blurred vision, urinary retention, poor memory, and impaired concentration. These can be caused by TCAs, MAOIs; low-potency antipsychotics such as thioridazine (Mellaril) and chlorpromazine (Thorazine), clozapine (Clozaril) (except dry mouth), and anticholinergic medications such as benztropine (Cogentin) and trihexyphenidyl (Artane). These disturbing side effects must be managed to enhance compliance with the treatment (Table 20–4).

Selective Serotonin Reuptake Inhibitors   The common side effects of these agents include insomnia, sexual dysfunction, and agitation or restlessness. These are mediated by their interactions with the serotonin neurotransmission system. SSRI-induced insomnia may respond to trazodone (Desyrel). The newer non-SSRI agents (bupropion, nefazodone, and mirtazapine) are associated with lower risks of sexual dysfunction. In akathisia-like restlessness, the dose may need to be reduced. Switching to another agent may be needed if the symptom is severe and persistent.

SSRI Discontinuation Syndrome   Abrupt discontinuation of paroxetine or fluvoxamine can result in dizziness, nausea, irritability, headaches, or cholinergic rebound symptoms (e.g., salivation, loose stools).

TABLE 20–3. COMPARING SIDE EFFECTS OF SSRIs AND TCAs-MAOIs

Side Effects	SSRIs	TCAs/MAOIs
Orthostatic hypotension	Low	High
Sedation, weight gain	Low	High
Anticholinergic effects	Low	High

TABLE 20–4. MANAGING ANTICHOLINERGIC AND OTHER COMMON SIDE EFFECTS OF ANTIDEPRESSANTS

Anticholinergic Side Effects	Management
Dry mouth	Use sugarless gums or candies. Carry a bottle of water and sip it frequently. Emphasize need for extra good dental and oral hygiene. Worse during the initial period of treatment.
Urinary retention	Report any problem on urination (e.g., dribbling, urgency, hesitancy, retention, etc). Monitor urinary patterns, especially for confused patients. Consult prescriber if the disturbance is persistent.
Constipation	Monitor bowel movement patterns. help patient to have a high fiber diet, maintain sufficient fluid intake, and exercise regularly. Consult prescriber for possible use of stool softeners.
Blurred vision	If persistent and disturbing, consult prescriber for possible medication adjustment.
Poor memory and concentration	If persistent and disturbing, consult prescriber for possible medication adjustment.

Other Side Effects	Management
Sedation	Symptom will usually subside with time. Monitor sleep patterns and related habits to eliminate factors adversely affecting sleep hygiene. May need to avoid driving.
Weight gain	Weigh patient monthly. Monitor diet patterns. Help patient to incorporate regular exercise in daily routines. Consult prescriber if weight gain is persistent despite application of practical measures as above.
Sexual dysfunction	Assess baseline sexual activity level and deviation from it. Consult prescriber if the deviation is too disturbing to tolerate.
GI upset	Take medications with or after meals.
Orthostatic hypotension	Monitor orthostatic BP regularly. Instruct patient to rise slowly when changing positions and to take sufficient fluid. Consult prescriber if BP is less than 90/60.

Other Side Effects of Specific Antidepressants

Agranulocytosis   Mirtazapine (Remeron) can cause agranulocytosis or neutropenia in 1 in 1000 patients. It should not be used with bone marrow suppressing agents such as carbamazepine (Tegretol) or clozapine (Clozaril).

Priapism   The incidence of priapism with trazodone (Desyrel) is 1 in 6000 patients. If the erection persists longer than 1 hour, emergency room treatment is required. If not treated promptly, priapism may result in permanent impotence.

Hypertension   Venlafaxine (Effexor) is associated with higher risks of hypertension.

Seizure Bupropion (Wellbutrin) and clomipramine (Anafranil) have been associated with higher risks.

Related Clinical Concerns

Elderly People TCAs are of particular concern because of their anticholinergic side effects in this age group. Urinary retention is a concern for men with enlarged prostates. The general rule is to start patient on very low doses and increase the dose slowly.

QRS Prolongation A 1-week supply of TCAs may be fatal if taken all at once to reach two to six times therapeutic levels in blood (i.e., 500–1000 ng/ml).

Depressive Episodes Caused by Medical Conditions Psychiatric symptoms of depression can be part of the clinical presentation of non-psychiatric illnesses such as Addison's disease, AIDS, asthma, heart failure, Cushing's disease, diabetes, hyper/hypothyroidism, infectious hepatitis, and malnutrition. Psychiatric medications may be tried to manage the symptoms while the underlying medical conditions are being treated.

Mania All antidepressants can cause mania in patients with bipolar disorder.

Monoamine Oxidase Inhibitors and Food Interactions MAOIs can cause high blood pressure, nausea, vomiting, and headaches as reactions with foods containing tyramine (Table 20–5). All perishable foods (vegetables, fruits, and meats) should be as fresh as possible. The special diet needs to be continued for 4 weeks after the medicine is discontinued.

Pregnancy TCAs and SSRIs have shown no statistically significant evidence of increased risks for congenital defects or teratogenicity. MAOIs are associated with higher risks.

TABLE 20–5. FOODS TO AVOID WHEN USING MAOIs

Food Categories	Foods to Avoid
Bread, cereals, pasta	Yeast extracts
	Brewer's yeast
Fruits	Overripe and spoiled fruits
Vegetables, beans	Broad bean pods. sauerkraut, Italian green beans
Meats, fish	All aged, dried, fermented, salted, smoked, and pickled meats and fish
	All processed meats
Milk, yogurt, and cheese	All aged cheese
	Soybean products (e.g., tofu, soybean milk)
Sweets, condiments, beverages	Meat and yeast extracts
	Sherry, vermouth, beer, ale, red wine
	Soy sauce

Use of St. John's Wort (Hypericum) St. John's Wort is an herbal product used for treatment of depression. Its mechanism is unclear. Not enough controlled studies have been done to support its efficacy. It is contraindicated in pregnancy, lactation, and cardiovascular disease. Because of its possible MAOI-like activity, caution is required regarding its adverse reactions with serotonergic or sympathomimetic agents and foods containing tyramine.

Patient and Family Education

- Teach patient that it may take several weeks before alleviation of target symptoms can be identified.
- Teach patient that the side effects tend to subside with time. The patient needs to work closely with the treatment team to minimize the discomfort during the early phase of treatment.
- Teach patient that the prescriber should be consulted before starting any other medications or dietary supplements while taking SSRIs or MAOIs.
- Advise patient that dietary precaution is crucial to avoid hypertensive crises while taking MAOIs.
- Teach patient that persistent symptoms such as headaches, nausea, insomnia, agitation, or rashes should be reported to the prescriber.
- Advise patient to report any sign of priapism to the treatment team or ER immediately.
- Advise patient to avoid alcohol while taking Bupropion (Wellbutrin) because of increased seizure risk.

MOOD STABILIZERS

Lithium is still the first-line choice for symptoms of manic episodes, although other agents are available from the category of anticonvulsants. When lithium is not tolerated because of its side effects, divalproex (Depakote) or carbamazepine (Tegretol) can be tried (Box 20–4). Other newer anticonvulsants such as gabapentin (Neurontin) or lamotrigine (Lamictal) are being tested. The anti-

---

BOX 20–4. Mood Stabilizers and Anticonvulsants

Mood Stabilizers	Dosage
lithium (Eskalith, Lithobid)	900–2100 mg/day
Anticonvulsants	
carbamazepine (Tegretol)	600–1200 mg/day
divalproex (Depakote)	1500–2500 mg/day
gabapentin (Neurontin)	900–3000 mg/day
lamotrigine (Lamictal)	100–400 mg/day

hypertensive agent verapamil (Calan) has also been used with some success when patients cannot tolerate the side effects of other mood stabilizers.

Hypotheses on Mechanisms of Action

Lithium (Eskalith, Lithobid)   Lithium's exact mechanisms of action are unknown. It appears to enhance the serotonergic transmissions. It also affects the norepinephrine system by increasing its function in some parts of the brain and decreasing it in others. It also affects membrane permeability and ionic transport. Its inhibition of intracellular enzymes is also studied as a possible mechanism of action.

Carbamazepine (Tegretol)   The mechanism of action of carbamazepine is unknown. It may be related to GABA level changes.

Divalproex (Depakote)   Divalproex decreases GABA metabolism to result in increased GABA in the CNS.

Efficacy in Treating Symptoms

Lithium (Eskalith, Lithobid)   The therapeutic effect of lithium may take 4 to 8 weeks to achieve. Serum levels of 0.5 to 1.2 mEq/L are recommended.

Carbamazepine (Tegretol)   The therapeutic effect of carbamazepine may take 2 to 4 weeks. The correlation between clinical responses and serum levels is not established, although plasma levels of 8 to 12 μg/ml are suggested.

Divalproex (Depakote)   The therapeutic effect of divalproex may take 2 to 4 weeks after plasma levels of 50 to 120 μg/ml are reached.

Common Side Effects

Lithium (Eskalith, Lithobid)   Toxic reactions to lithium can occur even within the therapeutic range (Box 20–5). It may produce toxic effects in patients who use diuretics or who have renal failure, hyponatremia, diarrhea, dehydration, and so forth. Long-term toxic effects can include diabetes insipidus, hypothyroidism, leukocytosis, hypotension, and so forth.

Carbamazepine (Tegretol)   Toxic effects with carbamazepine include leukopenia, aplastic anemia, gastrointestinal (GI) disturbances, sedation, blurred vision, vertigo, rash, arrhythmia, and hepatitis.

Divalproex (Depakote)   Toxic effects with divalproex include sedation, nausea, vomiting, tremor, GI upset, weight gain, ataxia, headache, hair loss, rash, clotting abnormalities, transient transaminase elevation, and false abnormality in thyroid function test.

BOX 20–5. Possible Side Effects and Toxic Effects of Lithium

- **Toxic effect from elevated blood level:** Persistent diarrhea, vomiting, coarse trembling of hands or legs, frequent muscle twitching in the arms or legs, blurred vision, confusion, severe discomfort, weakness, severe dizziness, seizure, coma, death.
- **Long term:** Hypothyroidism with swelling of the gland, sleepiness, feeling cold, unusual weight gain, headache, tiredness, cold fingers and toes, menstrual changes, dry puffy skin, constipation, muscle aches, slow thinking.
- **Initial adjustment period of several weeks:** Increased thirst, dry mouth, increased urination, mild nausea, worsening of acne or psoriasis, metallic taste, weight gain, occasional loose stools, mild dizziness, decreased sexual desire, slight muscular weakness, sleepiness, fine tremor in hands, mild stomach cramps.

Related Clinical Concerns

Managing Safety in Lithium Therapy   Lithium use must be monitored closely to prevent complications. Patients need an initial laboratory screening including complete blood count (CBC), thyroid levels, creatinine, blood urea nitrogen (BUN), electrolytes, glucose level, and an electrocardiogram (ECG). Then regular lithium blood levels need to be drawn to maintain a 0.5 to 0.8 mEq/L blood level after the acute phase is resolved. For the first month on lithium, blood levels are drawn weekly, then biweekly, and then every 2 to 3 months for maintenance once a stable level is achieved.

Causes of increased lithium levels include:

- Decreased intake of dietary sodium
- Sweating or dehydration
- Concurrent medications such as thiazides, amiloride, furosemide, ibuprofen, tetracyclines, methyldopa, and metronidazole

Contraindications include pregnancy, lactation, and history of myocardial infarction.

Managing Safety in Carbamazepine Therapy   For patients starting on carbamazepine therapy, the initial workup should include CBC with platelets, liver function tests, electrolytes and BUN, and an ECG in patients over 40 or with a history of cardiac problems.

Dosing should not increase by more than 200 mg/day until 800 mg/day is reached. These patients need to be monitored for possible blood dyscrasias and require periodic CBCs, liver function tests, and drug level tests. Many drugs contribute to increased blood levels of carbamazepine. Review other medications with a pharmacist. MAOIs should not be prescribed for 2 weeks before or after carbamazepine. Monitor closely for signs of infection.

Contraindications include a history of bone marrow suppression; glaucoma; cardiac, hepatic, or renal impairment; pregnancy and breast-feeding; and a history of allergic reactions to TCAs.

Managing Safety in Divalproex Therapy   Initial screening should include CBC, liver function tests, and prothrombin time/partial thromboplastin time. A major concern is the risk for hepatic failure; therefore, the patient needs to have periodic liver function tests and be monitored for symptoms such as jaundice and weakness during the first 6 months of therapy. Because clotting problems can also occur, patients need to be advised to avoid aspirin products and warfarin. In addition, some drugs such as cimetidine, fluoxetine, and amitriptyline can increase the blood levels of this drug. Divalproex is contraindicated during pregnancy and lactation and in the presence of any liver disease.

Patient and Family Education

- Teach patient to adhere strictly to lithium or carbamazepine therapy regimen.
- Advise patient to consult prescriber before starting any new medications or nutritional supplements.
- Teach patient how to avoid possible adverse interactions.
- Advise patient and family that lithium should be taken with food or milk to avoid GI irritation.
- Teach patient the lithium side effects that should be reported to the treatment team.
- Teach patient to avoid any significant changes in diet patterns or salt intake when taking lithium.
- Advise patient that, if a dose is missed, it is all right to continue with the next dose.
- Teach patient how to replace loss of fluids and electrolytes after diarrhea or vigorous exercise.
- Teach patient that OTC analgesics (e.g., ibuprofen and other nonsteroid anti-inflammatory agents) should be avoided while taking lithium.
- Advise pregnant patient that no mood stabilizers should be taken during pregnancy because of the risk of birth defects.
- Teach patient that flulike symptoms that occur while taking carbamazepine should be reported to the treatment team.
- Teach patient that easy bruising or bleeding, pallor, or weakness should be reported to the treatment team.

MEDICATIONS FOR PSYCHOTIC SYMPTOMS

Antipsychotic medications are divided into two primary categories, typical and atypical agents (Box 20–6).

Even though both groups are effective against the positive symptoms of schizophrenia, such as delusions and hallucinations, atypical agents are supposed to have greater efficacy against negative symptoms or deficits in function, such as social withdrawal and blunted affect. Atypical agents have a bet-

---

BOX 20–6. Antipsychotic Medications

Typical Agents	Dosage
chlorpromazine (Thorazine)	200–800 mg/day
thioridazine (Mellaril)	200–800 mg/day
fluphenazine (Prolixin)	10–40 mg/day
trifluoperazine (Stelazine)	5–60 mg/day
haloperidol (Haldol)	5–20 mg/day
perphenazine (Trilafon)	4–60 mg/day
fluphenazine decanoate (Prolixin Decanoate)	12.5–75 mg/2 wks
haloperidol decanoate (Haldol Decanoate)	50–300 mg/4 wks
pimozide (Orap)	1–10 mg/day (Note: Pimozide is indicated for suppression of severe motor and phonic tics in Tourette's syndrome.)
loxapine (Loxitane)	50–250 mg/day
molidone (Moban)	50–225 mg/day
thiothixene (Navane)	5–60 mg/day

Atypical Agents	
clozapine (Clozaril)	300–900 mg/day
risperidone (Risperdal)	2–8 mg/day
olanzapine (Zyprexa)	5–30 mg/day
quetiapine (Seroquel)	300–800 mg/day

---

ter side effect profile, with relatively less risk of extrapyramidal side effects (EPS) than typical agents (Table 20–6).

Most people with a first episode of psychosis respond to at least one of the typical or atypical agents. However, a patient may go through a period of trial and error for months or years to find the best available medication and dosage. A trial of any one medication should last for a substantial period, usually 6 to

TABLE 20–6. POTENCY OF TYPICAL ANTIPSYCHOTICS AND SIDE EFFECTS

		Side Effects			
Potency	Drug	EPS	Anticholinergic	Sedation	Seizure
Low	Chlorpromazine (Thorazine) (400–1000 mg/day)	Low	High	High	High
Low	Thioridazine (Mellaril) (400–800 mg/day)	Low	High	High	High
High	Fluphenazine (Prolixin) (20–60 mg/day)	High	Low	Low	Low
High	Haloperidol (Haldol) (20–60 mg/day)	High	Low	Low	Low

8 weeks, unless intolerable side effects occur early. Even though the atypical agents have a better side effect profile for long-term treatment, the typical or older agents may be chosen for short-term management of psychosis or long-term management of symptoms that do not respond to the atypical agents.

TYPICAL AGENTS

Typical antipsychotics treat the positive symptoms of schizophrenia (Box 20–7).

Hypotheses on Mechanism of Action

The effects of typical antipsychotics on positive symptoms have been thought to be associated with interactions with dopamine receptors in the brain. The medications' interactions with one type of dopamine may be associated with their antipsychotic efficacy, and interactions with another type of dopamine may be associated with side effects such as movement disorders. However, it is now hypothesized that other neurotransmitter systems than the dopamine are also involved in psychoses.

Efficacy in Treating Symptoms

All the typical antipsychotic agents are equally effective. However, the amounts of the medications required to exert a certain level of antipsychotic effect vary according to their potency or the degree of interaction with different types of dopamine receptors. A high-potency agent such as haloperidol (Haldol) in a dose of 2 mg may elicit the same level of antipsychotic effect as a low-potency agent such as thioridazine (Mellaril) in a dose of 100 mg.

BOX 20–7. Seven Categories of Positive Symptoms in Patients with Schizophrenia

1. **Hallucinations:** Perception of internal stimuli in auditory, visual, olfactory, or tactile forms.
2. **Delusions:** Beliefs that are groundless, idiosyncratic, and unreal.
3. **Conceptual disorganization:** Non–goal-directed flow of thinking process, loose associations.
4. **Excitement:** Excessive responsiveness to environment, accelerated motor behavior, hypervigilance.
5. **Hostility:** Verbal abuse, assaultive, sarcastic; nonverbal expression of anger or resentment.
6. **Grandiosity:** Unrealistic sense of superiority such as belief in extraordinary abilities, knowledge, power, wealth, or moral righteousness.
7. **Suspiciousness:** Excessive ideas of persecution resulting in guardedness, distrustful attitude, or verbalization of concern about being harmed.

Long-acting agents with average half-lives of 3 weeks (Haldol decanoate) and 2 weeks (Prolixin decanoate) are available in intramuscular forms. These lipophilic agents are injected into fatty tissues in muscles of the deltoid or gluteus maximus. In the case of Haldol decanoate, a daily oral dose of 10 mg or 300 mg/month can be replaced by a monthly injection of Haldol decanoate with 1/3 to 1/2 of the monthly oral dose (100 to 150 mg). The dosages for Prolixin decanoate can generally range from 12.5 to 75 mg every 2 weeks.

Common Side Effects

The low-potency typical agents have more side effects than the high-potency agents (see Table 20–6) because of the greater antagonism of cholinergic, adrenergic, and histaminergic receptor systems in the brain. However, high-potency agents have more risk for the development of extrapyramidal side effects (Table 20–7) because of the potent antagonism of the dopamine receptors that are associated with movement disorders.

The other common adverse effects of antipsychotic drugs may be minimized by the considerations listed in Table 20–8.

TABLE 20–7. SIGNS OF EXTRAPYRAMIDAL SIDE EFFECTS

Sign	Onset	Manifestations
Akathisia (motor restlessness)	Sudden or gradual	Pacing, shifting from one foot to another when standing, tapping feet while sitting, inability to sit still, rocking, feeling something jumping out of skin, feeling anxious, feeling physically tense, tossing and turning in bed, feeling wired up
Dystonia (involuntary muscle contraction with rigidity)	Sudden	Neck twisting (torticollis), back arching or head pulling backward (opisthotonos), clenched jaw (trismus), eyes fixed upward (oculogyral crisis), difficulty speaking and swallowing with hypersalivation, inability to close eyes (blepharospasm), protruding tongue
Tardive dyskinesia (muscle spasms with late onset)	After months or years of antipsychotic use	Rapid blinking of the eyes; wormlike tongue; chewing with nothing in mouth; lip puckering; facial grimacing; rhythmic involuntary movements of jaws, face, extremities, and trunk
Pseudoparkinsonism (signs similar to those of parkinsonism)	Sudden or gradual	Shuffling gait; coarse tremor; drooling; fixed facial expression; apathy; slowness of voluntary movement; cogwheel rigidity in arms, shoulders, and neck; lead-pipe rigidity in torso and extremities, which become unmovable; rabbit syndrome (tremor of the lips and mouth)

TABLE 20–8. MINIMIZING SIDE EFFECTS FROM THE TYPICAL AND ATYPICAL AGENTS

Type of Side Effect	Action
Cardiac problems	Use high-potency agents except pimozide (Orap) to avoid conduction abnormalities.
Hematologic disorder	Monitor CBC weekly for the first 6 months of clozapine treatment, then biweekly thereafter.
Parkinsonism	Low-potency agents may minimize parkinsonism because of their built-in anticholinergic property. The same is true of clozapine.
Prostatic hypertrophy	Avoid low-potency agents and clozapine (Clozaril), which exert high anticholinergic effects.
Seizure	Avoid loxapine (Loxitane) and clozapine (Clozaril) in clients with a history of seizure. Molidone (Moban) may have lower seizure risk than other antipsychotics.
Pregnancy	Avoid use of low-potency agents. Increased risk of anomalies is associated with use of the phenothiazines group, including chlorpromazine (Thorazine) and thioridazine (Mellaril). High-potency agents such as fluphenazine (Prolixin), haloperidol (Haldol), trifluoperazine (Stelazine), and perphenazine (Trilafon) are associated with lower risk during pregnancy.
Weight gain	Loxapine (Loxitane), molidone (Moban), and risperidone (Riperdal) are associated with lower risks.
Sexual side effects	Clozapine (Clozaril) and quetiapine (Seroquel) are associated with lower risks.

Related Clinical Concerns

Children   May be particularly vulnerable to the side effects of antipsychotics. In general, low doses of antipsychotic medications are found to be effective for many children with psychotic symptoms, autism, and vocal or motor tics.

Elderly People   Start with low doses of high-potency agents. Bedtime dosing may reduce the risk of problems associated with orthostatic hypotension, such as falling.

Psychotic Disorders Caused by Medical Conditions   Psychiatric symptoms of psychoses can be part of nonpsychiatric disorders such as Addison's disease, pernicious anemia, AIDS, CNS infection or neoplasms, Cushing's disease, delirium, dementias, lupus, and other conditions. It may be necessary to use antipsychotic medications to manage the symptoms while the underlying medical conditions are being corrected.

Reverse Epinephrine Effect   Certain antipsychotics such as clozapine, fluphenazine enanthate, chlorpromazine, and thioridazine can cause epinephrine reversal and a hypotensive response when epinephrine is used to increase blood pressure.

Skin Sensitivity to Sunlight   The skin needs to be protected from exposure to sunlight.

Heart Block   Overdoses of pimozide (Orap) or thioridazine (Mellaril) are associated with high risk.

Blindness   High doses of thioridazine (Mellaril) can cause pigmentation of the retina, which could lead to blindness.

ATYPICAL AGENTS

The medications in this category are used to treat both positive and negative symptoms of schizophrenia (Boxes 20–7 and 20–8). However, they can also be used to treat psychotic symptoms of other psychiatric disorders (schizoaffective disorders, major depression, and bipolar disorders).

Hypotheses on Mechanisms of Action

The mechanisms of action of atypical antipsychotics are unclear. It has been hypothesized that the atypical agents are more selective than the typical ones when they interact with different types of dopamine receptors. These dopamine receptors, which are associated with movement disorders, are less affected and minimize these side effects, especially with clozapine (Clozaril) or quetiapine (Seroquel). However, the atypical agents affect multiple neurotransmitter systems, making it difficult to understand their exact mechanisms of action. It has been proposed that, unlike the typical agents, all the atypical agents are antagonists of serotonin (5HT) receptors and also interact selectively with the dopamine receptors.

BOX 20–8. Seven Categories of Negative Symptoms in Patients with Schizophrenia

1. **Difficulty with abstract or logical thinking:** Difficulty in classification, generalization, conceptualization beyond concrete thinking.
2. **Lack of spontaneity and flow of conversation:** Diminished flow of productivity in verbal interaction with others.
3. **Blunted affect:** A reduction in nonverbal communicative cues or facial expressions.
4. **Social withdrawal:** Reduced activities of daily living or neglected interpersonal involvement.
5. **Poor rapport:** Inability to show interpersonal empathy, interest, sense of closeness or openness during conversation.
6. **Emotional withdrawal with difficulty identifying own feelings:** Lack of interest or involvement in life.
7. **Stereotyped thinking:** Rigid repetitive thought content.

Efficacy in Treating Symptoms

The positive symptoms respond faster to antipsychotics than the negative symptoms in general. Changes in negative symptoms or regaining of affect, social activities, or motivation may be observed over months and years of treatment when these agents are used along with psychosocial rehabilitation interventions.

Common Side Effects

All the atypical agents are generally less associated with extrapyramidal symptoms than are typical agents. However, the following side effects are reported:

Clozapine (Clozaril)   Excessive salivation during sleep, orthostatic hypotension, sedation, tachycardia, anticholinergic effects (constipation, blurred vision, urinary retention), seizure, agranulocytosis (0.4–1.0%), weight gain, urinary incontinence.

Risperidone (Risperdal)   Orthostatic hypotension, tachycardia, insomnia, headaches, weight gain. EPS are possible at higher doses. May cause elevation of prolactin.

Olanzapine (Zyprexa)   Weight gain, tachycardia, sedation, orthostatic hypotension. EPS are possible. May cause elevation of prolactin.

Quetiapine (Seroquel)   Sedation, weight gain, dry mouth.

Related Clinical Concerns

The Clozaril Patient Management System (CPMS)   Because of the possibility of granulocytosis, clozapine has been marketed under a unique system set up by the pharmaceutical company. All patients to be started on clozapine must be cleared through the CPMS before the treatment begins. The therapy can be initiated if the patient has:

- WBC>3500
- No history of clozapine-induced agranulocytosis
- No uncontrolled seizures

The physician and pharmacist are responsible for obtaining weekly WBC counts. Only a week's supply of clozapine will be dispensed after the WBC count is reported every week to the pharmacy. After 6 months of treatment with no hematologic problems, a 2-week supply of clozapine can be dispensed as the acceptable WBC count is reported biweekly (Table 20–9).

TABLE 20–9. MONITORING GRANULOCYTE COUNTS DURING CLOZAPINE THERAPY

WBC and Granulocyte Count	Action Plan

I. Reduced WBC within normal range:
    A. WBC count drops 3000 cells from
       previous test
    OR
    B. Three or more consecutive drops
       regardless of their counts
	I. (A) Monitor for infection; (B) CBC with
	   differentials if ordered by physician;
	   (C) continue clozapine.

II. Mild leukopenia: WBC = 3000–3500	II. (A) Monitor for infection; (B) CBC with differentials; (C) continue clozapine.

III. Granulocytopenia: WBC = 2000–3000
      Granulocytes = 1000–1500
	III. (A) Interrupt clozapine at once; (B) start
	     daily CBC with differentials; (C) observe
	     closely for infection; (D) resume clozapine
	     after normalization of granulocyte counts.

III. Severe granulocytopenia: WBC <2000
      Granulocytes <1000
      OR
      Agranulocytosis: Granulocytes <500
	IV. (A) Discontinue clozapine at once;
	     (B) consult with hematologist to consider
	     protective isolation in a medical unit;
	     (C) daily CBC with differentials; (D) cloza-
	     pine must NOT be restarted at all.

PATIENT AND FAMILY EDUCATION FOR TYPICAL AND ATYPICAL ANTIPSYCHOTICS

- Advise patient and family against stopping any medications without contacting the prescriber.
- Teach patient to recognize that it may take 2 to 12 weeks to experience any positive responses from antipsychotic medication.
- Teach patient to keep taking the medication consistently to avoid a return of the disturbing symptoms.
- Advise women patients that pregnancy should be avoided.
- Teach patient to report any exacerbation of target symptoms to the prescriber.
- Reinforce importance of following all drug monitoring to avoid long term problems.

MANAGING SIDE EFFECTS OF ANTIPSYCHOTIC AGENTS

Extrapyramidal symptoms are the major side effect of typical antipsychotic medications. The symptoms are very distressing and uncomfortable. Their presence will affect patient compliance with taking antipsychotic medications. Prevention and treatment of EPS is essential to keep patients taking their medications. Even medications that resolve EPS can cause their own side effects, particularly anticholinergic effects.

Parkinsonism and dystonia (see Table 20–7 for descriptions of symptoms) can be treated by antiparkinsonian drugs such as benztropine (Cogentin) or trihexyphenidyl (Artane), which are acetylcholine (muscarinic) receptor antagonists (anticholinergics). Akathisia can be resolved with beta-blockers such as propranolol (Inderal). Antihistamines and benzodiazepines are also used. No medication is available to treat tardive dyskinesia. High doses of vitamin E (1600–2000 IU) have been tried . See Table 20–10 for a list of the medications that treat these symptoms.

OTHER SIDE EFFECTS ASSOCIATED WITH SPECIFIC ANTIPSYCHOTIC MEDICATIONS

Neuroleptic Malignant Syndrome

Neuroleptic malignant syndrome (NMS) reactions to the typical antipsychotic agents can develop over a few days. This syndrome is uncommon, yet potentially fatal. Some risk is presented with risperidone (Risperdal) and olanzapine (Zyprexa). The signs include elevated temperature (>39°C [102°F]), severe EPS, autonomic instability, delirium, elevation of CPK, WBC, and liver enzymes. Medical interventions will be required. Cooling measures and hydration will be needed.

Autonomic Dysfunction

- *Tachycardia:* Beta blockers may be used if pulse exceeds 120 bpm.
- *Sialorrhea (excessive salivation):* Can be excessive with clozapine (Clozaril). Clonidine (Catapres) has been tested. No anticholinergic agents are recommended to control excessive salivation.
- *Dry mouth:* Extra care of the mouth and teeth is required because of higher risk of developing cavities.
- *Orthostatic hypotension:* Patients should be cautioned about the possibility of falling on abrupt change of posture.
- *Low-grade fever:* The homeostasis for body temperature may be affected by clozapine (Clozaril)

Other Categories of Side Effects

- *Elevated cholesterol and triglycerides:* Tends to occur in patients on antipsychotic agents. Type II diabetes may develop in association with the use of antipsychotics.

TABLE 20–10. MEDICATIONS FOR EXTRAPYRAMIDAL SYMPTOMS (EPS)

Drug Type	Drug and Dosage (mg/day)
Antiparkinsonian	Benztropine (Cogentin) (1–6 mg)
	Trihexyphenidyl (Artane) (1–15 mg)
Antihistamine	Diphenhydramine (Benadryl) (25–100 mg)
Beta-adrenergic blocker	Propranolol (Inderal (10–80 mg)
	Atenolol (Tenormin) (50–100 mg)
Alpha-2 adrenergic blocker	Clonidine (Catapres) (0.2–2.4 mg)

- *Weight gain:* Most psychiatric medications (antipsychotics, lithium, etc) are associated with the risk of weight gain.
- *Sedation:* Common with most psychiatric medications. This can be utilized for sleep problems.
- *Endocrine dysfunction:* Most antipsychotic agents (except clozapine and quetiapine) can elevate prolactin levels. This may lead to amenorrhea.
- *Liver enzyme elevation:* This elevation may be asymptomatic.
- *Hematologic dysfunction:* All antipsychotic agents can affect CBC values.

PATIENT AND FAMILY EDUCATION

- Review signs of EPS and reinforce the idea that treatment is available for these.
- Advise carrying water and hard candies to reduce dry mouth.
- Advise against stopping medications because of side effects or for other reasons.
- Encourage activity and monitor diet to avoid weight gain.
- Teach patient to report muscle stiffness or restlessness to the prescriber.
- Teach patient to report development of flulike symptoms while taking clozapine.
- Review drug-specific side effects with patient and family or caregivers.

COLLABORATIVE MANAGEMENT FOR ADVOCACY

Patients, families, psychiatrists, nurses, internists, pharmacists, and other related clinicians need to be involved in the management of the patient's medications. The patient and family can provide information on real-life experiences of the illness and the medication. Psychiatric clinicians can provide updated clinical information on the efficacy and safety of the medications. The other clinicians who are working with the patient can provide the data that can be utilized to assess the efficacy and safety.

One of the most common obstacles to advocacy is the patient's nonadherence to the treatment (Box 20–9). The reasons for this need to be addressed to encourage the patient's compliance with the treatment plan.

BOX 20–9. Factors that Contribute to Nonadherence to Pharmacologic Treatment

- Medication side effects.
- Medication not as effective as expected.
- Need to continue medication without patient sensing immediate improvement.
- Complicated drug regimes.
- Cost of medication.
- Patient feels worse when first starts medication; feels better when first stops medication.

The process of psychosocial rehabilitation (Box 20–10) provides the essential strategies to advocate for patients in the area of psychopharmacologic support. The minimum data set on the psychiatric medications can be applied for interventions with these strategies to develop partnership with patients and achieve the goal of valuing their medication in relation to their life goals.

CHARTING TIPS

The documentation should include information on the following five elements:

1. Target symptoms
2. The patient's understanding of the efficacy of the medication
3. The patient's adherence to the medication
4. Presence of side effects
5. Current mental status

COMMUNITY-BASED CARE

When a patient is discharged from an inpatient or outpatient setting, the written summary should include the names of all the medications that have been tried, the dosages, and the clinical responses. Make sure that the patient or family can verbalize the names of the medications, the dosages, and the

---

BOX 20–10. Use of Psychosocial Rehabilitation Process for Medication Management

1. **Mutual Understanding** (Diagnosis): Identifying symptoms and/or needs for help from a client's and/or family's perspectives.
2. **Collaborative Mapping** (Planning): Identifying a client's and/or family's strength or coping skills to manage symptoms that are interfering with their pursuit of life goals. The client or family can move faster for adjustment when their strength is acknowledged.
3. **Negotiated Support** (Intervention): Helping a client to clarify his or her concerns about medications and providing resources for decision making to choose pharmacologic therapy. Convey the idea that the medication can work only when the client or family takes charge of it.
4. **Interactive Appraisal** (Evaluation): Appraisal of pharmacologic therapy with client and family in terms of balancing benefits and adverse experiences.
5. **Guided Exploration** (Assessment): Identifying factors for possible nonadherence. Identifying possibility of better balance benefits and adverse experiences with new knowledge on available medications. The value of the medications for the client needs to be recreated at all times because it can become unclear during the treatment course.

Source: Adapted from Groenwold, 1996.

schedule for administration. If they cannot, instruct them to carry a card with all the information on it.

Any agencies that will be following patients need information on the psychiatric medications, resources to refill prescriptions, follow-up care, and emergency numbers for problems. Consider referring patient to psychiatric home care for medication and side effect management, blood level monitoring, and reinforcement of patient and family education.

APPENDIX A

Relaxation Techniques

Relaxation techniques can include any of the following:

- *Deep Breathing:* Take in several slow deep breaths by inhaling through your nose and exhaling slowly through your mouth. As you exhale, focus on relaxing your shoulders. Each time you take a deep breath, repeat a calming word to yourself such as "peace" or "one."
- *Muscle Relaxation:* After taking two slow deep breaths, raise your shoulders for 2 to 3 seconds and then let go. Do this 2 to 3 times. Then make a fist, hold it for 2 to 3 seconds, and then let go. Each time you let go, think of another part of your body becoming more relaxed. Imagine yourself going limp like a rag doll. You can continue to tense and relax other muscle groups in your body.
- *Imagery:* After taking several slow deep breaths and relaxing your muscles, create a pleasant image in your mind that you associate with relaxation. It can be a comforting memory or an image such as a garden or floating on a raft in the sunshine. Let your mind wander to whatever you find relaxing.

Tips on enhancing relaxation:

- Create a quiet environment.
- Sit in a comfortable chair.
- Give yourself permission to take this time for yourself.
- Devote enough time for practice.
- Every time your mind wanders to distracting thoughts, focus on your breathing.
- Practice regularly (relaxation is not always easy and often must become a learned skill).
- Consider the use of audio or video relaxation tapes with headsets.

APPENDIX B

Complementary and Alternative Approaches

Acupressure—Using massage on traditional acupuncture points.

Acupuncture—Using thin needles at designated points along meridians to balance the flow of energy. Used to treat uncomfortable symptoms and some conditions.

Alternative nutrition—Use of food to heal and maintain optimal health (e.g., macrobiotic diet).

Aromatherapy—Therapeutic use of odors from plant oils to treat illness and promote relaxation.

Biofeedback—Using electrical devices to record changes in body function to achieve relaxation and/or muscle control.

Folk remedies—Alternative health practices and therapies based on health beliefs and practices within cultural groups.

Guided imagery—Using the conscious mind to create images to evoke physiologic changes and promote healing and relaxation.

Healing touch—Healing method based on concept of human energy fields.

Herbal medicine—Use of plants for healing purposes.

Homeopathy—Therapy based on concept of "like cures like." Uses minute amounts of drug that normally would produce the same symptoms as the illness being treated.

Hypnotherapy—Creating a state of heightened awareness in which suggestions to improve health are made and are likely to be followed.

Light therapy—Use of alternative light (e.g., colored light, ultraviolet light) to treat various disorders.

Magnet therapy—Using electromagnetic frequencies emitting from the body to treat illness.

Massage—Manipulation of tissues and muscles to promote relaxation and healing.

Megavitamin therapy—Using higher doses of vitamins than usually recommended to prevent or cure illness.

Meditation—Ancient art of focusing one's attention on a single sound or image to promote relaxation and health.

Yoga—A philosophy and exercise system that combines movement and positions to promote health.

REFERENCES

Abramowicz, M (ed.): Drugs for psychiatric disorders. Med Letter Drug Therapy 36(933):89, 1994.

Agency for Health Care Policy and Research: Acute Pain Management: Operative or Medical Procedures and Trauma. Clinical Practice Guideline. Public Health Service, US Department of Health and Human Services (DHHS), Rockville, MD, February 1992.

Agency for Health Care Policy and Research: Depression in Primary Care, vol 1 and 2. Public Health Service, US Department of Health and Human Services (DHHS), Rockville, MD, 1993.

Agency for Health Care Policy and Research: Management of Cancer Pain. Clinical Practice Guideline. Public Health Service, US Department of Health and Human Services (DHHS), Rockville, MD, March 1994.

Agency for Healthcare Quality and Research: Outcomes for 19 Mental Diseases and Disorders web site. Available at http://hcup.ahrq.gov/hcupnet.asp. Accessed September 2001.

Agency for Healthcare Research and Quality: Improving Quality of Care for People with Depression: Translating Research into Practice Fact Sheet. Agency for Healthcare Research and Quality. Rockville, MD, 2000.

Aguilera, DC: Crisis Intervention Theory and Methodology, ed. 8. Mosby, St Louis, 1998.

Akiskal, HS: Mood disorders: Clinical features. In BJ Sadock and VA Sadock (eds.): Kaplan and Sadock Comprehensive Textbook of Psychiatry, ed. 7. Lippincott/Williams and Wilkins, Philadelphia, 2000.

Alcoholics Anonymous: Twelve Steps and Twelve Traditions. New York, 1953.

Alston, MH, and Robinson, BH: Nurses' attitudes toward suicide. Omega 25(3):205, 1992.

American Hospital Formulary Service (AHFS): Drug information. American Society of Hospital Pharmacists, Bethedsa, MD, 2000.

American Pain Society: Principles of Analgesic Use in Treatment of Acute Pain and Cancer, ed 4. Skokie, IL, 1999.

American Psychiatric Association (APA): Diagnostic and Statistical Manual of Mental disorders-Text Revision (TR). Washington, DC, 2000. (DSM-IV-TR)

American Psychiatric Association (APA): Diagnostic and Statistical Manual of Mental Disorders, ed 4. Washington, DC, 1994. (DSM-IV)

American Psychiatric Association: Practice guidelines for treatment of patients with substance abuse disorders. Am J Psychiatry 152(115):5, 1995.

American Psychiatric Association: Practice guidelines for treatment of patients with eating disorders (revisions). Am J Psychiatry 157:1 Supplement, 2000.

Antai-Otong, D: Psychiatric Nursing: Biological and Behavioral Concepts. WB Saunders, Philadelphia, 1995.

Antari-Otong, D: Helping the alcoholic patient recover. Am J Nurs 22:29, 1995.

Antari-Otong, D: The neurobiology of anxiety disorders: Implications for psychiatric nursing practice. Issues in Mental Health Nursing 21:71, 2000.

Barki, ZK, Kravitz, HM, and Berki, TM: Psychotropic medications in pregnancy. Psychiatric Annals 28:9, 1998.

Barry, PD: Psychosocial Nursing Assessment and Intervention, ed. 3. Lippincott-Raven, Philadelphia, 1996.

Bauer, B, and Hill, S: People who defend against anxiety through aggression toward others. In Varcarolis, EM (ed.): Foundations of Psychiatric Mental Health Nursing. WB Saunders, Philadelphia, 1994.

Beattie, M: Codependent No More. Harper-Collins, New York, 1992.

Beck, A: Cognitive Therapy and Emotional Disorder. New American Library, New York, 1979.

Beck-Little, R, and Weinrich, SP: Assessment and management of sleep disorders in the elderly. Journal of Gerontological Nursing 24(4):21, 1998.

Bergh, I, and Sjostrom, B: A comparative study of nurses' and elderly patients' ratings of pain and pain tolerance. Journal of Gerontological Nursing 25(5):30, 1999.

Berlinger, JS: Domestic violence: How you can make a difference. Nursing 31(8):58–63, 2001.

Bernstein, SB: Breaking the vicious cycle of noncompliance. Nursing 19(1): 74, 1989.

Bianchi, SM: The changing demographics and socioeconomic characteristics of single parent families . In SH Hansom, ML Jeins, DJ Julian, and MB Sussman (eds.): Single Parent Families: Diversity, Myths, and Realities. New York, Haworth Press, 1995.

Black, C: It Will Never Happen to Me. Ballantine, New York, 1987.

Blair, DT, and New, SA: Assaultive behavior: Know the risks. J Psychosoc Ment Health Serv 29:25, 1991.

Blair, DT, and New, SA: Patient violence in psychiatric settings: Risk identification and treatment as provocation. In Smoyak, SA, and Blair, DT (eds.): Violence and Abuse. Slack, Thorofare, NJ, 1992.

Borsook, D, McPeek, B, and Lebel, AA: The Massachusetts General Hospital Handbook of Pain management. Lippincott-Raven, Philadelphia, 1996.

Bowen, M: Family Therapy in Clinical Practice. Aronson, New York, 1978.

Brauner, DJ, Muir, JC, Sachs, GA: Treating nondementia illnesses in patients with dementia. JAMA 283(24) 3230, 2000.

Breitbart, W, and Holland, JC (eds.) Psychiatric Aspects of Symptom Management in Cancer Patients. American Psychiatric Press, Washington, DC, 1993.

Brentin, L, and Sieh, A: Caring for the morbidly obese. Am J Nurs 91(8):40, 1991.

Brown, TM, and Stoudemire, A: Psychiatric Side Effects of Prescription and Over-the-Counter Medications–Recognition and Management. American Psychiatric Press, Inc., Washington, DC, 1998.

Brownell, KD, and Wadden, TA: Obesity. In BJ Saddock and VA Saddock (eds.). Kaplan and Saddock's Comprehensive Textbook of Psychiatry, ed. 7. Lippincott/Williams & Wilkins, Philadelphia, 1999.

Burke, MM, and Walsh, MB: Gerontologic Nursing: Care of the Frail Elderly. Mosby, St Louis, 1992.

Cadoret, R: Antisocial personality. In G. Winokur and PJ Clayton (eds.) The Medical Basis for Psychiatry. Philadelphia, WB Saunders, 1994.

Caine, ED, and Lyness, JM: Delirium, dementia, amnestic and other cognitive disorders. In BJ Sadock and VA Sadock (eds.): Kaplan and Sadock Comprehensive Textbook of Psychiatry, ed. 7. Lippincott/Williams and Wilkins, Philadelphia, 2000.

Campbell, J, and Humphreys, J: Nursing Care of Survivors of Family Violence. Mosby, St Louis, 1993.

Campinha-Bacote, J: Cultural competence in psychiatric mental health nursing: A conceptual model. Nurs Clin North Am 29(1):1, 1994.

Carpenito, L: Nursing Diagnosis: Application to Clinical Practice, ed. 8. Lippincott/Williams & Wilkins, Philadelphia, 2000.

Carroll-Johnson, RM, Gorman, LM, and Bush, NJ: Psychosocial Nursing Care along the Cancer Continuum. Oncology Nursing Press, Pittsburgh, 1998.

Cassidy, K: How to assess and intervene in a domestic violence situation. Home Health Nurse 17(10):664, 1999.

Cassileth, BR: The Alternative Medicine Handbook. WW Norton and Co., New York, 1998.

Chenevert, M: STAT: Special Techniques in Assertiveness Training for Women in Health Professions, ed 4. Mosby, St Louis, 1994.

Chez, N: Helping the victim of domestic violence. Am J Nurs 94(7):33, 1994.

Chien, W: The use of physical restraints on hospitalized psychogeriatric patients. J Psychosoc Nurs 38(2):13, 2000.

Cochrane, CE Eating regulation responses and eating disorders. In GW Stuart and MT Laraia (eds.): Stuart and Sundeen's Principles and Practices of Psychiatric Nursing, 6th ed., Mosby, St Louis, 1998.

Collins, CE: Interventions with family caregivers of persons with Alzheimer's disease. Nurs Clin North Am 29(1):195, 1994.

Collins, GB: Contemporary issues in the treatment of alcohol dependence. Psychiatr Clin North Am 16(1):33, 1993.

Cooley, M: Bereavement care: A role for nurses. Cancer Nurs 15(2):125, 1992.

Copeland, LG: Caring for children with chronic conditions: Model of critical times. Holistic Nurse Pract 8(1):45, 1993.

Coward, DD: Self-transcendence: Making meaning from the cancer experience. Semin Oncol Nurs 13:248, 1995.

Davidizar, R: Meeting a client's spiritual needs. Caring 18(7):3,1999.

de Rond, ME, et al.: Daily pain assessment: Value for nurses and patients. J Adv Nurs 29(2):436, 1999.

de Rond, ME, et al.: (2000) A pain monitoring program for nurses: Effect on the administration of analgesics. Pain 89(1):25, 2000.

Decker, GM: An Introduction to Complementary and Alternative Therapies. Oncology Nursing Press, Pittsburgh, PA, 1999.

DeLaune, SC: Effective limit setting: How to avoid being manipulated. Nurs Clin North Am 26:3, 1991.

Devlin, BK, and Reynolds, E: Child abuse. Am J Nurs 94(3):26, 1994.

Doenges, ME , Townsend, MC, and Moorhouse, MF: Psychiatric Care Plans: Guidelines for Individualizing Care, ed 3. FA Davis, Philadelphia, 1998.

Dowd, MD: Consequences of violence. Pediatr Clin North Am 45(2):333, 1998.

Ebersole, P, and Hess, P: Toward Healthy Aging, ed 5. Mosby, St Louis, 1997.

Eisenberg, DM, et al.: Trends in alternative medicine use in the US: 1990–1997. JAMA 280(18): 1569,1998.

Ellis, JA, Blouin, R, and Lockett, J: Patient-controlled analgesia: Optimizing the experience. Clinical Nursing Research 8(3):283, 1999.

Falvo, DR: Medical and Psychosocial Aspects of Chronic Illness and Disability, ed 2. Aspen Publishers, Gaithersburg, MD, 1999.

Fein, ML: I.A.M.: A common sense guide to coping with anger. Prager Press, Westport, CT, 1993.

Fergusson, D: Is sexual orientation related to mental health problems and suicidality in young people? Arch Gen Psychiatry 56(10):876, 1998.

Ferrel, BJ, et al.: Beyond the Supreme Court decision: Nursing perspectives on end of life care. Oncol Nurs Forum 27(3):445, 2000.

Feske, U, et al.: Anxiety as a correlate of response to the acute treatment of bipolar 1 disorder. Am J Psychiatry 157(6):956, 2000.

Fillingham, RB: Sex, gender, and pain. Progress in Pain Research and Management, International Association for the Study of Pain Press. Seattle, WA, 2000.

Fincannon, JL: Analysis of psychiatric referrals and interventions in an oncology population. Oncol Nurs Forum 22(1):87, 1995.

Finger, WW, Lund, M, and Slagle, MA: Medications that may contribute to sexual disorders. Journal of Family Practice 41(1):33–43, 1997.

Fischer, C, and Hegge, M: The elderly woman as risk. Am J Nurs 100 (6):54, 2000.

Fitchett, G: Assessing Spiritual Needs: A Guide for Caregivers. Augsburg Fortress, MN, 1993.

Folstein, MF, Folstein, FE, and McHugh, PR: Mini-mental state: A practical method for grading the cognitive state of patients for the clinician. J Psychiatr Res 12:189, 1975.

Ford, DE, and Kamerow, DB: Epidemiological study of sleep disturbances and psychiatric disorders. JAMA 262:1479, 1989.

Fraser, K, and Gallop, R: Nurses' confirming/disconfirming responses to patients diagnosed with borderline personality disorder. Arch Psychiatr Nurs 7(6):338, 1993.

Freedman, NS, Kotzer, N, and Schwab, RJ: Patient perception of sleep quality and etiology of sleep disruption in the intensive care unit. Am J Respir Crit Care Med 159:1155, 1999.

Friedman, MM: Family Therapy: Theory and Practice, ed. 4. Appleton & Lange, Norwalk, CT, 1998.

Galanter, M, and Kleber, HD: Textbook of Substance Abuse Therapy. American Psychiatric Press, Washington, DC, 1994.

Galazis, RS, and Kempe, A: Therapy with clients with eating disorders. In Beck, CK, Rawlins, RP, and Williams, SR (eds.): Psychiatric Nursing. CV Mosby, St Louis, 1988.

Gallagher, S: Tailoring care for obese patients. RN 625:43, 1999.

Geary, SM: Intensive care unit psychosis revisited: Understanding and managing delirium in the critical care unit. Crit Care Nurs Q 17(1):51, 1994.

Gerner, RF: Treatment of acute mania. Psychiatr Clin North Am 16(3):443, 1993.

Giger, JN, and Davidhizar, RE: Transcultural Nursing: Assessment and Intervention ed. 3. Mosby, St Louis, 1999.

Glod, CA: Crisis Intervention. In CA Glod (ed.) Contemporary Psychiatric-Mental Health Nursing. FA Davis, Philadelphia, 1998.

Glod, CA: Long-term consequences of childhood physical and sexual abuse. Arch Psychiatr Nurs 7(3):163, 1993.

Goff, DC, Henderson, DC, and Manschreck, TC: Psychotic patients. In NH Cassem (ed.): Massachusetts General Hospital Handbook of General Hospital Psychiatry, ed. 4. Mosby, St. Louis, 1997.

Goldenberg, I, and Goldenberg, H: Family Therapy: An Overview, ed. 5. Brooks/Cole, Pacific Grove, CA, 1999.

Goldsmith, C: Obesity: Epidemic of the 21st century? Newsweek, May 8, 2000.

Goodwin, FK, and Jamison, KR: Manic-Depressive Illness. Oxford University Press, New York, 1990.

Gorman, JM, et al. Neuroanatomical hypothesis of pain disorder, revised. Am J Psychiatry 157(4):493, 2000.

Gorman, L, Sultan, D, and Luna-Raines, M: Psychosocial Nursing Handbook for the Nonpsychiatric Nurse. Williams & Wilkins, Baltimore, 1989.

Gray-Vickery, P: Combating abuse, Part 1: Protecting the older adult. Nursing 30(7):34, 2000.

Groenewold, L: Decreasing Readmission: The Comprehensive Role of Nursing in Psychosocial Rehabilitation. Presented at Contemporary Forums Psychiatric Nursing Conference in Hollywood, CA, 1996.

Grossman, D: Enhancing your cultural competence. Am J Nurs 94(7):58, 1994.

Haber, J, et al.: Comprehensive Psychiatric Nursing, ed. 5. St Louis, Mosby, 1997.

Haffner, L: Translation is not enough. Western Journal of Healthcare 157(3):255, 1992.

Hamolia, CC: Preventing and managing aggressive behavior. In GW Stuart and MT Laraia (eds.): Stuart and Sundeen's Principles and Practices of Psychiatric Nursing, ed. 6. Mosby, St Louis, 1998.

Hanna, VM, and Smith, JA: Helping a dependent patient help himself. Nursing '92 22(6):32c, 1992.

Harvath, TA, et al: Dementia-related behaviors. J Psychosoc Nurs Ment Health Serv 33(1):35, 1995.

Hatton, C, and Valente, S: Suicide: Assessment and Interventions. Appleton-Century-Crofts, Norwalk, CT, 1984.

Haven, E, and Piscitello, V: The patient with violent behavior. In Lewis, S, et al (eds.): Manual of Psychosocial Nursing Interventions. WB Saunders, Philadelphia, 1989.

Highfield, EF: Providing spiritual care to patients with cancer. Clinical Journal of Oncology Nursing 4(3):115, 2000.

Hingson, R, and Howland, J: Alcohol and nontraffic unintended injuries. Addiction 88:877, 1993.

Hoffman, NG, and Miller, NS: Perspectives of effective treatment for alcohol and drug disorders. Psychiatr Clin North Am 16(1):127, 1993.

Hospice and Palliative Nurses Association Statement on the Scope and Standards of Hospice and Palliative Nursing Practice. Kendall Hunt Publishing Co. Dubuque, IA, 2000.

Huart, S, and O'Donnel, M: The road to recovery from grief and bereavement. Caring 12(11):71, 1993.

Hudelson, E: Points to remember when caring for an obese patient. Nurs 22(10):62, 1992.

Jacob, SR: An analysis of the concept of grief. J Adv Nurs 18(11):1787, 1993.

Jacobs, DG: The Harvard Medical School Guide to Suicide Assessment and Intervention. Jossey-Bass Publishers, San Francisco, 1999.

Jefferson, LV: Chemically mediated responses and substance-related disorders. In GW Sundeen and MT Laraia (eds.): Stuart and Sundeen's Principles and Practices of Psychiatric Nursing, ed. 6. Mosby, St Louis, 1998.

Jensen, DP, and Herr, KA: Sleeplessness. Nurs Clin North Am 28(2):385, 1993.

Jimerson, DC, et al.: Medication in the treatment of eating disorders. Psychiatr Clin North Am 19(4):739, 1996.

Johnston, JE: Sleep problems in the elderly. J Am Acad Nurse Pract 6(4):161, 1994.

Joint Commission on Accreditation of Health Care Organizations (JCAHO): Accreditation Manual for Hospitals. Chicago, 2000, 2001.

Kahn, DM, et al.: Identification and modification of environmental noise in an ICU setting. Chest 114:535, 1998.

Kashani, J, et al.: Family violence: Impact on children. J Am Acad Child Adolesc Psychiatry 31(2):181, 1992.

Kelly, GL: Childhood depression and suicide. Nurs Clin North Am 26(3):545, 1991.

Kemp, C: Terminal Illness: A Guide to Nursing Care. Lippincott/Williams & Wilkins, Philadelphia, 2nd ed, 1999.

Kerfoot, K: Keeping spirituality in managed care: The nurse manager's challenge. Nurs Econ 13(1):49, 1995.

King, CJ, et al: Diagnosis and assessment of substance abuse in older adults: Current strategies and issues. Addict Behav 19(1):41, 1994.

Kluger, J: The battle to save your memory. Time, June 12:46, 2000.

Krach, P: Nursing implications: Functional status of older persons with schizophrenia. J Gerontol Nurs 19(8):21, 1993.

Kreisman, JJ, and Straus, H: I Hate You-Don't Leave Me: Understanding the Borderline Personality. Avon Books, New York, 1989.

Kubler-Ross, E: On Death and Dying. MacMillan, New York, 1969.

Laraia, MT, and Sundeen, SJ: (2001) Cognitive responses and organic mental disorders. In GW Stuart and MT Laraia (eds.): Stuart and Sundeen's Principles and Practices of Psychiatric Nursing, ed. 7. Mosby, St Louis, 2001.

Laumann, E: Sexual dysfunction in the US: Prevalence and predictors. JAMA 281:542, 1999.

Leach Mc Mahon, A: The nurse-client relationship. In J Haber, B Krainovich-Miller, A Leach McMahon, and P Price-Hoskins (eds.) Comprehensive Psychiatric Nursing, ed. 5. Mosby, St Louis, 1997.

Ledray, LE, and Arndt, S: Examining the sexual assault victim: A new model for nursing care. J Psychosoc Nurs Ment Health Serv 32(2):7, 1994.

Lego, S: Borderline personality disorders. In Varcarolis, E: Foundations in Mental Health Nursing. WB Saunders, Philadelphia, 1994.

LeMone, P, and Jones, D: Nursing assessment of altered sexuality: A review of salient factors and objective measures. Nursing Diagnoses 8(3):120, 1997.

Levenkron, S: The Best Little Girl in the World. Warner Books, New York, 1978.

Levine, S: The newly revised standards of care for gender identity disorders. Journal of Sex Education Therapy 24:121, 1999.

Lewis, A, and Levy, J: Psychiatric Liaison Nursing. Reston Publishing, Reston, VA, 1982.

Lewis, S: Verbal intervention. In Blumenreich, PE, and Lewis, S (eds.): Managing the Violent Patient. Brunner/Mazel, New York, 1993.

Liken, MA, and Collins, CE: Grieving: Facilitating the process for dementia caregivers. J Psychosoc Nurs Ment Health Serv 31(1):21, 1993.

Lilley, LL, and Aucker, RN: Pharmacology and the Nursing Process, ed 2. Mosby, St Louis, 1999.

Lindemann, E: Symptomatology and management of acute grief. Am J Psychiatry 101:141, 1944.

Lipson, JG, and Steiger, NJ: Self-care Nursing in Multi-cultural Context. Sage Publications, Thousand Oaks, CA, 1996.

Lipson, JG, Dibbie, SL, and Minarik, PA (eds.): Culture and Nursing Care. University of California San Francisco Nursing Press, San Francisco, 1996.

LiShiun, C, et al.: Empirical examiniation of current depression categories in a population-based study. Am J Psychiatry 157(4):573, 2000.

Luckman, J: Tanscultural Communication in Nursing. Delmar Publishers, Albany, NY, 1999.

Lynch, SH: Elder Abuse: What to look for, how to intervene. Am J Nurs 97(1):27, 1997.

Mace, NL, and Rabins, PV: The 36-Hour Day, rev ed. Johns Hopkins University Press, Baltimore, 1991.

Marks, RM, and Sachar, EJ: Undertreatment of medical inpatients with narcotic analgesics. Ann Intern Med 78:173, 1973.

Maslow, A: Motivation and Personality. Harper & Row, New York, 1954.

Massie, MJ, Gagnon, P, and Holland, JC: Depression and suicide in patients with cancer. J Pain Sympt Manage 9:325, 1994.

Matheny, KB, and Riordan, RJ: Stress—And Strategies for Lifestyle Management. Georgia State University Business Press, Atlanta, 1992.

Matthiesen, V, Sivertsen, L, and Foreman, MD: Acute confusion: Nursing intervention in older patients. Orthopaedic Nursing 13(2):21, 1994.

Mayfield, D, McLeod, G, and Hall, P: The CAGE questionnaire: Validation of a new alcoholism screening instrument. Am J Psychiatry 131:121, 1974.

McAndrew, M: People who depend on substances other than alcohol. In Varcarolis, EM (ed.): Foundations of Psychiatric Mental Health Nursing, ed. 2. WB Saunders, Philadelphia, 1994.

McCaffery, M: Nursing practice theories related to cognition, bodily pain and man–environmental interactions. UCLS Student Store, 1968.

McCaffery, M, and Ferrel, BR: Nurses' knowledge of pain assessment and management: How much progress have we made? J Pain Symptom Manage 14(3):175, 1997a.

McCaffery, M, and Ferrel, BR: Influence of professional vs. personal role in pain assessment and use of opioids. Journal of Continuing Education in Nursing 28(2):69, 1997b.

McCaffery, M, and Ferrell, BP: Understanding opioids and addiction. Nurs 94(8):56, 1994.

McCaffery, M, and Passero, C: Pain: Clinical Manual, ed. 2. Mosby, St Louis, 1999.

McCracken, AL: Aging and alcohol. Journal of Gerontologic Nursing 24 (4) 37, 1998.

McFarland, GK, and McFarlane, EA: Nursing Diagnosis and Intervention. Mosby, St Louis, 1993.

McGrath, PJ, and Finley, GA: Chronic and Recurrent Pain in Children and Adolescents. Progress in Pain Research and Management 17. International Association for the Study of Pain Press, Seattle, WA, 1999.

McGuire, L, and Graffam, S: Pain in the elderly. In M. Stanley and PG Beare (eds.) Gerontological Nursing. FA Davis, Philadelphia, 1995.

McKenry, LM, and Salernoe, E: Mosby's Pharmacology in Nursing, ed 21. Mosby, St Louis, 2001.

McMahan, AL: Substance abuse among the elderly. Nurs Practitioner Forum 4(4):231, 1993.

Mendlowicz, MV, and Stein, MB: Quality of life in individuals with anxiety disorders. Am J Psychiatry 157(5):669, 2000.

Miller, JF: Coping with Chronic Illness. ed. 3. FA Davis, Philadelphia, 2000.

Millison, M, and Dudley, JR: Providing spiritual support: A job for all hospice professionals. Hospice Journal 8(4):49, 1992.

Mokdad, AH et al: The spread of the obesity epidemic in the US 1991–1998. JAMA 282(16):1519, 1999.

Moller, M, and Murphy, MF: Neurobiological responses and schizophrenia and psychotic disorders. In GW Stuart and MT Laraira (eds.): Stuart and Sundeen's Principles and Practices of Psychiatric Nursing, ed. 7. Mosby, St Louis, 2001.

Morrison, EF: The evolution of a concept: Aggression and violence in psychiatric setting. Arch Psychiatr Nurs 8(4):245, 1994.

Morrison, EF: Toward a better understanding of violence in psychiatric settings: Debunking the myths. Arch Psychiatr Nurs 7(6):328, 1993.

Morrison, R, and Siu, AL: Survival in end-stage dementia following acute illness. JAMA 284(1): 47, 2000.

Moscicki, EK: Epidemiology of suicide. In DG Jacobs (ed.): Harvard Medical School Guide to Suicide Assessment and Intervention. Jossey-Bass, San Francisco, 1999.

Moscicki, EK: Identification of suicide risk factors in epidemiological studies. Psychiatric Clinics of North America 20:499–517, 1997.

Mulryan, K, Cathers, P, and Fagin A: Protecting the child. Nursing 30(7):39, 2000.

Myer, SA: Multisystem complications of bulimia: A critical care case. Dimensions in Critical Care Nursing 12(4):194, 1993.

National Council of Alcoholism and Drug Dependence Web Site. Available at www.ncadd.org. Accessed August 2001.

National Crisis Prevention Institute: Art of Setting Limits: Participant Manual. Brookfield, WI, 1991.

National Institute of Alcohol Abuse and Alcoholism web site. Available at www.niaaa.org. Accessed August 2001.

National Institute of Health (1998): First Federal Obesity Clinical Guidelines. Available at www.nhlbi.nih.gov. Accessed September 2000.

North American Nursing Diagnosis Association (NANDA): Nursing Diagnoses: Definitions and Classifications 2001. North American Nursing Diagnosis Association, Philadelphia, 2001.

Novello, AC, and Soto-Torres, LE: Women and the Hidden Epidemic. The Female Patient 17:17, 1992.

OBrien, ME: Spirituality in Nursing. Jones and Bartlett, Boston, 1999.

Occupational Health and Safety Administration (OSHA) web site. Available at www.oshaslc.gov. Accessed May 2000.

Pacquette, M: Anger. In RM Carroll-Johnson, LM Gorman, and NJ Bush (eds.): Psychosocial Nursing Care Along the Cancer Continuum. Oncology Nursing Press, Pittsburgh, 1998.

Palmer, AC and Withee, BM: Dementia care: Effects of behavioral intervention training on staff perceptions of their work in Veterans' Nursing home. Geriatric Nursing 17(3):137, 1996.

Pande, AC, et al.: Treatment of social phobia with gabapentin: A placebo-controlled study. J Clin Psychopharmacol 19(4):341, 1999.

Parker, B, and Campbell, JC: Care of Survivors of Abuse and Violence. In GW Stuart and MT Laraia (eds.): Stuart and Sundeen's Principles and Practices of Psychiatric Nursing. ed. 7. Mosby, St Louis, 1998.

Perdue, B, and Piotrowski, C: A nurse's guide to mental health: Assessment reference sources. J Psychosoc Nurs 38(2):40, 2000.

Perkins, K, and Tice, C: Suicide in Older Adults. J Appl Gerontol, 13:438, 1994.

Phipps, WJ: Chronic Illness and Rehabilitation. In WJ Phipps, JK Sandas, and JF March (eds.) Medical Surgical Nursing, ed. 6. Mosby, St Louis, 1999.

Pollack, MH, Mathews, J, and Scott, EL: Gabapentin as a potential treatment for anxiety disorders. Am J Psychiatr 155(7):992, 1998.

Poorman, SG: Sexual Responses and Sexual Disorders. In GW Stuart and MT Laraia (eds.): Stuart and Sundeen's Principles and Practices of Psychiatric Nursing, ed. 7. Mosby, St Louis, 2001.

Poster, E: A multinational study of psychiatric nursing students' beliefs and concerns regarding work safety and patient assaults. Arch Psychiatr Nurs 10:365, 1996.

Purnell, LD, and Paulanka, BJ: Transcultural Health Care : A Culturally Competent Approach. FA Davis, Philadelphia, 1998.

Raines, ML: Ethical decision-making in nurses: Relationships among moral reasoning, coping style and ethics stress. Journal of Nursing Administration Healthcare Law, Ethics, and Regulation 2(1):29, 2000.

Rando, T: Treatment of Complicated Mourning. Research Press, Champaign, IL, 1993.

Raudsepp, E: Six steps to becoming more assertive. Nursing 21(3):112, 1991.

Rawlins, RP, Williams, SR, and Beck, CK: Mental Health-Psychiatric Nursing. A Holistic Life-Cycle Approach, ed 3. Mosby, St Louis, 1993.

Redman, BK: The Practice of Patient Education, ed. 8. Mosby, St Louis, 1997.

Redman, BK: The Process of Patient Education, ed. 7. Mosby, St Louis, 1993.

Reed, MC, and Anderson, PA: Geriatric substance abuse disorders. Med Clin North Am 81(4):999, 1997.

Ripamonti, C, Zecca, E, and Bruera, E: An update on the clinical use of methadone for cancer pain. Pain 70(2–3):109, 1997.

Robert Wood Johnson Foundation: Chronic Care in America: A 21st Century Challenge. Robert Wood Johnson Foundation, Princeton, NJ, 1996.

Roper, JM, and Manela, J: Psychiatric patients perceptions of waiting time in the psychiatric emergency service. J Psychosoc Nurs 38(5):18, 2000.

Ross, L: Elderly patients' perceptions of their spiritual needs and care: A pilot study. J Adv Nurs 26(4):710, 1997.

Rouchell, AM, Pounds, R, and Tierney, L: Depression. In JR Rundell and MG Wise (eds.): Textbook of Consultation—Liaison Psychiatry. American Psychiatric Association Press, Washington, DC, 1996.

Ruby, RN, and Lydiard, RB : Management of side effects of anxiolytics. In R. Balon (ed.): Practical Management of the Side Effects of Psychotropic Drugs. Marcell Dekker, Inc., New York, 1999.

Saltzman, KB: Transforming the grief experience. In RM Carroll-Johnson, LM Gorman, and NJ Bush (eds.): Psychosocial Nursing Along the Cancer Continuum. Oncology Nursing Press, Pittsburgh, 1998.

Schatzberg, AF, and Nemeroff, CB (eds.): The American Psychiatric Press Textbook of Psychopharmacology. American Psychiatric Press, Inc. Washington, DC, 1998.

Schneider, JM: Clinically significant differences between grief, pathological grief, and depression. Patient Counseling and Health Education. Fourth quarter: p 276, 1980.

Schnelle, JF, et al.: The nursing home at night: Effects of an intervention noise, light, and sleep. J Am Geriatr Soc 46:430, 1999.

Schooler, NR: Negative symptoms in schizophrenia: Assessment of the effects of risperidone. J Clin Psychiatry 55(suppl):22, 1994.

Schultz, JM, and Videbeck, SD: Manual of Psychiatric Nursing Care Plans, ed. 5. Lippincott-Raven, Philadelphia, 1997.

Schuster, PM: Communication: The Key to the Therapeutic Relationship. FA Davis, Philadelphia, 2000.

Seligman, M: Helplessness: On Depression, Development and Death. WH Freeman, New York, 1975.

Selzer, JA, and Lieberman, JA: Schizophrenia and substance abuse. Psychiatr Clin North Am 16(2):401, 1993.

Sisney, KF: The relationship between social support and depression in recovering chemically dependent nurses. Image 25(2):107, 1993.

Shea, CA, Mahoney, M, and Lacey, J: Breaking the barriers to domestic violence interventions. Am J Nurs 97(6):26, 1997.

Smith-Dijulio, K, and Holzapfel, SK: Families in crisis: Family violence. In Varcarolis, EM (ed.): Foundations of Psychiatric Mental Health Nursing, ed 2. WB Saunders, Philadelphia, 1994.

Smythe, E: Surviving Nursing. Addison-Wesley, Menlo Park, CA, 1984.

Soloff, PH, et al.: Characteristics of suicide attempts of patients with major depressive episode and borderline personality disorder: A comparative study. Am J Psychiatry 157(4):601, 2000.

Stanley, KJ: Silence is not golden: Conversation with the dying. Clinical Journal of Oncology Nursing 4 (1):34, 2000.

Stanley, M, and Beare, PG: Gerontological Nursing. FA Davis, Philadelphia, 1995.

Stephens, ST: Patient education materials: Are they readable? Oncol Nurs Forum 19(1):83, 1992.

Stepnick, A, and Perry, T: Preventing spiritual distress in the dying client. J Psychosoc Nurs Ment Health Serv 30(1):17, 1992.

Stolley, JM, et al: Managing the care of patients with irreversible dementia during hospitalization for comorbidities. Nurs Clin North Am 28(4):7, 1993.

Stratton, L: Evaluating the effectiveness of a hospital's pain management program. J Nurs Care Qual 13(4):299, 1999.

Strauss, AL, et al.: Chronic Illness and the Quality of Life, ed. 2. CV Mosby, St Louis, 1984.

Stuart, GW: Anxiety responses and anxiety disorders. In GW Stuart and MT Laraia (eds.): Stuart and Sundeen's Principles and Practices of Psychiatric Nursing, ed. 7. Mosby, St Louis, 2001a.

Stuart, GW: Self-protective responses and suicidal behavior. In GW Stuart and MT Laraia (eds.): Stuart and Sundeen's Principles and Practices of Psychiatric Nursing, ed. 7. Mosby, St Louis, 2001b.

Stuart, GW: Emotional responses and mood disorders. In GW Stuart and MT Laraia (eds.): Stuart and Sundeen's Principles and Practices of Psychiatric Nursing, ed. 7. Mosby, St Louis, 1998.

Stuart, GW, and Sundeen, SJ: Principles and Practices of Psychiatric Nursing, ed. 7. CV Mosby, St Louis, 2001.

Sullivan-Marx, EM: Delirium and physical restraint in the hospitalized elderly. Image 26(4):295, 1994.

Surgeon General of the US: Mental Health: A Report of the Surgeon General. US Government Printing office. Washington, DC. Available at www.nimh.nib.gov/mhsgrpt, 2000.

Taylor, B: "Coming Out" as a life transition: Homosexual identity formation and its implications for healthcare practice. J Adv Nurs 30:523, 1999.

Taylor, EJ: Spirituality and the cancer experience. In R.M Carroll-Johnson, LM Gorman, and NJ Bush (eds.): Psychosocial Nursing Care along the Cancer Continuum. Oncology Nursing Press, Pittsburgh, 1998.

Taylor, EJ, Amenta, M, and Highfield, M: Spiritual care practices of oncology nurses. Oncol Nurs Forum 22(1):31, 1995.

Topf, M, Bookman, M, and Arand, D: Effects of critical care unit noise on the subjective quality of sleep. J Adv Nurs 24:545, 1996.

Torkelson, D, and Dobal, M: Sexual rights of people with serious and persistent mental illness. Journal of the American Psychiatric Nurses Association 5(5):150–63, 1999.

Torrey, EF: Surviving Schizophrenia: A Family Manual. Perennial Library, New York, 1988.

Townsend, MC: Psychiatric/Mental Health Nursing: Concepts of Care, ed. 3. FA Davis, Philadelphia, 2000.

Tunnessen, WW: Signs and Symptoms in Pediatrics, ed. 3. Lippincott/Williams & Wilkins, Philadelphia, 1999.

Turnbill, J, et al: Turn it around: Short-term management of aggression and anger. J Psychosoc Nurs Ment Health Serv 28(6):1, 1990.

Tweed, SH: Intervening in adolescent substance abuse. Nurs Clin North Am 33(1):29, 1998.

Twycross, A: Pediatric Pain Management: A Multidisciplinary Approach. Scovill-Patterson, Inc., 1998.

Twycross, A: Pain management: A nursing priority? Journal of Child Health Care 3(3):19, 1999.

Valente, S, and Saunders, J: Diagnosis and treatment of major depression among people with cancer. Cancer Nurs 20(3):168, 1997.

Valente, SM, et al: Understanding grief after suicide. Nurseweek 6:10, 1993.

Valente, SM, Saunders, JM, and Cohen, MZ: Evaluating depression among patients with cancer. Cancer Practice 2:65, 1994.

Valente, SM: Recognizing Depression in the Elderly. Am J Nursing 94(12):18, 1994.

Varcarolis, EM: Foundations of Psychiatric Mental Health Nursing, ed. 3. WB Saunders, Philadelphia, 1998.

Walker, L: The Battered Woman. Harper & Row, New York, 1979.

Weiner, D, et al.: Pain in nursing home residents: An exploration of prevalence, staff perspecitives, and practical aspects of measurement. Clin J Pain. 15(2):92, 1999.

Wells, A: Cognitive Therapy of Anxiety Disorders: A Practice Manual and Conceptual Guide. John Wiley, New York, 1997.

Wessman, AC, and McDonald, DD: Nurses' personal pain experiences and their pain management knowledge. Journal of Continuing Education Nursing 30(4):152, 1999.

Wolfe, BE: Eating disorders . In CA Glod (ed.): Contemporary Psychiatric-Mental Health Nursing. FA Davis, Philadelphia, 1998.

Wong, DL, and Hockenberry-Eaton, M: Wong's Essentials of Pediatric Nursing, ed. 6. Mosby, St Louis, 2001.

Wong, DL, et al.: Whaley and Wong's Nursing Care of Infants and Children, ed. 6. Mosby-Year Book, St Louis, 1999.

Wynne, CF, Ling, SM, and Remsburg, R: Comparison of pain assessment instruments in cognitively intact and cognitively impaired nursing home residents. Geriatric Nursing, 2000.

INDEX

Numbers followed by an "f" indicate figures; numbers followed by a "t" indicate tabular material.